COMPUTING IN ANESTHESIA AND INTENSIVE CARE

DEVELOPMENTS IN CRITICAL CARE MEDICINE AND ANESTHESIOLOGY

COMPUTING IN ANESTHESIA AND INTENSIVE CARE

edited by

OMAR PRAKASH, MD
Thoraxcentrum, Academic Hospital Dijkzigt,
Erasmus University, Rotterdam

associate editors

SIMON H. MEY M.Sc and **RICHARD W. PATTERSON MD**
Thoraxcentrum,   *University of California Medical Center,*
Rotterdam   *Los Angeles*

1983 **MARTINUS NIJHOFF PUBLISHERS**
a member of the KLUWER ACADEMIC PUBLISHERS GROUP
BOSTON / THE HAGUE / DORDRECHT / LANCASTER

Distributors

for the United States and Canada: Kluwer Boston, Inc., 190 Old Derby Street, Hingham, MA 02043, USA
for all other countries: Kluwer Academic Publishers Group, Distribution Center, P.O.Box 322, 3300 AH Dordrecht, The Netherlands

Library of Congress Catalog Card Number 83-17301

ISBN 0-89838-602-0 (this volume)

P R E F A C E

This volume represents selected topics in Computing in
Anesthesia and Intensive Care and contains the proceedings
of the Second International Symposium, held in Rotterdam,
September 6-10, 1983.

This monograph provides the role of Computing in Anesthesia and Intensive Care, covering a wide range of topics:

Education, Monitoring, Innovative Techniques, Computer
Assisted Intravenous Anesthesia, Data Management and Closed
Loop Systems.

At the outset, I must thank the keynote speakers and
others for submitting their manuscripts promptly. I express
my gratitude to R.W. Patterson, Simon Meij and Bas van der
Borden for helping me to edit this volume. Finally, thanks
are due to E.N.R. Rulf, Norma van Toornburg and Claudia
Dijkstra for their help and cooperation.

July, 1983   Omar Prakash, M.D.

CONTENTS

Contributors

Angers, D. Department of Anesthesiology, Yale University School
    of Medicine, New Haven, CT 06510, USA.
Arena, L. Department of Anesthesiology, UCLA School of Medicine,
    Los Angeles, USA.
Baehrendtz, S. Department of Medicine I, South Hospital, Stock-
    holm, Sweden
Bellville, J.W. Department of Anesthesiology, UCLA School of
    Medicine, Los Angeles, USA.
Bender, H.J. Department of Anaesthesiology, University of
    Heidelberg, Mannheim, West Germany.
Beneken, J.E.W. Division of Medical Electrical Engineering,
    University of Technology, Eindhoven, The Netherlands.
Bernauer, J. Department of Anaesthesiology, University of
    Heidelberg, Mannheim, West Germany.
Blom, J.A. Division of Medical Electrical Engineering, University
    of Technology, Eindhoven, The Netherlands.
Borden, S.G., van der. Thorax Centrum, Erasmus University,
    University Hospital Dijkzigt, PO Box 1738, 3000 DR Rotterdam,
    The Netherlands.
Bormann, B., von. Department of Anaesthesiology and Intensive
    Care, Justus Liebig University, Giessen, West Germany.
Brovko, O. Department of Anesthesiology, UCLA School of Medicine,
    Los Angeles, USA.
Bshouty, Z. Intensive Care Department, Rambam, Medical Center and
    Technion School of Medicine, Haifa, Israel.
Bursztein, S. Intensive Care Department, Rambam, Medical Center
    and Technion School of Medicine, Haifa, Israel.
Chance, B. Department of Biophysics, University of Pennsylvania,
    Philadelphia, PA 19104, USA.
Cluitmans, P. Division of Medical Electrical Engineering,
    University of Technology, Eindhoven, The Netherlands.
Corenmen, J. Department of Anesthesia, Stanford University School
    of Medicine, Stanford, CA 94305, USA.
Davies, W.L. Nuffield Department of Anaesthetics, John Radcliffe
    Hospital, Oxford OX3 9DU, United Kingdom.
Daub, D. Department of Anaesthesiology, University of Technology,
    Aachen, West Germany.
Delemarre, J.B.V.M. Department of Cardiovascular Surgery, St.
    Antonius Hospital, Utrecht, The Netherlands.
Dickinson, C.J. Anaesthetics Laboratory, St. Bartholomew's
    Hospital, West Smithfield, London EC1A 7BE, United Kingdom.
East, T.D. Department of Anesthesiology, University of Utah,
    Salt Lake City, UT 84132, USA.
Edmonds, H.L.,Jr. Department of Anesthesiology, University of
    Louisville, Louisville, Kentucky 40292, USA.
Evans, J.M. Nuffield Department of Anaesthetics, The Radcliffe
    Infirmary, Oxford OX2 6HE, United Kingdom.
Fraser, A. Nuffield Department of Anaesthetics, The Radcliffe
    Infirmary, Oxford OX2 6HE, United Kingdom.

Gyulai, L. Department of Biophysics, University of Pennsylvania, Philadelphia, PA 19104, USA.

Harrison, B.J. Nuffield Department of Anaesthetics, John Radcliffe Hospital, Oxford OX3 9DU, United Kingdom.

Hartung, H.J. Department of Anaesthesiology, University of Heidelberg, Mannheim, West Germany.

Hayes, J.K. Department of Anesthesiology, University of Utah, Salt Lake City, UT 84132, USA.

Hedenstierna, G. Department of Clinical Physiology, Huddinge Hospital, Stockholm, Sweden.

Hempelmann, G. Department of Anaesthesiology and Intensive Care, Justus Liebig University, Giessen, West Germany.

Hengeveld, S.J. Department of Instrumentation and Automation, St. Antonius Hospital, Utrecht, The Netherlands.

Hilberman, M. Department of Anesthesia, University of Pennsylvania Philadelphia, PA 19104, USA.

Hinds, C.J. Anaesthetics Laboratory, St. Bartholomew's Hospital, West Smithfield, London EC1A 7BE, United Kingdom.

Jordan, W.S. Department of Anesthesiology, University of Utah, Salt Lake City, UT 84132, USA.

Keefer, J.R. Department of Anesthesiology, Yale University School of Medicine, New Haven, CT 06510, USA.

Kerr, J.H. Nuffield Department of Anaesthetics, John Radcliffe Hospital, Oxford, OX3 9DU, United Kingdom.

Kessel, H.M. van. Department of Anesthesiology, Leyden University Hospital, Leiden, The Netherlands.

Kling, D. Department of Anaesthesiology and Intensive Care, Justus Liebig University, Giessen, West Germany.

Korsten, H.H.M. Department of Anaesthesiology, St. Antonius Hospital, Utrecht, The Netherlands.

Lehmann, K.A. Department of Anaesthesiology, University of Technology, Aachen, West Germany.

Leusink, J.A. Department of Anaesthesiology, St. Antonius Hospital Utrecht, The Netherlands.

Maguire, H.T. Department of Anesthesiology, University of Louisville, Louisville, Kentucky, 40292, USA.

McGraw, C.P. Department of Surgery, University of Louisville, Louisville, Kentucky, 40292, USA.

McIntyre, J.W.R. Department of Anaesthesia, University Hospital, Edmonton, Alberta, Canada.

Meij, S.H. Thorax Centrum Erasmus University, University Hospital Dijkzigt, PO Box 1738, 3000 DR Rotterdam, The Netherlands.

Meijer, J.H. Department of Medical Physics, Free University, Amsterdam, The Netherlands.

Meijler, A.P. Division of Medical Electrical Engineering, University of Technology, Eindhoven, The Netherlands.

Miller, P.L. Department of Anesthesiology, Yale University, School of Medicine, New Haven, CT 06510, USA.

Nandorff, A. Department of Anesthesiology, Leyden University Hospital, Leiden, The Netherlands.

Naqvi, N.H. Department of Anaesthetics, Bolton Royal Infirmary, Bolton, Lancashire, United Kingdom.

Nijhuis, R. Department of Anesthesiology, Leyden University Hospital. Leiden, The Netherlands.

Olsson, G.L. Department of Paediatric Anaesthesia, St. Görans Hospital, Stockholm, Sweden.

Osswald, P.M. Department of Anaesthesiology, University of Heidelberg, Mannheim. West Germany.

Pace, N.L. Department of Anesthesiology, University of Utah, Salt Lake City, UT 84132, USA.

Peters, R.M. Department of Surgery, School of Medicine, University of California, San Diego, CA 92103, USA.

Poppers, P.J. Department of Anesthesiology, Health Sciences Center, State University of New York at Stony Brook, Stony Brook, NY 11794, USA.

Prakash, O. Thorax Centrum, Erasmus University, University Hospital Dijkzigt, PO Box 1738, 3000 DR Rotterdam, The Netherlands.

Pronk, R.A.F. University Hospital, Free University, Amsterdam, The Netherlands.

Rampil, I.J. Department of Anesthesia, University of California, San Diego, CA 92161, USA.

Ream, A.K. Stanford University Medical Center, Department of Anesthesia, Stanford, CA 94305, USA.

Reves, J.G. Department of Anesthesiology, University of Alabama, Birmingham, Alabama 35294, USA.

Ritchie, G. Department of Anesthesiology, University of Alabama, Birmingham, Alabama 35294, USA.

Russ, W. Department of Anaesthesiology and Intensive Care, Justus Liebig University, Giessen, West Germany.

Schneider, H. Department of Medical Physics, Free University, Amsterdam, The Netherlands.

Schurink, G.A. Department of Anaesthesiology, St. Antonius Hospital, Utrecht, The Netherlands.

Shepard, L.S. Departments of Anesthesiology and Biometry, Cuyahoga County Hospital and Case Western Reserve University School of Medicine, Cleveland, Ohio, USA.

Shoemaker, W.C. Department of Surgery, Harbor/UCLA Medical Center, Torrance, CA 90509, USA.

Simons, A.J.R. Department of Clinical Neurophysiology, St. Antonius Hospital, Utrecht, The Netherlands.

Sjogren, S.I. Department of Anesthesiology, University of Louisville, Louisville, Kentucky 40292, USA.

Skaredoff, M.N. Department of Anesthesiology, Health Sciences Center, State University of New York at Stony Brook, Stony Brook, NY 11794, USA.

Spain, J. Department of Anesthesiology, University of Alabama, Birmingham, Alabama 35294, USA.

Spierdijk, Joh. Department of Anesthesiology, Leyden University Hospital, Leiden, The Netherlands.

Staden, R. van. Department of Anaesthesiology, St. Antonius Hospital, Utrecht, The Netherlands.

Stanley, T.H. Department of Anesthesiology, University of Utah, Salt Lake City, UT 84132, USA.

Subramanian, V.H. Department of Biochemistry, University of Pennsylvania, Philadelphia, PA 19104, USA.

Sudan, N. Department of Anesthesiology, Yale University School of Medicine, New Haven CT 06510, USA.

Sullivan, S.F. Department of Anesthesiology, UCLA School of
    Medicine, Los Angeles, USA.
Tanner. G. Department of Anesthesiolgy, Yale University School
    of Medicine, New Haven, CT 06510, USA.
Ty Smith, N. Department of Anesthesia, University of California,
    San Diego, CA 92161, USA.
Voigt, E. Department of Anaesthesiology, Eberhard-Karls-University,
    Tübingen, West Germany.
Westenskow, D.R. Department of Anesthesiology, University of Utah,
    Salt Lake City, UT 84132, USA.
Wiberg, D.M. Department of Anesthesiology, UCLA School of Medicine
    Medicine, Los Angeles, USA
Wiley, R.S. Department of Anesthesiology and Biometry, Cuyahoga
    County Hospital and Case Western Reserve University School of
    Medicine, Cleveland, Ohio, USA.
Wise, C.C. Nuffield Department of Anaesthetics, The Radcliffe
    Infirmary, Oxford OX2 6HE, United Kingdom.
Wolfenson, L.B. Department of Anesthesiology and Biometry,
    Cuyahoga County Hospital and Case Western Reserve University
    School of Medicine, Cleveland, Ohio, USA
Yelderman, M. Department of Anesthesia, Stanford University
    School of Medicine, Stanford, CA 94305, USA.
Yoon, Y.K. Department of Anesthesiology, University of Louisville,
    Louisville, Kentucky 40292, USA.

Computer Operating Systems for Patient Monitoring

Allen K. Ream

Computer monitoring systems have obvious application to the management of
acutely unstable patients.   However, in designing such systems, attention is
usually given to the hardware and the user programs.   I'd like to discuss
another essential element, the operating system, both to demonstrate its importance, and to document significant trends which are of great value to users.
Our underlying thesis is that the character of the operating system can have an
enormous influence on the effectiveness of the monitoring system, and its ability to adapt to changes in clinical practice.

1.0 Historical Influences

   I first learned to write instructions for a computer, to program, in 1960
using MIT's TX-0; a forerunner of the first product of Digital Equipment Corporation. As students, we had low priority, and we executed our programs late
at night.   The program was sent to the computer via a teletypewriter which
punched paper tape; one mistake meant that the entire program had to be
retyped.   The commands which we entered were primitive; each represented a
single operation of the central processor. Many instructions had to be written
to accomplish a very simple result.

   We knew that speaking to the computer in its own language of 1's and 0's
was not useful; human thinking does not easily associate meaning with strings
of numbers. So we wrote our commands with simple abbreviations, like ADD and
MPY (multiply), and a program assembled them into the 1's and 0's, of machine
language, which the computer could recognize and execute.

   Assembly languages were widely accepted, but still difficult to use, and
much effort went into developing more complex commands, which could then be
compiled into machine language. These higher level languages were useful
because a set of commands making up a program could be more concise, and therefore more easily written and understood.   The compiling programs were made
progressively more elaborate, and additional features were added which checked
for errors, as dividing by zero, or using the commands in ways that the
designers forbade.   FORTRAN is one of the most famous inventions of that
period; it is presently the most widely used compiling high level scientific
programming language in the world.

   To compute (i.e. run a program) with this approach, one coded the problem
in FORTRAN, punched it into cards or paper tape, and submitted the cards to the
computer operator. He fed the cards into the computer, and activated the com-

piling program which translated one's program into machine language. The computer then executed this machine language program. The result of the first several tries would often be a set of messages indicating that the program had failed to compile because of an error in programming language syntax.

This was a generally acceptable approach because computers were new and expensive, and far better than the manual alternatives. But the process of entry and compiling introduced delays in obtaining a program that would execute properly. This approach also separated the user from the computer.

Then John Kemeny and his colleagues at Dartmouth College developed the BASIC language. It was a simple language and not intended for serious application. But it was on-line; i.e. a user could type in material at a terminal and immediately execute his program. Because each line of instructions was separately interpreted or translated into machine code, the programs did not run as quickly, but the user could rapidly test code sequences without a long wait for compiling, and most users found failures reported by this mode easier to correct than failures reported via messages from a compiling program.

It is generally believed that more individuals have learned BASIC than any other programming language; human conveniences have outweighed many serious (and valid) limitations of the language. Perhaps another way to express its attractiveness is to note that in many simple computer applications the greatest cost is the time and effort required to write the program, not the cost of executing it.

Initially, computers were used to automate manual calculations. But as experience was acquired, it became apparent that the speed of the computer allowed a new activity: real-time operation. This term has been used in many ways; a widely accepted definition is a response time so fast that the information is available before the user needs it. It is obvious that speed is a crucial attribute of a successful real-time system.

Real-time systems were applied very early to physiologic modeling and monitoring; Homer Warner at the University of Utah was one of the first, initially with an analog computer, then with a digital computer (when one big and fast enough could be funded). However, these early computer systems were extremely expensive and bulky, leading to the concept of a remote computer. And compared to multiple users through terminals they were inefficient. I recall the ACME system used at Stanford in 1967. It could support multiple terminals with keyboard input, but monitoring one dog experiment with the help of an auxiliary computer required the entire system!

In the United States, the National Institutes of Health funded several major projects to develop computerized patient monitoring. Certain attributes seemed universal. A system was built around specific hardware. Specific tasks such as measurement, data storage and report generation were defined. Specific programs were written to accomplish these tasks for a particular application, such as hemodynamic monitoring. As more experience was acquired, repetitive activities were collected into separate programs, which could be used by each program which required them. These collected programs formed the nucleus of what became known in other contexts as an operating system. The programs which were directly concerned with specific measurements and projects could be considered applications programs.

2.0 Definition of an Operating System

A typical dictionary definition of an operating system is the set of programs which have to do with translation, supervision, maintenance, control and execution of computer programs. I find this definition too abstract. The distinctions are functional, and of great practical importance. We will develop this definition by considering our monitoring application.

Some of the specific tasks which an operating system must accomplish include communication with the user via a terminal, driving a printer or other output device, and supporting information storage. Storage includes files and their directories, as well as the means of modifying, copying, and transferring them. While these tasks are quickly listed, the complexity of mature operating systems demonstrates that they are not simple.

We have noted that early computer applications did not involve real-time. This meant that speed of execution and coordination of input and output with program execution were not given adequate consideration. The primary concern was manipulation of data, to balance a ledger, or to complete a mathematical calculation or fitting of a curve. Getting the data into or out of the system was considered a separate problem. A characteristic of early languages was the failure to provide adequate high level commands for input and output.

This separation persists in most modern languages. Two widespread examples are BASIC, a favorite of users, and PASCAL, a favorite of computer science teachers. To state the same view in different terms; VISICALC, the proprietary program which is said to have contributed more to the sales of Apple computers than any other proprietary software, was successful because input and output were integrated into the language. Previous languages were perfectly acceptable mathematically for solving these applications, but even we old timers prefer the spreadsheet (VISICALC) approach. It's easier, faster, and leads to fewer mistakes.

Also, in many early commercial applications, the persons who controlled the design of the system did not directly put in or receive data. While batch methods for input were sometimes frustrating for users, they were easier to design, and in applications like accounting, to control. However, all programs running on a given machine had certain tasks in common; they had to be entered, used a particular language, and left results which had to be returned in some manner to the user.

To collect these tasks, job control programs were written. They grew by accretion, as system tasks were recognized and added. One needs to know how long each program executes to charge fees, and to remove a program which has been caught in an endless loop, is badly written, or whose execution time exceeds the user's budget. It is necessary to control memory access for each user based on credentials, need, account size, etc. The programs to store on disk or tape, print, or plot should not be unique to each user; memory is wasted, and it is better to devote resources to one good solution in which all can share. As these programs grew, their collective identification as an operating system became accepted.

3.0 Early Real-time Operating Systems

Developers of computer applications which met real-time requirements found gaps in early operating system design. These systems were slow, difficult to change, lacking in essential features and often executed tasks in an order which led to delays. Thus developers wrote their own real-time operating systems. However, a community of users developed more slowly, and many solutions were specific to a given application. Approaches tended either to unique solutions, often in assembly language for speed of execution, or to central time sharing systems, building on the attributes found effective in the financial and scientific worlds.

Initially, central systems had a number of attractive attributes. They permitted the sharing of a costly resource, and provided access to a common data base in applications where this was vital. However, with the decrease in cost of computers, financial pressures no longer favored centralization. Major data base access does not need to be a frequent activity of monitoring, and the cost of communication equipment has become a significant part of the cost of a central system.

Central systems have other undesirable attributes. Software, the major system expense, is more complex. Failures have more widespread effects. And in many central systems, the design allows the number of interactions to increase more rapidly than the number of users, preventing economies of scale.

While the complexity of centralized systems is not immediately obvious, it has effects which are of profound interest to users. The system is isolated from users, changes are more difficult to implement, and the increased complexity means that changes often have unintentional side effects.

In many large monitoring systems, growth has proceeded to the point where no one user fully understands the system. (This was graphically demonstrated to me some years ago, when government funding was provided to duplicate a well-known patient monitoring system, using one of the principal developers, on a new computer system. The project ran significantly over time and budget and was abandoned.)

In the short term, increasing the size of the computer may compensate for inefficiency (a tactic which suggests an explanation as to why such operating systems have not been rapidly replaced by computer manufacturers), but the underlying difficulties remain.

Attempts have been made to solve these problems by providing complex constraints for programmers, and by formal approaches to timesharing which partition activities. However, as we shall see below, timesharing techniques developed for keyboard real-time applications are usually inefficient when used for monitoring.

A major concern is the effect of isolating users from program function and maintenance. When we speak of patient care, the user is often the most expert in analyzing available information. Creating a system which hides the basis on which calculations are made and the way data is combined is not a sound practice. These mechanisms need to be accessible to users in a way which relates to their clinical needs. It is difficult to fully convey the degree of isolation which these programming practices assure without multiple detailed examples. However, I am confident that most readers have, at one time or another, experienced the feeling of helplessness associated with such practices.

4.0 Modern Trends in Real-Time Operating Systems

In designing a modern monitoring operating system, a number of concepts appear attractive. In the available space, we discuss only examples.

For the reasons previously identified, a computer should be dedicated to a single monitoring application. A central system may be used for data storage, but with proper design the rate of data transfer between it and the dedicated system should be relatively low. [1]

The operating system should be written in a higher level language, so that changes can be made and understood without introducing unexpected side effects. A higher level language also permits portability: the ability to move the system to a new computer, extending the life of the software. The computer language also must execute efficiently, since timing is a critical concern in these applications. If this need cannot be met, assembly language may be used, but the practical limitations are severe.

The system must be broken into pieces, modules, which are separate in the sense that they can be changed individually. An excellent example of a simple operating system is CPM, which is presently the most widely used system for microprocessors in the world. It is broken into three major modules: the command interpreter, which translates commands from the user into actions, the portion which deals with input and output (which is different for each computer), and the remaining operating system functions. When CPM is moved to a new computer, only the input/output portion needs to be changed. I am not aware of an operating system for monitoring applications, using a similar approach, which is generally available.

In the same way, the application programs which run under the operating system for a particular monitoring application should be modular, so that they are simple enough to understand, and can be changed without unexpected effects. For example, a user may wish to change the way heart rate is calculated. This change should not affect the way other data is averaged or recorded.

There is one critical area, however, where the attributes of a monitoring system for this application are unique: timing.

Clock time is necessary, not only for calendar functions, but for precise timing of measurements. If the system controls patient monitoring, a whole new set of complex tasks must be implemented: frequent sampling of the transducer outputs; accumulation of data in some area of memory; and what may be called final calculations, in which manipulation is performed before storage and display. While these routines can be written entirely into the application programs, it is becoming apparent that many of them belong in the operating system.

Many operating systems evolved from the batch processing mode. Each user had a job; the operating system executed them serially. Each job ran to completion, or until it exceeded a preset time, and was replaced by the next in line. Execution was speeded up by writing to memory, and another processor handled output to the printer or other media.

When languages like BASIC became available, a compromise was necessary. The computer serviced others while a user was deciding what to type at his console. At present, the time between the characters sent to or received from his console can be used! Partitioning of workspace in the computer is usually straightforward. Most systems reserve dedicated space for the user, and he is not allowed to exceed this allotment. Partitioning of time is more complex, because each user must share the same central processor.

When an activity literally cannot wait (usually when making a measurement), an interrupt is programmed. A signal generated by an electronic clock or the measuring device interrupts whatever is currently being executed, saves one or two key registers, and gives control to a small program associated with the interrupt. When this program has executed, the registers are restored, and control is returned to the program which was executing. This approach works well if the interrupt program is short and simple, usually only saving acquired data for later use.

Partitioning tasks which behave like users is more difficult, and extensive literature has accumulated around solutions developed for multiple users. Without becoming too detailed, it is sufficient to note that a common approach is timesharing. After a specified time has elapsed, the previously executing program is saved in midstream, and the next task is started. However, requiring the system to transfer at an arbitrary time makes the process complex. It is not uncommon for a multiuser operating system to consume half of the available computer time in overhead, i.e. switching between tasks.

In a simple system, with only one task executing, this problem is avoided. Instead, considerable programming effort is necessary to accomplish multiple activities with different time constraints, such as completing averaging for data just acquired over an interval, writing to a display screen, and providing calculations in response to a keyboard request. This solution is even less satisfactory if the tasks become complex; the program becomes a specialized operating system.

However, there are some advantages to the timesharing approach. The software can be maintained and is relatively successful in protecting other tasks from programming errors in one task. Constraints can usually be relaxed by moving to a larger computer, an approach which is not unattractive to computer manufacturers. But, overhead is high and memory is not always used efficiently.

Multitasking is an approach used early in the development of computers because of its efficiency. The fundamental difference is that the exchange of the task being executed occurs when a task is completed instead of at a predetermined time. The changeover can be quite simple; a handful of status variables is all that needs to be retained. In our multitasking system written in polyFORTH, swapping tasks requires less than 30 millionths of a second, using a relatively slow processor!

Using a multitasking system does introduce some restraints. It is the responsibility of the programmer to design programs that finish tasks often enough to avoid monopolizing the computer. The total time of execution is not a problem; because overhead is enormously reduced, the effective capacity of the computer is increased.

A careless programmer can have a significant effect on a multitasking system. However, in a monitoring system, all of the programs are already interrelated. Further, the partitioning between tasks separates functions which are asynchronous, as writing to disk, plotting, printing, and terminal communications. This results in simpler programs.

Another consideration is that the value of data decays with time. The greatest detail is required immediately after measurement. The minimum detail is that required for the permanent record. Our data suggests that the decay from initial to final detail is exponential. Accurately characterizing this process and building it into the monitoring system can enormously reduce the size of the computer and data storage required, compared to that required with the historical technique of preserving the originally measured level of detail. Never postpone processing which can be immediate; delay usually slows execution by introducing additional steps.

A related issue is that the value of code which executes efficiently is relative. Minor inefficiencies in code which executes each time measurements are obtained can have a relatively enormous effect on the speed of program execution. Conversely, routines executed infrequently can be relatively inefficient without adding significantly to the time required for program execution. This latter group includes most of the code. Thus, careful attention to design permits writing much code in relatively inefficient ways, to make it easier to understand and to change, with little penalty. But the exceptions are of crucial importance. When possible, the exceptions should be protected in the operating system.

5.0 The Partition Between the Operating System and Applications Programs

We began with three elements, the hardware, the applications programs, and the operating system. The operating system, like a programming language, is fixed, but the applications programs can be changed as one learns more about the problem and its interpretation. To be successful, the operating system should be simple, consistent, and easily understood. It must also have sufficient flexibility to provide software tools powerful enough to allow simple and understandable applications programs.

Functions which relate to a particular application, or to understanding of the physiology, should not be built into the operating system. For example, the software which detects heart rate and makes it available for other calculations should be part of the applications programs. Conversely, functions which are generic should be part of the operating system. There is no advantage to including code to operate the system clock or the analog to digital converter in applications programs. When and if specific physiologic calculations become so generally accepted as to become truly universal, they may be added to the operating system as trigonometric functions are added to most computer languages. However, if the mode of calculation is uncertain or based on the application or physiologic insights, it does not belong in the operating system. To include it is to guarantee a fatal weakness.

Most physiologic monitoring systems available today do not meet these goals. Sometimes the operating system and the application are a single program. Often they are partially separated, but co-mingled, making evolution difficult or impossible. And often functions which should be in one area are in the other. Because the systems are designed for a specific application and configuration of hardware, these weaknesses mean that they cannot be transferred to other computers and institutions. And around the world, a relatively enormous degree of duplication of effort has resulted.

My method of dramatizing the proper boundary between the operating system and application programs is to use the analogy of the alphabet and words created from it. The operating system is analogous to the alphabet; adherence to a common system with sufficient flexibility offers enormous advantages. Applications programs are analogous to words. Standardization is essential-- to communicate meaningfully, we must agree on the definition of left ventricular end-diastolic pressure-- but definitions evolve with time and our understanding. Appropriate standards must allow a means for this drift to occur, and to be noted. [2] Applications programs contain this flexibility; operating systems do not.

6.0 The Uses of Operating Systems

The history of monitoring reveals a fascination with technique. However the primary incentive of monitoring is to acquire, order, and present the information in a way which eases decision making and allows it to occupy a bigger fraction of the user's time.

The first step is to acquire the data. When this is done, choices must be made. Only a fraction of the possible measurements are useful, and sophistication is necessary to determine which measurements are to be used. [3]

Results should be ordered by reference to underlying goals, as outcome; and by reference to implementation, as alternative therapies. (The issue of whether or not to apply the therapy is clarified by this kind of linkage.) It is apparent that the appropriate structure will evolve with the user's understanding. [4] Why then do so many on-line operating systems make this aspect of the approach inflexible? A needed attribute is the ability of motivated users to change the mode of presentation. Changeable attributes should be part of the application program, and accessible to review.

Recent trends emphasize these considerations. Monitoring is an activity which is improved by the application of machine intelligence. Achieving computer intelligence requires knowledge, and accessible rules for using that knowledge. The ability to provide understandable explanations is one of the most important attributes of this approach. The lack of this ability is a major reason why physicians have refused to embrace programs performing clinical diagnosis, even when excellent performance has been demonstrated in clinical trials. [5] It is necessary for users to understand and appreciate the approach in order to trust the results and use them effectively.

In this way, the monitoring system can be used to reinforce or teach good practice. It has been suggested that personnel who learn to use a well designed monitoring system subsequently demonstrate an improved ability to manage patients without it.

Recent studies of scientific learning appear relevant to this clinical application. Students approach learning with extensive internal models of reality. After instruction in new concepts, they tend to return to prior theories to solve problems which vary from the examples studied. Learners look for meaning, and will try to find order and regularity in their observations. Bits of information isolated from these ordered mental structures are forgotten, or become inaccessible to memory. Naive theories are inevitable, and must be confronted directly to be reconciled with more appropriate or reliable concepts. [6]

These results suggest that an interpretive monitoring system which does not make its decision rules accessible cannot be easily reconciled with the user's concepts of reality. It certainly cannot be easily used to improve those perceptions, nor to stimulate discovery of inadequacies in its own decision rules.

This is a powerful argument for making operating systems more modular; so that specific changes can be made without destroying the integrity of the system, and so that specific applications, as the calculation of rate, averaging interval, or such indices as the viability ratio or S/DR (supply/demand ratio) [3] can be easily implemented, reviewed, altered, or rejected as experience grows. Decision rules which are both appropriate and isolated from other parts of the system are easier to understand, and the effects of changing them are clearer, and more easily implemented.

The capability of evolution is an essential attribute. Structures and attributes reserved for the operating system should be those regarded as most basic, widely applicable, and generally accepted. Capabilities which are likely to evolve should be in the applications programs which run under the operating system. And the system should favor both modular intellectual structure, and portability to other hardware systems.

Most presently used operating systems for patient monitoring are less modular and general than is desirable. This has led to the same problems being solved repeatedly by different investigators, and different groups, even by the same individuals at different times for slightly different applications. It is evident that substantial benefits will accompany the development of operating systems for monitoring which are general, modular, maintainable and portable. Attributes which appear highly desirable include multitasking, the use of high level programming languages, and rules of data analysis which are accessible and understandable to clinical users, while the system is in use.

By necessity, this discussion has been brief. Our companion presentation, defining the development of a specific real-time operating system which is now in its second generation, provides insight into our biases in implementing the proposed techniques.

REFERENCES

1. Prakash O, Meij S, Zeelenberg C, van der Borden B: Computer-based patient monitoring. Crit Care Med 10(12):811-822, 1982

2. McCleary GF Jr: An effective graphic "vocabulary". IEEE CG&A 46-53, April, 1983.

3. Gravenstein JS, Newbower R, Ream AK, Smith NT: Integrated Approaches to Monitoring. New York: Butterworths, 1983

4. Osborn JJ: Computers in critical care medicine: promises and pitfalls. Crit Care Med 10(12):807-810, 1982

5. Duda RO, Shortliffe EH: Expert   systems   research.   Science   220:261-268, 1983.

6. Resnick LB: Mathematics and science learning: a new conception.   Science 220:477-478, 1983

On the Use of Computers in the Practice of Anaesthesia

D. Daub and K.A. Lehmann

1. Introduction

Computers are entering every sector of our daily and professional life and they won't spare Anaesthesiology. Administration, stock-keeping, documentation are already partially done,
and, in the very near future, will surely be performed exclusively, by means of computers. Other tasks like medical corre-
spondence and similar secretarial work will be performed by
text editor systems,and even our scientific papers will be
typed, corrected, edited and printed by such a system. There
is no need to discuss those applications in detail because
they will follow the extramedical development, and we will
have to accept the solutions which are worked out in other
disciplines and other sectors of human life.

A special design, however, is needed for specific medical
problems such as the monitoring of critically ill patients.
Although industry and business have already taken the leading
position and the forces of the free market are active in di-
recting further moves, we are able to influence the future
development in monitoring. But the range of our influence is
limited. As a matter of fact, most problems regarding data
acquisition, data-base or computing facilities have been
solved and we have to acknowledge the fact that the technical
tool we are provided with by the industry is on a much higher
level than our medical knowledge, i.e. we are rarely able to
use to their full extent all the possibilities which are incorporated in a well-designed system.(4)There are indeed
some aspects which can be improved in the design of man - machine interface regarding data input and also data representation, both problems not being specifically medical ones,
which are sure to be solved in the near future. For the monitoring purpose the development is also proceeding and the
computer will be an integrated part of every future monitoring system - like it or not, and there is no use discussing
problems which have already been solved, or are just on the
point of being solved. We shan't stop the process in progress
and our possibilities to interfere, or even merely influence
it, are limited. The question we really should be concerned
with, and the solution of which will demand the utmost effort,
is: How can computers be implemented into anaesthesiology,
and is it worthwhile doing it? Will the introduction of that
new technology really improve our daily routine work as an-

aesthesiologists? The answer is that there is a lot of work
to be done to make anaesthesiology ready for the data-process-
ing approach. This paper will report on our 10-year endeav-
ours, our successes and failures in establishing a model
ready for the computer to assist us in performing anaesthesia.

2.1. Descriptive Approach

The first attempt at structuring the rather amorphous knowledge in anaesthesiology was based on documentation.(3) The
fundamental concept of that first approach was to gather data
of all anaesthesias performed in the department, to process
them and by that to make available to every single member of
the department the full extent of experience gained by the
whole staff. This approach, which today can only be judged
when reviewing the situation of medical data processing as
it used to be ten years ago, was considered promising because
no phase im the period of hospitalization and illness is as
well-documented as anaesthesia. A real-time on-line documentation and monitoring system was installed all over our hospital and every site of action was equipped with a colour
visual display and a keyboard, over which all data could be
entered during anaesthesia and intensive care. A special data
bank was established and a self-learning programme system
processed all data entered. We had our specially designed
text editor and sophisticated presentation devices to make
access and handling as comfortable as possible to the un-
trained user.

The results were disenchanting. It was an illusion to believe
that we could gain a much clearer insight by processing all
the data gathered. We could only show the incoherent variability of actions leading to the well-defined state of anaesthesia. There was not even the faintest aspect which was
common to all anaesthesias reported and there was not a
single fact extracted out of the data bank which we didn't
know before. One fact was obvious: we did not collect the
data concerning anaesthesia itself but only the possible
side-effects. Most of our documented data did not reflect
the process of anaesthesia proper but the physical state of
our patients regarding their basic functions. These data
used to be crucial in the days when anaesthesia was a balanced intoxication but were not essential for a modern university department.

The only information extracted out of the data bank which
actually concerned anaesthesia proper revealed the dosage
habits of the staff members, and that, at least, was considered to be helpful to newcomers. The analysis of the drug
administration led to the anaesthetic time-dose curves as
introduced by KEERI-SZANTO (9) for every single drug. However, the injection of the different drugs according to those
curves did not effect a more stable or efficient anaesthesia.
We ended up concluding that only one half of the anaesthesias
performed following that scheme were satisfactory. This was
probably an averaging effect, and it re-occurred when analyzing sub-sets of our patients according to the type of oper-

ation and anamnestic data. The result of five years of work was the realization that anaesthesia is too complex a process to be described by documentation only, that the mapping of that process onto the records is poor and that the variability of response for every individual is enormous.

2.2. Pharmacokinetic Approach

The second attempt towards an optimated anaesthesia was based on the commonly accepted conception that there are plasma levels of drugs which - being above a certain level - ensure a stable anaesthesia. Thus, the ideal anaesthesia would be achieved by using a fixed regimen for every drug under consideration, which can easily be controlled and simulated by a computer. But before the implementation of this concept into the existing system, those plasma and organ levels would have to be defined for each of the drugs whose cooperation results in clinical anaesthesia. Therefore a programme was started to establish the pharmacokinetic data which were needed to evaluate that concept. But those threshold concentrations could not be found, neither could, for example, the analgesic plasma level of fentanyl (13) nor the sleeping level of diazepam (5). These findings are in contrast to some other results published (7,8,20), and a certain evaluation of these divergences must be inserted in this context, even if leading away from the subject in question, namely computer application.

Since the beginning of the 1970s, pharmacokinetics has gained considerable importance in anaesthesiology.(12,19) With the methodological tool provided by this discipline, conclusions have been drawn regarding the uptake, distribution and elimination of drugs, but attempts were also made to predict how the effects and side-effects would progress over a period of time on the basis of representative groups of measured data. (19) This concept can yield substantial success: not only can half-life values, distribution, clearance and bioavailability be calculated, but they can also be used as variables for any extrapolation. Such sets of curves seem so relevant and plausible to most observers that two fundamental prerequisites are often forgotten:

First, the parameters for the kinetic calculations are averages of numerous individual data, often with considerable scattering, which usually makes an average curve irrelevant for clinical cases (problem of biological variability). Secondly, the desired predictions appear conceivable only when the site of action coincides with one of the compartments represented (problem of receptor theory).

The pronounced biological variability, demonstrated for fentanyl consumption and fentanyl plasma concentration during routine neuroleptic anaesthesia in fig. 1 and 2, is the reason why attempts to optimize dosage on the basis of pharmacokinetic parameters have been unsuccessful. The attempts to use drug concentrations in plasma or in specific compartments have failed because

14

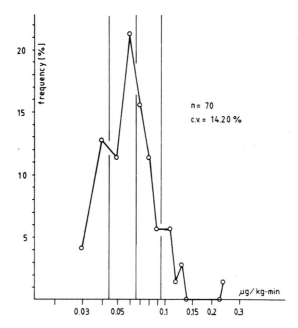

Fig. 1: The use of fentanyl in routine neuroleptanaesthesia
normalized to kg body weight and minute

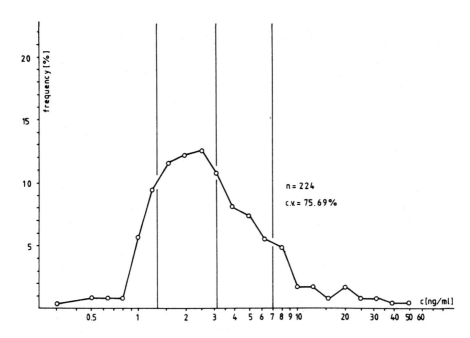

Fig. 2: Plasma level of fentanyl at the point of clinically
necessary follow-up injection (analgesic titration)
in routine neuroleptanaesthesia

- there is no generally valid correlation between plasma level
  and pharmacodynamic effect;
- the subdivision of tissues of the human body into compartments is not related to real organs, but their number or
  size is varied in such a way that a mathematical approximation of the model to the more readily accessible blood
  level measurements can be achieved by the simplest possible
  means;
- there is no proven and constant relation between brain concentrations and pharmacodynamic effect either.

The good correlation between plasma level and effect, which
is required for the practical use of that concept, is certainly shown in the case of medications which work in the
plasma itself, like heparin. It is questionable in the case
of drugs that non-specifically affect all cells, like halothane, and is extremely improbable in those whose operation
is mediated by receptors. Nevertheless, even for diazepam or
fentanyl have such correlations been confirmed repeatedly in
experiments. We ourselves have found such correlations for
diazepam (5) and fentanyl (fig. 3), HUG (7) found a good
correlation of fentanyl level and respiratory depression,
and so did others. However, this is only valid when the pharmacodynamic and kinetic parameters are compared in a group
under the same limiting conditions at the same time. If equal
concentrations are set in relation to their effect at different times, they generally correlate no longer (fig. 4).

Numerous other factors, like additional drugs administered,
psyche, circadian rhythms, eating, may modify the pharmacodynamic effect without any connection with plasma levels.
But even the plasma levels are extremely variable. The plasma
concentrations to be expected after i.v. administration of a
dose of fentanyl, standardized according to body weight or
even blood volume, can be predicted only within an order of
magnitude. Thus, already in this very first step, a certain
variability is inherent. Those variations alter any pharmacokinetic modelling considerably as they are the basis on which
the whole system is established.

If individual groups of patients are observed separately,
significant differences appear: for example, fig. 5 shows
that the plasma level during halothane anaesthesia at any
time after a bolus injection of fentanyl is twice as high as
in ethrane anaesthesia. KORTILLA (10) was able to show that,
without injecting another dose, serum diazepam levels rise
after the patient's having a meal and that this rise is significantly higher after a carbohydrate-enriched meal than
after one containing a lot of fat. These are only two examples
showing how difficult it is to really ensure equal conditions
for every member of your set about to be tested. In a clinical study this prerequisite will never be fulfilled regarding all the aspects which should be considered, namely the
different drugs, infusion and nutrition regimens, individual
drinking habits, physical and psychological conditions.

There are, however, some explanations for the variability in
serum concentrations after application of a normalized dosis

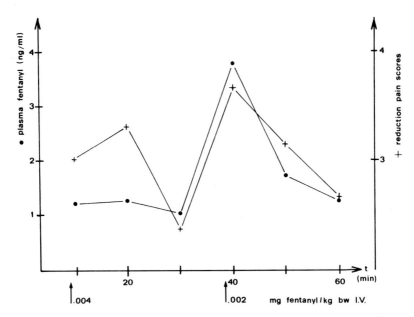

Fig. 3: Pain reduction, scored by a visual analogue scale, in relation to plasma fentanyl levels

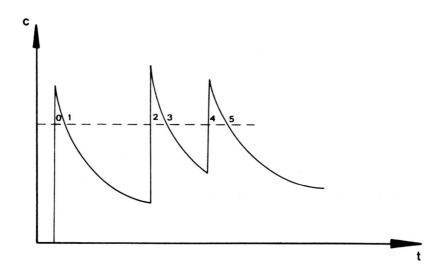

Fig. 4: Equal plasma concentrations of fentanyl in the course of neuroleptanaesthesia do not necessarily indicate equal pharmacodynamic effects. Correlation is good at t_o or t_n, but over-all correlation is poor

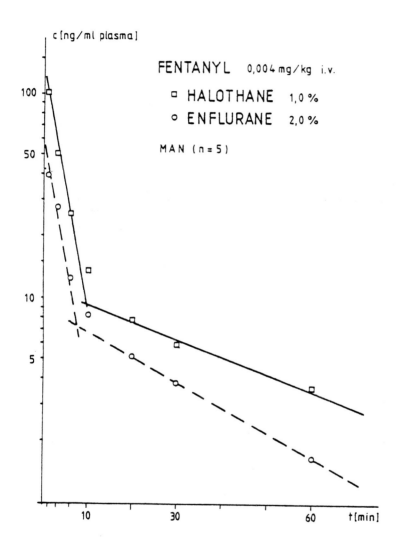

Fig. 5: Plasma level after I.V. bolus injection of 0.004 mg
        fentanyl per kg body weight during halothane and
        enflurane anaesthesia

of an anaesthetic drug. The smaller volume of distribution
under halothane is partially due to the reduced blood flow
through the liver as demonstrated by THULIN (21). Our group
has been able to show that also the metabolism of fentanyl,
whose importance for the kinetics has been underestimated in
favour of redistribution mechanisms, is altered by halothane
and a lot of other different drugs used in anaesthesia and
the perioperative period.(14) Great attention has been lav-
ished on pH changes or pH gradients at interfaces, which result in iron trapping of the easily diffusable weak bases.
This phenomenon is well supported (19) for the secretion of
fentanyl into the acid gastric juice. But pH gradients, which
admittedly are not so pronounced as in the area of the stomach wall, also appear in other organs during anaesthesia.
However, the greater mass of the organs is definitely able
to hold back large quantities of drugs, as shown by our group
for the muscle tissues in rats. (15) This leads us to the
problem of depot formation, which plays a considerable role
in the variability of plasma concentrations. Various studies
(15) show that large quantities of intravenously injected
drugs are temporarily stored in tissues with good blood circulation such as the lungs, but are also easily and flexibly
released again. Every change in tissue perfusion can thus
result in a change in blood level.

Blood pharmacokinetics, which is at present employed univer-
sally, is certainly not able to describe the characteristic
effects of drugs which act via receptors. Significantly deeper insights into the actual events are expected from the
study of receptor kinetics, although there presently exist
only model concepts, especially in the area of opiate and
benzodiazepin receptors. The diffusion of anaesthetic drugs
through the various membranes from the capillaries to the
receptors is obviously possible without interference. The
rapid onset of effects confirms this. Our own investigations
on erythrocyte membranes show an equalization of concentrations between intra- and extracellular spaces through the
membranes almost immediately. The erythrocyte membrane (and
this should also serve as an example for other membranes)
thus represents no obstacle for the diffusion of the free
base fentanyl.

The stability of the specific bonding of fentanyl to the
opiate receptor is unknown. It is certain (as has been shown
by the radiographic studies of LADURON (16))that the fentanyl
receptor complex can again dissociate, in contrast to lofentanil, which undergoes irreversible bonding. Consequently,
among other things, the rate of association of the molecule
to the receptor and that of the dissociation of the fentanyl
receptor complex are of importance for receptor kinetics:

$$fentanyl + receptor \rightleftharpoons fentanyl\text{-}receptor\ complex$$

This simple relation describes only very unsatisfactorily the
interrelation of the molecule and the receptor since we must
regard the receptor not as a static system, which is solidly
and unchangeably localized on a membrane, but as a dynamic

process. The receptor molecule is synthesized in the Golgi apparatus, brought by intraneuron transport to the membrane, where it has the capacity to react with the opiate molecules for a limited time and under limited circumstances, and then is again transported away and transformed or decomposed. This process can be affected by various mechanisms. For example, a high concentration of opiate molecules or antagonists can lead to internalization of the receptor molecule, thereby liminating the pharmacodynamic effect. This is only one explanation for how the receptor can be present either in an active or inactive form. The factors that influence the process at the receptor are essentially unknown, but they may play a role in the variability in the effect of fentanyl. Which mechanisms appear after activation of the receptor and mediate the intrinsic activity is completely unidentified.(11)

Receptor kinetics is an area where intensive research has been carried out because it promises to explain the receptor-mediated effect of opiates. This hope will probably not be fulfilled because there are too many findings which cannot be explained by pharmacokinetics, including receptor kinetics. Thus, for example, the time of action of lofentanil, which does indeed undergo irreversible bonding with the recptor, is not identical with the conjectured turnover of the receptor molecule. In our above-mentioned investigation of the effect of diazepam, we were able to determine that with increasing occupancy of the receptors the pharmacodynamic effect decreases.(5) We explain this discrepancy between pharmacokinetics and pharmacodynamics on the basis of the pronounced capacity of the central nervous system for autoregulation. Our medications do not act on a rigid system, as when a sheet is rolled from a block of steel, but on a highly flexible system, which has the ability to correct any intrusion (= medicinal effect) within a certain amount of time. It is this adaptive power of the central nervous system,and the speed with which it is able to adjust to altered conditions, which appear to determine the duration of effect of drugs that act on the central nervous system. The duration of effect is not determined by pharmacokinetics, which at best can explain only how the drug reaches the receptor. It is thus inevitable that,in research on such complex processes as the effects of drugs which act on the central nervous system, pharmacokinetic methods must be combined with pharmacodynamic ones.

For this reason, HULL (8) introduced a pharmacodynamic compartment into his pharmacokinetic model, which enables him to adapt his model to the effect which is observed. Our group proceeded one step further, neglecting all mathematical modelling and pharmacokinetics and solely relying on pharmacodynamics. The pharmacodynamic approach is based on clinical experiences, which have already enabled anaesthesiologists to provide a reliable service for some decades. We are all able to recognize conditions in which an additional injection of fentanyl is necessary to restore a steady-state anaesthesia, which means there must have been signs that previously analgesia was insufficient. The statement is similarly true for the other components of anaesthesia like cortical depression or muscular relaxation.

2.3. Pharmacodynamic Approach - Steps towards a Model of Anaesthesia

Our extensive investigations on pharmacokinetics were planned to establish a computer model for the process of anaesthesia. This approach failed - not because of inadequate technical facilities but exclusively because of the unrealistic expectations we placed in pharmacokinetics. Starting out from this realization, we remembered the clinical basis of our daily work and concentrated on the measuring of the desired effects (which are variable, too). Most of these more recent investigations also make use of computers, but in the more limited form of single purpose processors integrated in a monitoring device,such as an averaging processor for evoked potentials and similar devices.

In the studies to be described next, the testing conditions were kept as constant as possible and only one parameter was changed in every new phase. We studied the components cortical depression and analgesia - both elements of a balanced anaesthesia - in awake young male volunteers, students of the Aachen Technical University, aged 25 $\pm$ 2.2 years, with comparable intelligence, motivation, physical fitness, psychological situation. None of them had a history in any psychological impairment, they never took psychopharmacological or any other drugs over a longer period. None was addicted to alcohol, heavy smokers were also eliminated. The investigations were performed in an identical manner, in the same environment, and started at the same time of day. The volunteers were requested to have a normal sleeping period in the night preceding the tests and, after that, to have only a light meal. Summing up, we can say that we really tried hard to establish as nearly identical testing conditions as possible, which it had been impossible to ensure in the clinical set-up we had used to do our previous studies.

A set of tests was used in the investigations on cortical depression: electrophysiological tests such as acoustically evoked potentials of the brain stem and cortex, as well as a smoothed RMS-voltage of the EEG and of the HF-activity (100-3000 Hz) of the biosignal gained from a P_z - A_2 lead from the skull. Apart from this collection of objective data, subjective tests were conducted to evaluate the volunteer's mood during the different testing phases including activation, desactivation, state anxiety, concentration, depression, self-confidence, and so on. In addition, the test also included the flicker fusion frequency and the d_2-test (18,22, 5). Sedation was induced by two normed doses of diazepam according to bodyweight (6), the blood concentration of which was determined at relevant points of time in the course of the test procedure, and, in a follow-up study, by acupuncture of the sedation points Neiguan and Sanyinjao on both sides.

The results of this investigation on cortical depression showed that diazepam produces another effect than acupuncture, which makes the two incomparable: diazepam produces desactivation and a reduction of cortical functions whereas acu-

puncture more specifically produces relaxation. None of the
elements of this set of tests enabled us to distinguish the
effect of classical acupuncture and electro-acupuncture from
placebo-acupuncture; only the oral examination of the volunteers revealed a relaxing effect.

In the diazepam group there were only few significantly different test results in relation to plasma concentration or
dose administered. We found that the smoothed voltage of the
HF-activity as introduced into that test setting by us (one
experiment with cats and implanted electrodes has been reported so far (17)) proved to be a clinically applicable technique to evaluate the component cortical depression, which
we need to perform an adequate anaesthesia.

There has indeed been done a lot of work to introduce electrophysiological methods into anaesthesia, the EEG being a fa-
vourite one. But the aim of the investigations always was to
measure the complex process of anaesthesia itself, and not
one specific component. For that reason, most of the literature cannot really be compared with our results and consequently a comparison is not attempted here.

Contrary to our expectations, we found a fairly good correlation between plasma diazepam level and our new parameter.
This was, however, only the case when effect was correlated
to plasma levels at given times during the fixed course of
the procedure. If you generally compare plasma level with
effect at any chosen time, then the two parameters no longer
correlate. This might be one explanation for the contradictory reports in literature: Some scientists rely on data
gained within a fixed frame of an experiment - others ran-
  domly measure blood levels in a clinical setting and compare them with clinical effect.

Similarly contradictory results are obtained when one exam-
ines the second component of our vector anaesthesia, namely
analgesia, in a comparable test set-up (same restrictions
in choice of volunteers etc.). Fig. 3 shows the time-courses
of awake male volunteers, displaying a rather parallel shape
of pain reduction course (scored by an analogue visual scale)
and fentanyl plasma concentration course. These findings contrast with most of our other investigations, especially with
those where the data were sampled within a clinical setting.
We were not able to define an "analgetic plasma-fentanyl
level", neither during anaesthesia nor in the post-operative
period when we used the on-demand-analgesia computer. Also,
the correlation between fentanyl plasma concentration and
respiratory depression, as expressed by arterial pCO_2, is poor.

We are now trying to develop a technique to measure objectively the noxious input into the CNS, well knowing that pain
is too subjective a phenomenon to be described by neurophysiology. But so far, our numerous studies on evoked responses
- noxiously evoked or not - have not provided us with the
reliable tool we need to optimize balanced anaesthesia.

Muscle relaxation, the third essential component of balanced anaesthesia, was not investigated in a single-drug study because this is not feasible in living organisms. But the Train of Four method (1) of measuring the function of the neuromuscular junction is a reliable tool and easily applicable in the clinical setting. The tests make it evident that muscle relaxation is also variable and is influenced by a number of other factors, for example by other medication. This suggests the conclusion that the different components of anaesthesia cannot simply be reassembled in an additive process since anaesthesia evidently is partially due to synergisms. So our way of establishing a pharmacodynamically based model of anaesthesia must be viewed with certain reservations.

3. Future Developments of Computer Application in Anaesthesiology

The prospective development concerning the implementation of computer technology into anaesthesia is bound to be ambiguous. Considerable improvement in solving detail problems of clinical anaesthesia is to be expected. But the fundamental solution - providing a reliable model of the process of anaesthesia - will not be reached in the foreseeable future. The reason for this is that there is no commonly accepted theory, not to mention a common practice, of anaesthesiology itself and therefore even the most refined technical equipment cannot be fully put to use. Anaesthesiology has to provide its scientific basis first before anaesthesia can be operated by a computer. Therefore, basic research - perhaps of the kind we have just reported about - must illuminate the obscure fundamentals of our "art". At the time when this will be accomplished, all problems we had to cope with regarding response-time, man-machine interface, problem-oriented presentation of data and results will surely have been solved for other fields of medicine, which will then provide the computer with reliable and accepted models. At present, anaesthesiology must rely more on experience and skill than on science.

References

1. ALI, H.H.; SAVARESE, J.J.
   Monitoring of the Neuromuscular Function
   Anesthesiology 45(1976), 216

2. BRICKENKAMP, R.
   Test d_2 - Aufmerksamkeits-Belastungstest
   in: DER, C.J. Hogrefe, Göttingen 1972

3. DAUB, D.; DESTUNIS, S.; HALBACH, M.; HÖVEL, R. vom;
   KALFF, G.
   First Experiences with a Documentation System via Display
   Terminals
   Acta anaesth. belg. 26(1975), suppl. 200

4. DAUB, D.
   Data Processing in the Course of Anaesthesia
   in: E. Rügheimer, M. Zindler (editors):Anaesthesiology
        Excerpta Medica, Amsterdam,Oxford, Princeton 1981

5. DAUB, D.
   Eine multifaktorielle Untersuchung zur Diazepam-Wirkung
   Fortschr. Medizin 100(1982), 2068

6. GAMBLE, J.A.S.; DUNDEE, J.W.; ASSAF, R.A.S.
   Plasma Diazepam Levels After Single Dose Oral and Intra-
   muscular Administration
   Anaesthesiol. 30(1975), 164

7. HUG, C.C.jr.; McCLAIN, D.A.
   Ventilatory Depression by Fentanyl in Anesthetized
   Patients
   Anesthesiology 53(1980), suppl. 56

8. HULL, C.J.
   The Role of Pharmacokinetics in the Development of New
   Drugs: Narcotic analgesics
   Sixth European Congress of Anaesthesiology 1982

9. KEERI-SZANTO, M.
   Anesthetic Time/Dose Curves II: The Limiting Factor in
   the Utilisation of Intravenous Anesthetics During Surgical
   Operations
   Clin. Pharm. Therap. 2(1961), 45

10. KORTTILA, K.; KANGAS, L.
    Unchanged Protein Binding and the Increase of Serum
    Diazepam Levels After FOOD Intake
    Acta Pharmacol. Toxicol. 40(1977), 241

11. KOSTERLITZ, H.W.
    Opioid Peptides and Pain - an Update
    in: J.J. Bonica et al. Advances in Pain Research and
         Therapie, Vol. 5. Raven Press, New York 1983

24

12. LEHMANN, K.A.; DAUB, D.
    Opioide - das Beispiel Fentanyl
    Klin. Anästhesiol. Intensivther. 24(1982), 44

13. LEHMANN, K.A.; GENSIOR, J.; DAUB, D.
    "Analgetische" Fentanyl-Blutkonzentrationen unter
    Neuroleptanalgesie
    Anaesthesist 31(1982), 655

14. LEHMANN, K.A.; WESKI, C.; HUNGER, L, HEINRICH, C.; DAUB,D.
    Biotransformation von Fentanyl. II. Akute Arzneimittel-
    interaktionen - Untersuchungen bei Ratte und Mensch
    Anaesthesist 31(1982), 221

15. LEHMANN, K.A.; HUNGER, L.; BRANDT, K.; DAUB, D.
    Biotransformation von Fentanyl. III. Einflüsse chroni-
    scher Arzneimittelexposition auf Verteilung, Metabo-
    lismus und Ausscheidung bei der Ratte
    Anaesthesist 32(1983), 165

16. LADURON, personal communication

17. RODIN, E.; WASSON, S.; TRIANA, E.; RODIN, M.
    Hochfrequenzableitung: Wert und Grenzen der Methode
    Z. EEG-EMG 4(1973), 9

18. SCHMIDTKE, H.
    Über die Messung der psychischen Ermüdung mit Hilfe des
    Flimmertestes
    Psychol. Forschung 23(1951), 409

19. STÖCKEL, H.; HENGSTMANN, J.H.; SCHÜTTLER, J.
    Pharmacokinetics of Fentanyl as a Possible Explanation
    for Recurrence of Respiratory Depression
    Br. J. Anaesth. 51(1979), 741

20. STÖCKEL, H.; SCHÜTTLER, J.; MAGNUSSEN, H.; HENGSTMANN, J.H.
    Plasma Fentanyl Concentrations and the Occurence of
    Respiratory Depression in Volunteers
    Br. J. Anaesth. 54(1982), 1087

21. THULIN, L.; ANDREEN, M.; IRESTEDT, L.
    Effect of Controlled Halothane Anaesthesia in Splanchnic
    Blood Flow and Cardiac Output in the Dog
    Acta Anaesthesiol. Scand. 19(1975), 146

22. TURNER, P.
    Critical Flicker Frequency and Centrally Acting Drugs
    Br. J. Ophthal. 52(1968), 245

COMPUTERIZED DATA ACQUISITION AND DISPLAY IN ANESTHESIA

Beneken[x], J.E.W., Blom[x], J.A., Meijler[x], A.P., Cluitmans[x], P.
Spierdijk[+], Joh., Nandorff[+], A., Nijhuis[+], R., van Kessel[+], H.M.

      x : Division of Medical Electrical Engineering,
           Eindhoven, University of Technology, the Netherlands
      + : Department of Anesthesiology
           Leyden University Hospital, the Netherlands

SUMMARY

In a collaborative effort to investigate the impact of computer supported
and centralized data acquisition and display in anesthesia on the quality
of care and on the task performance of the anesthesist, such a system has
been designed and this will be described. A total of 32 primary variables
can be handled. After data reduction and feature extraction a maximum of
64 derived variables are stored on floppy disk every 15 seconds.

A variety of display formats are available showing subsets of all signals
on two color displays in numerical or graphical form.

Selecting these subsets and their respective alarm limits is done by
means of a standard keyboard using simple statements and is supported by
a so called helpfile.

Interventions and other relevant information can be entered using the
same keyboard, thus opening the possibility for eliminating manual record
keeping.

A standard or special anesthesia record can be generated for accompanying
the patient or for documentation.

The different approaches to the evaluation of the system will be
described.

It is recognized that coupling of such bedside units both for remote
surveillance and for communicating administrative and other not
continuously available information, improves the versatility of the
system.

ACKNOWLEDGEMENT

These investigations were supported in part by the Netherlands Foun-
dation for Technical Research (STW), future Technical Science Branch/
Division of the Netherlands Organization for the advancement of Pure
Research (ZWO) and the Honeywell and Philips Medical Electronics Group.

INTRODUCTION

There is a tendency of an increasing number of signals and derived
variables to be incorporated in the monitoring of patients during
anesthesia and in intensive care units. The addition of new signals
hardly ever leads to the deletion of other signals. This is probably
based on a feeling of insecurity.
We must realize that each new signal that is being monitored brings
along its cost, in terms of risk to the patient, investment and time.
It is therefore essential to assess the relative contribution of this
new signal to the quality of the monitoring process; i.e. given the set
of signals already in use, what is the improvement when a new signal is
added? Beyond a certain point the addition of new information leads to
new uncertainty and degrades the result (Ream, 1981)
In the diagnostic process, it is possible to evaluate "result" in an
objective, qualitative way. The changes in the sensitivity and
specificity of the diagnosis as a result of the addition or deletion
of a certain variable can be calculated on the basis of false negative,
false positive, correct negative and false   negative scores. Different
methods for multiple regression analysis have been implemented on
computers (Gelsema, 1981) which can support such decision processes.
In monitoring, the situation is much more complex. Many definitions of
monitoring have been given; the common denominator is that monitoring
is a continuous diagnostic process based upon a (semi)continuous flow
of information. This makes simple assessment methods useless. From
failure analysis (Gravenstein et al, 1980, section 4, Failure to monitor)
some conclusions can be drawn with respect to the importance of measuring
certain variables. A similar conclusion can be drawn from mortality
studies.(Lunn and Mushin, 1982) Such approaches yield useful information
but not specific enough to support decisions as to what should we monitor.
A different aspect, which in general terms is not related to the choice
of a particular set of signals, is the degree of signal processing.
Depending on the type of signals, its processing will yield a set of
derived variables. In some cases, this set consists of a large number of
new signals, e.g. following frequency- or power spectral analysis.

However, in most cases the derived variables represent certain features
of the signal, such as maxima, minima and mean values, intervals between
events (R-R) or values sampled at certain instants such as end-expiration
(Blom et al.,1982).

Essential for the proper functioning of a patient-monitoring system is
a good quality of the measured signals. This quality control can be
performed on the derived variables. Error detection algorithms have been
developed that use the statistics of the individual variable to detect
sudden changes of unexpected magnitudes or duration (Jorritsma et al.,1979)
By looking at simultaneous changes in a number of variables, it may
become feasible to distinguish between equipment failure and a change
in the state of the patient. Some degree of self-assessment of the
equipment becomes possible, however the saying, "garbage in, garbage out"
is still a fundamental and valid statement.

It is a fact that human visual perception is very well trained to perform
pattern recognition, while it becomes a very laborious task if performed
by a computer. On the other hand, numerical operations, comparisons and
memory functions are very well performed by computers. Based on such
considerations, it is felt that the initial quality control of the
signals should be done by the anesthesist using an analog display. This
is not a time-consuming task, since no numeric evaluation of the curves
is needed that can reliably be done by the computer.

Once reliable information is available, the automatic detection of trends
in (derived) variables is an important extension of the power of
monitoring systems. Trends can be caused by changes in the state of the
patient or they can be induced, in which case they represent responses
of a patient to treatment (Beneken et al., 1983). In both situations one
is interested in an early detection with an estimation of the time of
onset and an indication of the accuracy of the estimated slope. Coincidences in the onset of trends is important diagnostic information.

Where feature extraction and trend detection are operations performed
on a single variable or a signal, the next important step is the study
of (inter)relations between different variables and/or their characteristics. Many of these relations can be treated in an heuristic way,
using as much a priori information as possible; e.g. peripheral resistance can be calculated from mean arterial pressure and cardiac output;
lung- and thoracic cage compliance can be derived from respiratory
pressure and -flow.

Many variables will show a high degree of correlation, indicating the presence of redundancy in the available information. This may lead to omission of one of the variables, unless this redundant information is utilized to improve the reliability of the data acquisition system as a whole. Two examples: 1. A discrepancy between heart rate derived from the ECG and from the arterial pulse may uncover loose electrodes or a clogged arterial line. 2. A high correlation between end-expiratory gas concentrations and bloodgas values is normally present. Yet, an increase in the difference between the two sets of values contains important diagnostic information about ventilation, perfusion and diffusion.

A more systematic approach to the study of interrelations leads to mathematical formulations of models. Such models will, in general, represent only a part of the patient's behaviour since only a limited set of variables is available. This leads to the design of so called input-output models, where inputs are drug dosage, infusion rates and other quantifiable interventions; the outputs are the measured signals and their derived variables. Such models can be used for the prediction of the effect of planned interventions and support the development of an optimal treatment. The degree of predictability is a measure of the completeness of the model i.e. of the completeness of the set of measured variables. This way, we have an objective indicator for the quality and completeness of the monitoring process.

Besides quality and information content of the available signals, the information transfer between the monitoring devices and the human supervisor (nurse, intensivist, anesthesist) is at least equally important.

Fundamental aspects, such as visual perception, readability, use of colours and lay-out should be considered in the design of displays. From the functional point of view, the mixture of momentary values, time history and visualisation of relations between different quantities is certainly not unique. There is a large subjective element in the design of displays and of man-machine interfaces. A thorough clinical evaluation of proposed solutions is therefore a great challenge.

THE DEVELOPED SYSTEM

When developing a monitoring system one can choose between two possible
configurations:
  1: A central computer, which processes the data of several beds or
     operating rooms;
  2: A stand alone system.
The system we developed is a stand alone system. Data collection,
processing and displaying are done at the bedside, without the need of
a central system. There are two advantages of this design:
  1: Processor time is fully available for processing the data of one
     patient. Time need not be shared with other patients. More signals
     can be monitored and more processing can be done at shorter inter-
     vals;
  2: A connection between bedside apparatus and the central processor
     is not needed, eliminating one possible source of error which may,
     in case of failure, disrupt the entire bedside monitoring.

For most of the measured signals the usual front-end equipment is present
and performs some specific preprocessing: e.g. from the arterial
pressure, the front-end equipment determines diastolic, mean and systolic
pressure. The latter three are fed into our system. Our data acquisition
and display system is therefore supplementary to the front-end equipment.
The system configuration is shown in fig. 1. The input signals of the
system are analog electric signals. A maximum of 32 of these signals are

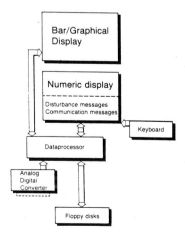

Fig.1. configuration.

digitized by the Analog to Digital Converter. These are sampled by the dataprocessor with a frequency of 50 Hz. The dataprocessor calculates derived variables and after some data processing every variable gets its own status. Every 15 seconds variables with their status are stored on floppy disk. At regular intervals variables and status are sent to two display processors ; they take care of the data presentation. The way of presentation is discussed later.

A keyboard is attached to one of the display-processors for man-machine interaction.

Everything that is typed in, is also stored on floppy disk.

DATA PROCESSING.

Data processing is performed to determine the dynamic properties of the signal. Subsequent processing assigns a status to the variables; basically we distinguish between: invalid, valid and stable.

Initially, all signals are invalid. When a connection is made, the corresponding signal can be declared valid. It will then receive the status: learning. On this signal some disturbance detection is performed. During monitoring the running average $x(K)$ and the running deviation $d(K)$ from a signal are calculated (Jorritsma et al., 1979). Whenever a new input sample $x(K+1)$ is greater then $x(K)+4\ d(K)$ the processing routines will give the signal the status "sudden change up". When $x(K+1) < x(K)-4\ d(K)$ the signal will get the status "sudden change down". This we call "dynamic error detection".

It is also detected if a signal is exceeding static alarm limites, if so, the appropriate status (above higher or below lower alarm) is given. These alarm limits can be set by the anesthetist.

Whenever one of the above mentioned fault conditions lasts longer than 15 seconds, also an error message is generated as well as presented on the lower display screen.

When no fault condition is present, the signal has the status "stable".
The following schematic sums up the different signal conditions; a signal
has always one status out of the seven underlined possibilities.

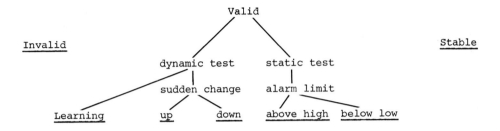

INTERACTIONS BETWEEN SYSTEM AND USER.

Users interact with the system by means of a keyboard and two colour
display screens. A pervasive design decision has been, that use of the
keyboard should be minimal: inexperienced users will nicely get along
with a minimum of effort. Another design decision was to enable
experienced users to have access to all information in their own
preferred format, though this may require some more effort.
Two categories of keyboard entries exist: commands and data. Commands
order the system to perform some function, e.g. to start processing a
new signal or to generate a new display. Data entered at the keyboard
consists of drug dosages, infusion rates, surgical events etc. We cannot
fully explain our keyboard entry method here, but we want to mention
some of its features:
- dedicated function keys allow entry with a minimum of keystrokes.
  For instance, the command "ON CO2 PART", which tells the system that
  the capnograph and the arterial line are connected and that their
  signals must be processed, takes four keystrokes: three function keys
  and the "ENTER" key.
- experienced users can enter a command in one line, while novice users
  will be prompted for each following entry with a question as long as
  the command is not complete. The latter method, though initially
  slower, is virtually self-learning.

- at any time pressing the "HELP" key provides the user with detailed information on how to proceed.
- in case of erroneous entry the system pinpoints the error and shows the valid alternatives. Pressing "HELP" gives a more complete explanation on how to proceed.

The two colour screens serve three purposes. In the first place, part of one screen serves as a terminal, that echoes keyboard characters, prints prompting questions and in general serves the interaction between system and user. A second part of this screen serves as the alarm system: it provides static alarms, dynamic alarms and computer errors (a full floppy disk, a cable disconnection, etc.) Alarm messages are as specific as possible. Lastly, the major part of both screens is dedicated to the presentation of the state of the patient. This information presentation is organized in a hierarchical fashion, as is shown in figure 2.

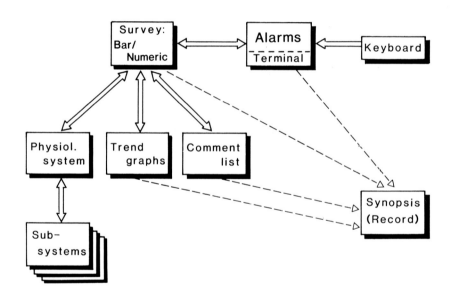

Fig. 2. Organisation of the presented information.

There, the full drawn lines connect optional display formats. The interrupted lines indicate that the anesthesia record can be generated either
on-line, during the operation or off-line, after the operation.
In some of the more complicated operations a tremendous quantity of
information is potentially available, which can only be assimilated
if presented orderly. The default presentation is a survey of the state
of the patient. Two fields are visible. Upto 40 variables or derived
quantities are presented numerically on what we call the numeric display,
which shows momentary values only.
In figure 3 a possible lay-out of the numeric display is represented.
Four columns and ten rows and separation lines that can individually be
placed, facilitate grouping of variables into functionally related
blocks of numeric values.
The variable name and value are not shown when their status is invalid.
When an alarm condition of one or more variables is detected, the back
ground colour of the corresponding name area turns red.
Below the numeric field, two area's of the screen are reserved for alarm
messages; one serves as terminal in relation with the key board.

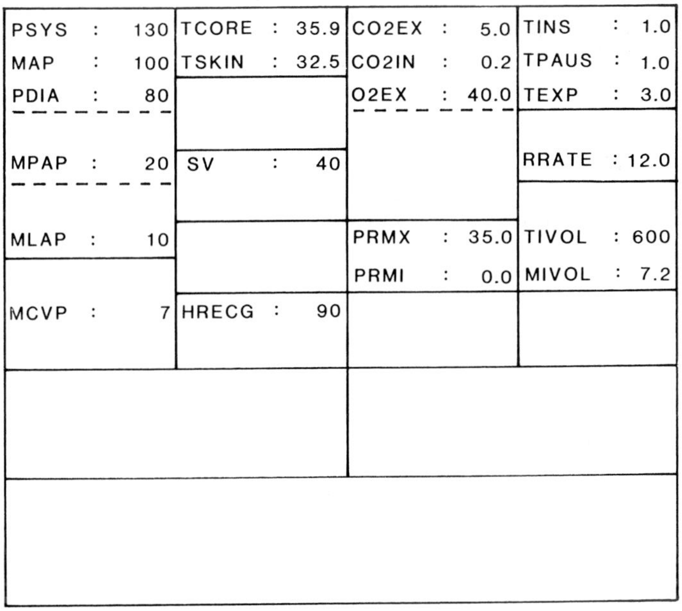

PSYS : 130	TCORE : 35.9	CO2EX : 5.0	TINS : 1.0
MAP : 100	TSKIN : 32.5	CO2IN : 0.2	TPAUS : 1.0
PDIA : 80		O2EX : 40.0	TEXP : 3.0
MPAP : 20	SV : 40		RRATE : 12.0
MLAP : 10		PRMX : 35.0	TIVOL : 600
		PRMI : 0.0	MIVOL : 7.2
MCVP : 7	HRECG : 90		

Fig. 3. Numeric Display.

The second screen shows as bar display the ten most important variables
in a therapy-oriented way: is the variable in its normal range, how far
is it from the alarm limits, how is the trend and is it stable now?
One glance at this display gives this quick overall picture. We expect
that this survey, together with the alarms, will be the most relevant
display most of the time, Therefore, we will describe the display in
more detail.
Fig. 4 gives one of the bars showing core temperature data. Every bar
gives the behaviour of one variable over the last three hours on a
logarithmic time axis. The present value is shown flashing.

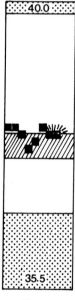

var T.core
nrm 37.0
prv 37.2

interval

1'	(0 – 15 sec)
2'	(15 – 45 sec)
3'	(45 sec – 2¼ min)
4'	(2¼ – 6¾ min)
5'	(6¾ – 20¼ min)
6'	(20¼ – 60¾ min)
7'	(60¾ – 182¼ min)

Fig. 4 Bar graph display. The six data points on the left
represent the behaviour of the variable over the past three hours.
The corresponding time intervals are given. The data point on the
right represents most recent 15 sec. interval.

The value of the variable is presented on a linear vertical axis. The upper and lower fields represent two red alarm area's. In the middle of the bar the blue normal area is presented. The space between the blue and red bands are black attention area's. Below the bar the name of the variable, its normvalue and its present value are displayed.

When a proper choice of the 10 variables has been made this display gives in one glance a survey of the status of the patient.

Sometimes more detailed information is necessary. In that case the survey display is (partially) removed and a more specific display is generated. First of all, trend graphs of selected signals will be important. A default trend display exists, but the user can choose any combination of signals, and their scaling and the scaling of the time axis can be selected from 15 min. to 4 hrs. full scale.

The comment list will present (all or a selection of) the data entered at the keyboard. Entries can then be added, deleted or changed.

The development of the organ oriented displays is still in a planning stage. This system type will group all relevant information about a system, e.g. the circulation, on one screen. Even more detailed information, e.g. about the mechanical heart function, will be provided by the sub system displays. These displays will in general provide their information in a mixed format: partially graphs, numerical values of variables and derived, calculated quantities (e.g. indices), events, relevant injections and infusions, etc., if available.

At this time our system does not handle the analog displays of the raw signals like ECG and blood pressures, because the front end equipment provides those. We do recognize the great importance of these displays because of the signal quality control that they provide and therefore (parts of) these curves will need to be integrated with the more specialized display types.

A synopsis, which is as yet not implemented, will show the anesthesia record as it is being built up using a plotter. It will have the same format as is used for the manual record and is meant to replace it. At the end of the operation it is complete.

An off-line editing program allows each user to specify his own defaults
for the layout of the various displays. With relatively little effort
this allows adjustment of the data presentation to different groups of
patients, type of surgery, available operating room front end equipment
and individual preferences, thus minimizing peroperative data entry
effort and maximizing the usefulness of the displays.

AUTOMATED RECORD KEEPING

Documentation of anesthetic data is needed under a number of distinctly
different circumstances and for different purposes, such as:

- pre-operative	- for recording of pre-operative information
- during anesthesia	- to show preanesthetic information
	- for recording of measurement results
	- to discover trends, inconsistencies etc.
	- for recording observations and interventions
	- to assess responses to treatment
	- to force attention to the patient
- post operative	- for transfer of information to the I.C.U. or recovery room
	- to assess complications, immediate or delayed
	- to reveal information for future anesthesia
	- for legal purposes
- general use	- clinical research, e.g. technique, drugs
	- medical statistics
	- teaching

Each of these applications may require a different record with different
degrees of detail. Should we be able to reconstruct the course of events
from the recorded information? The opinions differ. If the answer is yes,
the discussion about which information should go on record, runs parallel
with the discussion about which signals should be monitored during

anesthesia. However it is good to realize that personal observations remain extremely important. Subtle changes may be observed without realizing it. Yet, they play their role in decision making but will never go on record.

Irrespective of the importance of personal observations, assessment of the condition of a patient, only on the basis of the monitored variables, both continuous and intermittent, is impossible if not at the same time the inputs to the patient (drugs, ventilation, other interventions) are recorded properly with the same degree of accuracy with respect to timing and quantity (Beneken et al., 1983).

Reasons for automation have often been listed; relevant for the anesthesia record are:

- reduction of administrative load
- more time available for patient care
- improvement of the quality of the document

It is obvious that automatic generation of anesthesia records is only possible in the presence of a certain sophistication level of the monitoring equipment.
Signals and information from all further sources that are being surveyed during anesthesia, should be stored in some memory.

When an adequate and interactive display system is available, the presence of an anesthesia record during anesthesia is no longer necessary. All relevant information can be retrieved from memory and be displayed upon request. Most of the above listed purposes can be performed automatically and different solutions are available for entering non-numeric data and observations (Baetz et al., 1979). Attention to the patient can be drawn in many different ways.

Nothwithstanding the degree of automation in the O.R., the patient who is being transferred to the post-operative care unit should always be accompanied by a written or printed information sheet, unless a fully integrated patient data management system is operational which encompasses both the O.R. and the post-operative unit.
During the transition period from manual to automated record keeping one is likely to find differently equiped O.R.'s in the same department. It is believed to be essential that during this period the automated systems

produce (e.g. at the end of the operation) an anesthesia record that is highly similar to the manually completed record, both with respect to general lay-out and information content. This is an important safety measure. The lay-out of such a standard record will thus be determined by the local circumstances and procedures.

In addition to this standard record, the full exploitation of the power of automated, computer supported data acquisition systems can yield an extension of the standard record while keeping the general design of the lay-out. Such an extended record can show more details, such as pre- and post-event time plots of any number of variables, or numeric values at shorter intervals, etc. Such a record can be made as a patient-tailored anesthesia record by handling the data interactively at a computer terminal; each patient and/or each situation requires different data for assessment.

The future then will show no record keeping during anesthesia. Data acquisition systems will store all information into memory devices (e.g. floppy disks) and will produce records containing only the information needed for the transfer of the patient and for other post-operative purposes.

Additional information, e.g. for research or teaching, is, at all times, available and can be edited and printed in accordance with the specific purposes.

EVALUATION.
Many technicians and anesthetists are engaged in the development of systems for the automation of several tasks of the anesthetist. Most progress on this subject is made independently and thus different aspects are being emphasized in the different designs.
The automatic generation of the anesthesia record is a starting point for some of the designers (Frazier et al., 1981).
Others favour the centralized registration of their patients' state and the therapy (Kontron Ltd.). Optimal man machine interaction that is, the facility to easily enter and recall interventions and information is also considered an important aspect (Rau 1982). On line monitoring is the main interest for again another group (Demeester 1982).

In the development of the DADS system described above, priority was given to the aspect of on-line monitoring. It was tried to stimulate pattern recognition by implementing special display facilities and hierarchical alarm structures.

All those various systems will have their impact on the functioning of the anesthetist and thus (possibly) on patient care. It is clear from the effort being put forth in the development of those systems that there is perhaps a need for them. Or, if not really a need, the evolution in intensive care units and operating rooms is in a state ready for the introduction of this kind of system. In the first part of this paper certain as ects, such as the number and quality of signals and their degree of processing, which have led to this evolution, were mentioned. For the introduction of these systems to be justified it has to be proven that they are a necessity from a medical point of view and economically acceptable. The criteria for assessment used by people differ:

- an improvement of morbidity and/or mortality of the patients,
- a significant decrease of incidents and
- the improvement of the work situation of the anesthetist,

are the different gradations.

The directly visible design demands are mostly directed toward a lower workload for the anesthetist (by recordkeeping for instance), better monitoring of patients (especially when one anesthetist serves more than one operating room), or more efficient registration of patient data. Besides the justification, it will be very valuable to test the performance as such, to find achilles heels and loose ends so as to carry out essential improvements.

At present our DADS is being evaluated (Meyler et al., 1983). The objective is in particular to make judgements with respect to incidences and worksituation. In addition the performance is tested. The approach to the evaluation procedure is based upon both literature and practice.

= A review of incidents and their associated factors can provide items for investigating whether the system helps in obviating or detecting them and if that is not the case whether it is possible to implement such a possibility as yet. Cooper et al.,(1978) show that most of the preventable incidents involve human error (82%) with amongst others, drug-syringe errors being a frequent problem. If, for instance, one

could attach a barcode to all syringes which would have to be read
before administration, some inadvertent swaps could be prevented. As
associated factors they mention amongst others: fatigue, failure to
perform a normal check and distraction. These can certainly be
improved by systems which reduce workload and present the essential
information in an ergonomic fashion.

- With respect to the worksituation (carriage, fatigue of the eyes etc.)
a thorough literature study on ergonomics in connection with the
system is essential.

- A study on the task analysis of the anesthetist is done to get to
understand the decision processes. This is a necessity to find out
for instance whether the correct variable set is presented in an
optimal way. Besides, it can function to detect weakness in the
anesthetic procedure and workload.

For instance 10-15% of the time is spent on recording (Kennedy et al.,
1976)

The studies will result in a checklist of items against which the DADS
is being tried. If unavoidable, items will have to be checked with the
anesthetists, but unobtrusive methods will have preference. (for instance
the use of data on disk).

The intention is to get results that are generally applicable and if
possible, statistically significant. In the future one could hope that
all the different systems could melt into a few standardized types.
Perhaps followed over a longer period of time something can be said as
well about morbidity and/or mortality which in fact are of the utmost
importance for the patient.

DISCUSSION.

The Eindhoven-Leyden data acquisition and display system was designed
as a flexible system to study the usefulness of such apparatus in the
operating room and the intensive care unit.

Although we chose to make a stand-alone system, we do recognize the
usefulness of communication between systems. We forsee a network of
independently operating bedside units (or O.R. units) with options

for data communication to other bedside units for remote surveillance
or consultation and for data communication with the clinical laboratory
and an administrative information system. Because of bedside processing
and -storage, a high reliability is obtained which is not dependent upon
this network.

The described system offers many facilities in terms of displays, alarms,
user interactions and patient- or specialist tailored records. Such a
system is basically not realistic for every day use in a peripheral
hospital, nor even in a university hospital.

The built-in, software based, flexibility allows for a systematic study
of the wishes and needs of the clinicians and attending personnel, and
of the benefit of such systems in terms of improvement in the quality
of care. The results of this study will yield design criteria for future
monitoring systems.

The following ten demands sum up the conditions that have to be met by
a clinically useful data acquisition and display system:

1. Measurements of continuous variables should be performed
   automatically and not manually.

2. Intermittently available quantities and non-numeric information
   should be easy to enter.

3. A rapid and easy check on the quality of the inputsignals should be
   supplemented by automatic tests on quality and internal consistency
   of the data.

4. Easy access to subsets of data concerning one or more organsystems.

5. Hierarchical alarming structure, based upon both fixed and variable
   alarm limits.

6. Facilities should be available to reveal interrelations, coincidences
   and other systematic patterns.

7. Lay-out of displays, the use of colours and other features should be
   consitent.

8. The system should monitor its own performance.

9. All interactions between the user and the system should be stored
   and saved.

10. It should be simple to learn how to operate the system.

42

REFERENCES.

Baetz, W.R. Schneider, A.L.J., Apple, H., Fadel, J. and Katona, P.
    The anesthesia keyboard system
    in: Monitoring Surgical Patients in the Operating Room.
    Eds. J.S. Gravenstein et al.
    Ch. Thomas, Springfield Ill. 1979 P. 197 - 212

Beneken, J.E.W. Blom, J.A.
    An integrative patient monitoring approach
    in: Integrated approaches to monitoring Ed. J.S. Gravenstein et al
    Butterworth 1983 (in press)

Beneken, J.E.W., Blom, J.A. Saranummi, N.
    Accuracy in trend detection
    in: Integrated approaches to monitoring Eds. J.S. Gravenstein et al
    1983 in press Butterworth

Blom, J.A., Beneken, J.E.W.
    On line information and data reduction in patient monitoring
    in: Computing in medicine Eds. J.P. Paul et al. McMillan Press
    1982

Cooper, J.B., Newbower, R.S. Long, C.D., Buknam McPeek
    Preventable Anesthesia mishaps : A Study of human factors
    Anesthesiology 49 : 399 - 406, 1978

Demeester, M.
    Chronider = Système versatile de collecte automatique de
    memorisation et de monitoring de données physiologiques et de
    données cliniques.
    Personal communication.

Frazier, W.T. Paulsen, A.W, Harbort, R.A. Odom, S.H., Haygood, W.F.,
    Integrated Anesthesia Delivery/Monitoring System with computer
    assisted anesthetic record generation.
    Presented at Scientific exhibit, 55th congress of the International
    Anesthesia Research Society, Atlanta, Georgia. March 8 - 12, 1981

Gelsema, E.S.   ISPAHAN users manual (4th edition)
    Dept. of Medical Informatics, Free University Amsterdam   1981

Gravenstein, J.S., Newbower, R.S., Ream, A.K., Smith, N.Ty.
    Essential non invasive monitoring in anesthesia
    Grune and Stratton   New York   1980

Jorritsma, F.F., Gieles, J.P.M., Blom, J.A., Beneken, J.E.W. Nandorff, A.
    Bijnen, A. van, Spierdijk, J.
    Error detection in patient monitoring
    Biomedizinische Technik   Band 24, 50 - 51, 1979

Kennedy, P.K., Feingold, A., Wiener, E.L., Hosek, R.S.
    Analysis of tasks and human factors in anesthesia for
    coronary-artery by pass.
    Anesthesia and Analgesia 55 : 374-377,   1976

Kontron medical ltd.
    DPS 100 Data processing system for critical care
    Bernerstrasse süd   169,
    CH-8048   Zürich   Switzerland

Lunn, J.N., Mushin, W.W.
    Mortality Associated with Anesthesia
    Nuffield Provincial Hospitals Trust, London 1982

Meijler, A.P., Beneken, J.E.W., Nandorff, A., Spierdijk, J.
    A data acquisition and display system for improved medical
    pattern recognition.
    in: Objective Medical Decision-making; systems approach in
    acute disease.   Eds. J.E.W. Beneken and S.M. Lavelle
    Springer Verlag, 1983   in press.

Rau, G. Ergonomic design aspects in interaction between man and
    medical systems.
    in: Proceedings world congress on medical physics and biomedical
    engineering. 1982 sept. 5-11 Hamburg nr. 4.01.

Ream, A.K. Computer Assisted Multivariate Analysis in Cardiovascular
    Measurements. Presented in Punta Ala, Italy. September 1981
    Frontiers for Cardiology in the Eighties.

MICROCOMPUTER BASED AUTOMATIC CAPTURE OF SIGNALS FROM NON-INVASIVE INSTRUMENTS.

N. H. NAQVI, F.F.A.R.C.S.
DEPARTMENT OF ANAESTHETICS,
BOLTON ROYAL INFIRMARY, BOLTON, LANCASHIRE, U.K.

Development of microprocessors during recent years and their extensive use has significantly improved the performance of electronic instrumentation. One such example is the recent increased availability of non-invasive blood pressure recorders for measuring systemic, systolic and diastolic arterial blood pressure, heart rate and mean arterial pressure. Such a device incorporating a microprocessor and using oscillometric principle was described in 1978 (Tompkins and Webster, 1981). Since then, significant developments in integrated circuit technology have refined and enhanced their performance. One important advantage of this new generation of instruments is that the required parameters can be measured and documented automatically, with accuracy and consistency. Many problems which are inherent in the manually operated simple blood pressure apparatus are removed. Their acceptance has been slow as physicians are traditionally conservative and cautious in accepting a new development. There is no doubt that micro-processors are here to stay, not as the latest vogue but on the merit of sophistication and cost effectiveness. This is one development where prospective users cannot afford to delay acceptance. Any hesitation, or further delay, might deny them a very useful tool. One problem facing medical users of the microprocessor-based medical equipment is the same as that facing users outside medicine. The manufacturers due to severe competition, are not developing uniform standardised products. They are striving to outdo each other rather than help the consumer by producing equipment which in inter-changeable and machines that can 'talk' to each other.

Unfortunately medical users have been unable to influence this but have to spend their limited funds to acquire recorders and printers for their monitors if they want to keep and maintain accurate recordings. Freedom of choice among clinicians to use whatever equipment they choose must remain. Any restriction in this respect would hinder further developments and therefore would be strongly opposed by the profession.

The value of accurate record-keeping is well established and this is always desirable for good patient care. Any form of technological help which can contribute to accuracy and automation in record-keeping deserves examination. Hesitation and unwillingness of doctors to produce medical records for self-audit has been criticised (Lunn and Mushin, 1982). This hesitation would be unnecessary if records are automatically prepared and preserved. For medico-legal purposes, legible and accurate records of events are always advisable. Some doctors are notorious in preparing notes and records using illegible writing. Any records prepared in such a way that are not legible and cannot be understood by others have limited value.

Invasive monitoring of vital signs during anaesthesia and intensive care is now widely practised. It has its own advantages, disadvantages and dangers. Invasive monitoring is generally considered to be accurate and more comprehensive. But it is also true that accuracy is dependent upon diligent maintainance of equipment and correct application of transducers. This problem is multiplied when mainframe computers are used with invasive monitors for data collection and processing. These systems require continuous technical back-up which greatly increases expense. Such justified restrictions make invasive ystems only suitable for large institutions where technical help is available.

Non-invasive monitors are in common use both in general hospitals and in specialised centres, and no doubt this type of monitoring is most suitable for the needs and requirements of routine day-to-day work in most hospitals. These techniques should be employed more often, on the merit of simplicity,

safety, and consistent performance. To fulfil the increasing
need for reliable, cost effective non-invasive monitors,
sophisticated hardware is now available. Manual collection
of data which is displayed by non-invasive monitors at desired
intervals is quite laborious and time consuming. If this task
is automated it will release the medical and nursing staff
for other more important duties in patient care. Moreover
such automation would also improve accuracy, consistency and
legibility in medical records. Since the manufacturers do
not conform to a uniform standard, problems arise when data
needs to be processed for storage and recall, if a range of
non-invasive devices are in use. At present it is difficult
to find a way to integrate signals from different non-invasive
devices for display in real time, and also to store the data
for future retrieval and reference. Such a need can be fulfilled by using a suitable microcomputer and interfacing it
with various non-invasive monitors of choice. The signals
from monitors are captured, integrated and communicated to
microcomputer for display in real time in a suitable format
and can also be stored. A facilty based on this principle
can easily overcome many problems of incompatibility of
medical instruments, produced by various manufacturers.
Microcomputer interfacing would also be useful for some of
the non-invasive instruments used in doctors' offices and
laboratory for simple investigation, but such tailor-made
interfacing hardware is not yet available. One manufacturer
has recently introduced a dedicated interface which only
displays respiratory parameters captured from an electronic
ventilator. Some other users of microcomputers have designed
and built their own interface. Table 1 offers examples in
which non-invasive monitors and other devices have been
successfully interfaced with a microcomputer utilising
hardware available off the shelf. Some of these systems are
commercially available and can be purchased with all
facilities of backup services and maintainance. They are
flexible enough to be updated in future if required. Others
are still at research and development stage.

TABLE 1

1. VITAL SIGNS MONITORS
   a) Blood pressure monitor.
   b) Thermometer.
   c) Carbon dioxide analyser.
   d) Respiratory monitor.

2. GAS AND ANAESTHETIC VAPOUR MONITORS.
   a) Oxygen analyser.
   b) Anaesthetic vapour monitor.

3) LABORATORY AND OFFICE INVESTIGATIONS
   a) Computed spirometry.
   b) Computerised obstetric measurements.

4) QUALITY CONTROL
   a) Instruments "Watch Dog"

VITAL SIGNS MONITORS

It has been mentioned earlier that microprocessors have been used extensively in non-invasive blood pressure monitors, to measure display and record systolic, diastolic, blood pressure, heart-rate and mean arterial pressure. Quite a few of these machines have appeared in the market. Some of them provide the facility of built-in recorder or printer, while others offer these as an option. The format of hard copy varies from a digital print-out to a variety of trend recordings. These machines utilise various physical principles to sense or detect systolic and diastolic arterial pressure. A large majority of them are based on an oscillometric principle, while others utilise doppler, infrasound and audio-frequency sensors. Since most of these provide the facility to be connected with recorders, it is possible to make use of the analogue signals available at the output sockets and interface them with a suitable microcomputer. Some of the very latest models also incorporate a standard interfacing facility like a RS 232 (Electronic Industry Association Standard) to make interfacing a lot easier.

Apart from blood pressure monitors other non-invasive vital signs monitors commonly used during anaesthesia and intensive care are: thermometers, respiratory monitors to measure respiratory parameters like rate of respiration, tidal volume and airway pressure. Gas analysers to display end expired carbon dioxide concentration and oxygen analysers which monitor oxygen percentage in fresh gas flow.

Microcomputer based capture and processing of signals related to above mentioned parameters, using a range of monitors, has been described (Naqvi, 1982). The system is built around a compact computer, Hewlett-Packard 85 (HP 85). The computer is small enough to be accommodated on an anaesthetic machine and can display the data in real time during the intra-operative period. Figure 1 shows computer and various monitors assembled on an anesthetic machine. It provides a printout in graphic and digital form and also stores the data for future retrieval. Communication between computer and monitors is achieved by an electronic system or interface specially designed for this purpose. The hardware components of this interface are enclosed in a small box or can be accommodated inside the computer after some modification. The interface is assembled by using printed cards which can be purchased. A six channel analogue to digital converter is used to receive signals from an electronic thermometer, carbon dioxide analyser and ventilator. The respiratory parameters are captured from output socket of an electronic ventilator like Servo 900 B. Software is designed to process these signals to display the data on computer screen in a traditional graphic form. A printout in digital form is produced simultaneously by the built-in printer (Figure 2). The data can be stored either on built-in cassette or floppy disc. The hardware in the interface can also be adapted to read a suitable electronic ventilation monitor. This makes it possible to use a non-electronic mechanical ventilator. The respiratory values are monitored electronically with a separate less expensive instrument. A prototype, soon to be marketed, of such a respiratory monitor has been interfaced in

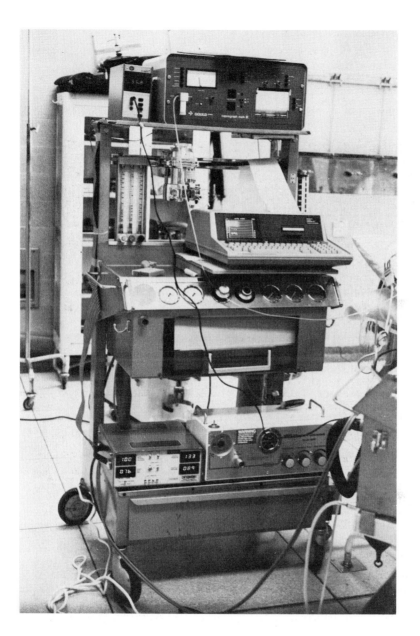

Fig. 1. Photograph of H.P. 85 and
various monitors assembled
on an anaesthetic machine.

50

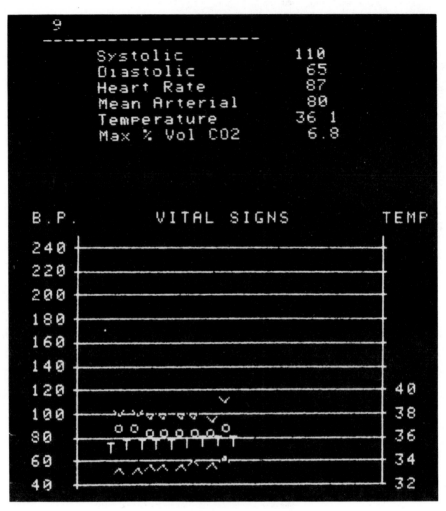

Fig. 2. A typical hard copy of
graphic and digital record
of vital signs.

place of the electronic ventilator, with the system described above.

In order to receive signals from a non-invasive blood pressure monitor a two-channel RS 232 is used. Two commercially available blood pressure monitors Dinamap and Sentry have been successfully interfaced and some others can be used without major alteration in software and hardware. The building blocks of this interface are shown in Figure 3. Apart from the cards which receive signals other ready made circuit cards required to process the signals and interpret them in a format suitable for HP 85 are Intel 8085 and a card with small random access memory (RAM). Intel 8085 is used as buffer and sets flag for the RAM whenever the HP 85 is ready to receive data. This system is connected with the computer through an industry standard interface called microface. The microface is a specially designed communication device producing logical communication between monitors and HP 85. Software is designed for this system to process data in real time. The visual display unit displays a chart which is traditionally prepared by anaesthesiologists, when they prepare anaesthetic record manually. Six digit hospital number for identification, patient's description and other information regarding pre-op assessment, premedication and breathing system, etc., can be entered using the computer keyboard. The drugs used and post-operative comments are entered by resetting the menu for relevant data in a question answer sequence. Retrieval of any one stored record is extremely quick and easy. A program for statistical analysis can be prepared and added as sub-routine to the existing system. Hard copy of a comprehensive anaes-thetic record can be prepared with the help of a plotter, using a preprinted blank record form. This offers a complete anaesthetic record in a matter of seconds. Moreover this system can help to organise storage and retrieval of anaesthetic records within the department, utilising minimum space. Manual filing of records is always a difficult problem, specially in a small general hospital. Using a system where data is automatically acquired, recorded and stored in a small

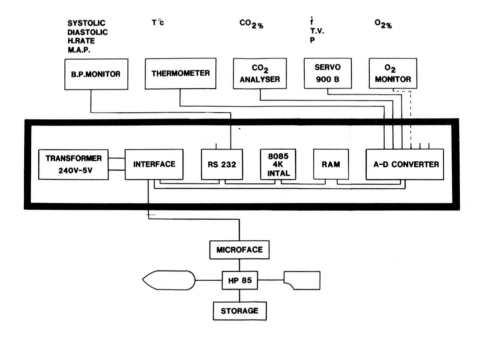

Fig. 3. Diagrametic representation of
the interface used with H.P. 85
and non-invasive vital signs monitors.

space would greatly enhance not only patient care, but help research and self-audit. There is no doubt that such a system would prove to be cost effective. The system is particularly suitable for a small general hospital, where non-invasive monitoring is commonly used and preferred to invasive techniques. The computer is not dedicated and can be used for other purposes within the department.

Work is in progress to interface a neuromuscular monitor, and a suitable anaesthetic vapour monitor to measure percentage of volatile anaesthetic agents.

COMPUTED SPIROMETRY

Many dedicated systems for computed spirometry are available, not only for use in the office of respiratory physician but also for use in pulmonary function laboratory (Robischon, 1982). The cost and limited lifespan, at present prohibits wider use of these dedicated systems. They can be cost effective if a large number of tests related to spirometry are requested. At present the overall picture of computerised spirometry still confuses most potential users. But the value of such non-invasive investigations is accepted.

A relatively cheap and workable system has been designed and marketed by Vitalograph. It is based on a popular micro-computer, Apple II, which is interfaced with the standard spirometer. Spirotrac II has achieved acceptability among respiratory technicians. There are several reasons for this ready acceptability. It provides the analogue trace of the test in the way which technicians were accustomed to watch before the computer was added to it. It does not provide a jargon of numbers and calculated results, as some of the dedicated systems are built to do. The system has volumetric discrimination of 0·0025 litres. Its reasonable cost is also a strong factor. The microcomputer used is a popular model and its large memory is available for many other additional needs. Software for this system is designed to make calculations and present them on the screen and store the data on floppy disc. A hard copy can be produced by printer. The data can be subjected to statistical analysis if desired.

The system is extremely useful when respiratory parameters
are being studied under controlled conditions using different
drugs. It makes an extremely useful research tool for quick
controlled comparisons. The system has the flexibility to
be updated according to the developing future needs in
respiratory therapy. The software can be enhanced to
individual requirements. Figure 4 shows the system used
in a respiratory laboratory and Figure 5 gives schematic
details of the interface.

COMPUTER OBSTETRIC MEASURING SYSTEM

Use of ultrasound equipment in the obstetric department
to monitor the well being of mother and foetus has been a
success story. The foetal heart monitors and sensor of
uterine contractions have been in use for over a decade, in
all obs tetric hospitals. Such non-invasive monitoring
during labour has significantly contributed towards the
safety of mother and quality of foetus. Monitors based on
ultrasonic detection are in common use but linking these
timetested monitors with a microcomputer has received little
consideration as yet. But microcomputers have been interfaced
with the static ultrasound scanner, which is widely employed
for monitoring foetal development.

The system is designed by Sonicaid Limited and called
Sonicomp. Again an Apple microcomputer is used. The software
and hardware is designed to display a static scanning picture
on the computer visual display unit. Its 8 - bit digital
converter can be used in conjunction with many earlier linear
array real-time scanners and smaller, low cost scanners
without a frame freeze facility. It can be used to upgrade
older scanners to the standard of modern ones at a fraction
of the replacement cost. The image is displayed on the
computer screen and can be frozen whilst measurements are made.
Accuracy is enhanced because the measurements are made directly
on to this frozen image with the help of an electronic graphic
tablet with stylus and computer generated small cursor. This

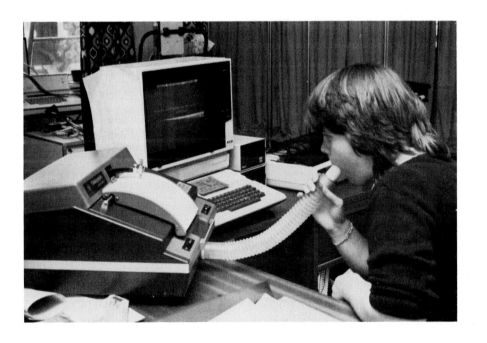

Fig. 4. SPIROTRAC II used in a
respiratory laboratory.

56

VITALOGRAPH SPIROMETER/APPLE INTERFACE

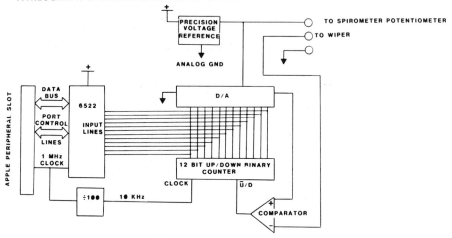

Fig. 5.   Schematic diagram of
          Vitalograph spirometer
          interface.
          (Courtesy of Vitalograph).

removes errors due to parallex or picture distortion. It is
simple to use and no special training is required to operate
the system. It allows essential obstetric measurements extremely
fast and high degrees of accuracy. More than 20 separate
measurements can be made at one examination, which are stored
and can be retrieved for comparisons with others taken at
later visits. In this way the Sonicomp provides accumulated,
accurate and comprehensive information to the obstetrician
regarding foetal development. The user can review and edit
the data if necessary. One floppy disc can accommodate
obstetric records of over 500 patients. Hard copy can be
produced at any time by a silent printer. The hardware
remains non-dedicated and offers as a bonus the advantage of
48K Apple memory for any other use within the obstetric unit.
Figure 6 shows a hard copy of various obstetric measurements
obtained from the Sonicomp.

QUALITY CONTROL

Microcomputers are extensively interfaced with all types
of electronic instruments in industry for quality control.
Their use for this particular purpose in medical field is not
yet popular. In laboratory environment quality control is
fairly easy. If a delicate instrument, like blood gas
analyser is used in an isolated way, like an intensive care
unit, operation room or a baby care unit, its performance
needs to be watched with strict standards. In these circumstances a microcomputer using a suitable software can provide
the essential requirements to maintain quality control,
acting as "Watch-Dog".

DISCUSSION

Sophisticated mainframe computers are only available to a
few medical centres with a reputation of excellence. Their
use and maintainance requires highly trained and skilful
personnel. They are not considered suitable for small general
hospitals where routine and day-to-day work is carried out
using simple and less expensive equipment. For the purpose

58

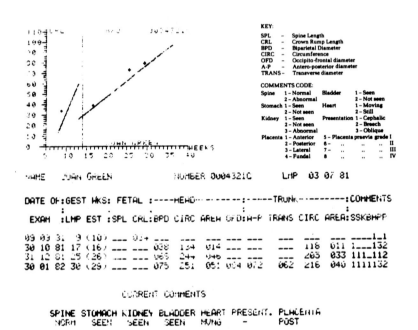

NAME   JOAN GREEN   NUMBER 0004321C   LMP 03 07 81

DATE OF:GEST WKS: FETAL :----HEAD---------:-----TRUNK---------:COMMENTS
   EXAM :LMP EST :SPL CRL:BPD CIRC AREA OFD:A-P TRANS CIRC AREA:SSKBHPP

09 03 31 9 (10) ___ 03+ ___   ___ ___ ___   ___   __   ___ ___-1_1
30 10 81 17 (16) ___ ___ 038 134 014 ___ ___   ___ 118 011 1___132
31 12 81 25 (26) ___ ___ 065 244 045 ___ ___   ___ 205 033 111_112
30 01 82 30 (29) ___ ___ 075 251 051 004 072   062 216 040 1111132

CURRENT COMMENTS

SPINE STOMACH KIDNEY BLADDER HEART PRESENT. PLACENTA
NORM SEEN   SEEN   SEEN   MVNG   –   POST

Fig. 6.   A sample hard copy of
          obstetric record obtained
          using Sonicomp.
          (Courtesy of Sonicaid Ltd.)

of monitoring and investigations, non-invasive techniques are safer and advisable unless indicated otherwise. If non-invasive devices are employed, which are designed by different manufacturers it becomes a difficult problem to prepare automatic records for data management. This task can be made easy if a suitable microcomputer is selected and interfaced to these devices for real time display and data processing. Some of these applications have been described in this chapter. Although the microcomputers are extensively used in medicine for data collection, management and statistical analysis etc., those described here are chosen specially on the basis where microcomputer directly communicate with monitors and instruments through skilfully designed hardware and software, and parameters are measured and tested non-invasively. These systems are developed fairly recently and have not gained wide acceptability. It is observed that such a system needs highly motivated staff to make maximum use. A lot of effort and time is required to train the staff. Maybe in the near future system based on "turn-key" principle are introduced which need minimum effort and understanding to operate. Microcomputers do not conform to various recommendations of medical standards of safety, although they are safe devices to be used in offices and homes. If microcomputers are interfaced with medical instruments then safety regulations might be endangered. This problem is worrying those who want to interface the microcomputer with instruments. No doubt it needs further examination by recognised bodies. The non-invasive monitors and other equipment **which have** been interfaced are isolated from patients and conform to International Electrotechnical Commission 601 and its equivalent British Standard 5724. If microcomputers are interfaced with these equipments then the computers are not connected to the patient directly. Even after these precautions the micro-computer can also be isolated with the help of an isolating transformer.

Another problem is of the inter-changeability of medical
instruments. It is highly desirable that manufacturers should
start providing uniformity at output signal. It would be
extremely helpful to the users of various monitors if a
standard interface like RS 232 may be provided as standard
device, so that interfacing for the purpose of collecting
data is made easy with microcomputers. They are extremely
useful tools available at low cost compared to mainframe
computers. They can be used with minimal technical expertise
and can fulfil many needs of anaesthetic department and
intensive care units.

REFERENCES
1. Lunn J.H., Mushin W.W. 1982. Mortality associated with anae-
    sthesia. London. The Nuffield Provincial Hospital Trust.
2. Naqvi N.H. 1982. Proceedings of VI European Congress of
    Anaesthesiology. Paper 393. Association of Anaesthetists
    of Great Britain and Ireland.
3. Robischon T. 1983. Computed Spirometry. Respiratory
    Therapy. Jan/Feb.
4. Tompkin W.J., Webster J.G. 1981. Design of Microcomputer
    based Medical Instrumentation. Englewood Cliffs. New
    Jersey. Prentice Hall Inc.

PHYSIOLOGIC MONITORING OF CRITICALLY ILL PATIENTS: Computerized data acquisition, outcome prediction, organization of therapy and prospective clinical trials.

William C. Shoemaker, M.D.

INTRODUCTION

Postoperative patients often develop sudden, unexpected circulatory problems in the perioperative period. The urgency of these unanticipated life-threatening emergencies should require our most serious scientific effort. Various studies have claimed improved efficacy in resuscitation, but these studies were often seriously flawed because they have not rigorously developed an appropriate experimental design; e.g., use of historical rather than concurrent control values, prospective allocation of patients, etc. Physiologic criteria of therapy and measurement of the relative efficacy of specific clinical management would be greatly facilitated by the development of an accurate, reproducible index of severity (or outcome). This severity index also could be used as a "proxy outcome" to evaluate various therapeutic modalites.

DEVELOPMENT OF PREDICTIVE OR SEVERITY INDICES

Several severity or prognostic indices have been developed for various conditions including trauma (1-5), myocardial infarction (6), and intensive care (7-16). These have recently stimulated considerable interest in this subject as feasible and effective approaches to the management of critically ill patients.

Many predictive indices are based either on retrospective correlations or normative standards generated by panels of experts. Sophisticated approaches to pattern recognition involve cluster analyses and other complex computer programs; others require only hand-held calculators for calculation of their predictions. The present paper summarizes our attempts to evaluate the critically ill postoperative and post-trauma patient in the surgical ICU setting, to develop and apply predictors in a systematic therapeutic approach, and to evaluate the effectiveness of this approach to improve ICU patient care.

Evaluation of Various Monitored Variables

Because shock is common to cardiovascular diseases, fatal accidental and surgical trauma, and all fatal acute illnesses, cardiorespiratory variables are an appropriate basis for study. Moreover, hemodynamic and oxygen delivery (DO_2) measurements can be frequently and repetitively monitored. Finally, these monitored variables were found to provide crucial information on underlying physiologic mechanisms useful for prognosis and therapy.

The usefulness of invasive cardiorespiratory monitoring has been compared with the conventional monitoring using as the criteria the capacity to anticipate death or cardiopulmonary arrest. For example, preliminary studies showed that the conventionally monitored variables (ECG, mean arterial pressure (MAP), heart rate (HR), hematocrit (Hct), central venous presure (CVP), urine output, and blood gases) may be useful descriptors of the end stage of circulatory failure. However, they have not been found to be as sensitive or accurate in early warning of death in critically ill postoperative patients (17,18).

TABLE 1

NUMBER AND PERCENT OF PATIENTS WITH
TWO OR MORE VALUES IN THE NORMAL RANGE

	NONSURVIVORS		SURVIVORS	
	Number	%	Number	%
Mean arterial pressure	29	78	68	89
Heart rate	30	81	66	87
Central venous pressure	35	95	72	95
Pulmonary wedge pressure	11	30	21	28
Cardiac index	35	95	64	84
Mean of these variables		76		75

Values of the most commonly monitored variables (vital signs, MAP, HR, CVP, pulmonary artery wedge (WP) and cardiac output (CO)) are shown for survivors and nonsurvivors in a series of critically ill post-operative survivors and nonsurvivors of life-threatening conditions (Table 1). With vigorous therapy, we were able to bring the values of the nonsurvivors back into the normal range in 76%, but they still went on to die. By comparison, the survivors had two or more normal values in 75%. Clearly, either we were measuring inappropriate variables, or we had the wrong criteria for separating survivors from nonsurvivors (17-19).

Criteria for Evaluation of Physiologic Variables

Although a few controlled studies have been performed, the major problem in this area is to determine criteria for: (a) which variables are most relevant to biologic endpoints, such as survival or death; (b) in what circumstances are these variables appropriate; (c) what combination of variables are most useful for the initial resuscitation as well as subsequent monitoring in critical periods; (d) which variables are valuable for clinical decision-making, such as institution of specific therapy and titration of therapy to optimal goals; and (e) which variables are needed for routine surveillance of noncritical, uncomplicated patients (18).

Correct prediction of outcome for each cardiorespiratory variable is the most rigorous criterion of its biologic significance as well as its relevance to clinical management. Thus, if a variable is unable to differentiate the dying patient from the patient who survives, it is not very useful or appropriate. However, if it is a good predictor of outcome, it may reflect an important pathophysiologic problem and, therefore, is relevant to therapeutic decision-making. The percentage of correct outcome predictions for each cardiorespiratory variable was evaluated at each stage and over all stages (20-22). Unfortunately the most commonly measured variables were the poorest, least relevant predictors. The advantage of the outcome predictors is that they are heuristically or phenomenologically determined and do not depend on "clinical opinion" or "party line". They are not dependent on a given probability distribution; in this sense, the statistical analyses are "distribution-free".

The cardiorespiratory variables with the largest and smallest capability of predicting outcome at each stage were evaluated as the percentage of correct predictions (20). These percentages changed from stage to stage, indicating their stage-specificity. For example, pulmonary vascular resistance index (PVRI) is a good predictor in the early stage (B, low), but not in the middle or late stages; MAP is a poor predictor in the early stages, but a good predictor in the late stage. In the late stage, most variables predict outcome well, but clinical judgment at this time also may be excellent and the clinical usefulness of predictions is less (20).

Physiologic Basis for Prediction

Physiologic reactions that provide compensations to maintain circulatory integrity must be identified, described, and evaluated. For example, physiologic responses, such as increased cardiac output, may be a compensation for reduced Hct, reduced PaO_2, or reduced tissue oxygenation. If it is established that increased cardiac output is a compensation with survival value, then therapy might better be directed toward augmenting this response rather than returning circulatory values to the normal range. Thus, it is of major importance to understand the interactions of physiologic variables that are common to surgical trauma as well as other critical illnesses.

Maintenance of general physiologic responses to stress may have great relevance to all, or most all, critically ill patients. Even though particular mechanisms are known to be directly concerned with the origin of a specific disease, it may be necessary to provide general support to the physiologic compensatory responses. The ICU provides an opportunity to provide ancillary support.

The Traditional Approach

The traditional approach to therapy of shock and trauma states has been focused on relatively superficial manifestations of shock, such as BP, HR, CVP, Hct, PaO_2, etc. When physiologic measurements are made, the conventional approach is often simply to correct physiologic deficits after their appearance is detected, rather than to direct early or preventative therapy toward the most likely underlying pathophysiologic mechanisms. This approach generally ignores the pathophysiology and underlying regulatory mechanisms of shock and trauma syndromes.

Description of Cardiorespiratory Patterns in Survivors and Nonsurvivors

The basis for prediction and other pattern recognition systems is a description of the natural history of the disease. The patterns of changes on hemodynamic and oxygen transport variables were retrospectively surveyed in a large series of critically ill postoperative patients to define the sequential physiologic patterns of survivors and nonsurvivors during periods remote from therapy (19). When the data were separated in temporal stages by objective criteria, there were clearly defined cardiorespiratory patterns in each etiologic category of shock. Moreover, the sequential cardiorespiratory patterns of survivors were found to be different from those of nonsurvivors despite a wide variety of illnesses and an even wider spectrum of operations. We observed that in the early period of shock and trauma syndromes, there was usually a normal or high cardiac output (unless limited by hypovolemia or myocardial functional impairment) as well as inadequate oxygen transport.

These data and other experimental findings led us to conclude that the basic physiologic defect in shock states is not low flow, as cardiac output may be high, normal or low; rather, it is a maldistribution of flow that results in inadequate oxygen transport. By contrast, the late period of shock (terminal and preterminal stages) had hypotension and low cardiac output. We have used oxygen transport variables as measures of tissue perfusion, and changes in oxygen transport as measures of the therapeutic effectiveness in comparative studies of various agents; in the studies evaluating therapeutic efficacy, the patients act as their own controls.

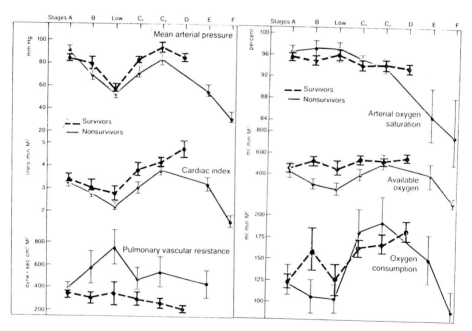

TABLE 2

CARDIORESPIRATORY VARIABLES: ABBREVIATIONS, UNITS, CALCULATIONS,

Volume-Related Variables	Abbreviations	Units
Mean arterial pressure	MAP	mm Hg
Central ven. pressure	CVP	cm H_2O
Central blood volume	CBV	ml/M^2
Stroke index	SI	ml/M^2
Hemoglobin	Hgb	g/dl
Mean pulmon. art. press.	MPAP	mm Hg
Wedge pressure	WP	mm Hg
Blood volume	BV	ml/M^2
Red cell mass	RCM	ml/M^2

Flow-Related Variables		
Cardiac index	CI	liter/min•M^2
Left vent. stroke work	LVSW	g•M/M^2
Left cardiac work	LCW	kg•M/M^2
Right vent. stroke work	RVSW	g•M/M^2
Right cardiac work	RCW	kg•M/M^2

Stress-Related Variables		
System. vasc. resist.	SVR	dyne•sec/cm^5•M^2
Pulmon. vasc. resist.	PVR	dyne•sec/cm^5•M^2
Heart rate	HR	beat/min
Rectal temperature	temp	°F

Oxygen-Related Variables		
Hbg saturation	SaO_2	%
Arterial CO_2 tension	$PaCO_2$	torr
Arterial pH	pH	---
Mixed venous O_2 tension	PvO_2	torr
Arterial-mixed venous O_2 content difference	$C(a-v)O_2$	ml/dl
O_2 delivery	DO_2	ml/min•M^2
O_2 consumption	VO_2	ml/min•M^2
O_2 extraction rate	O_2 ext	%

Perfusion-Related Variables		
Red cell flow rate	RCFR	---
Blood flow/volume ratio	BFVR	---
O_2 transport/red cell mass	OTRM	---
Tissue O_2 extraction	TOE	---
Efficiency of tissue O_2 ext	ETOE	---
O_2 transport/red cell flow	OTRF	---

[a] Hct corrected for packing fraction and large vessel hematocrit/total body hematocrit ratio.

[b] Venous pressures expressed in mm Hg.

NORMAL VALUES, PREFERRED VALUES, AND PREDICTIVE CAPACITY

Measurements or Calculations	Normal Values	Preferred Values	Percent Correct
Direct measurement	82 - 102	> 84	75
Direct measurement	1 - 9	< 5	62
CBV = MTT x CI x 16.7	660 - 1000	> 925	61
SI = CI ÷ HR	30 - 50	> 48	67
Direct measurement	12 - 16	> 12	66
Direct measurement	11 - 15	< 19	68
Direct measurement	0 - 12	> 9.5	70
BV = PV ÷ (1-Hct)^a x SA	men 2.74	> 3.0	76
	women 2.37	> 2.7	
RCM = BV - PV	men 1.1	> 1.1	85
	women 0.95	> 0.95	
Direct measurement	2.8 - 3.6	> 4.5	70
LVSW = SI x MAP x .0144	44 - 68	> 55	74
LCW = CI x MAP x .0144	3 - 4.6	> 5	76
RVSW = SI x MPAP x .0144	4 - 8	> 13	70
RCW = CI x MPAP x .0144	0.4 - 0.6	> 1.1	69
SVR = 79.92 (MAP-CVP)^b ÷ CI	1760 - 2600	< 1450	62
PVR = 79.92 (MPAP-WP)^b ÷ CI	45 - 225	< 226	77
Direct measurement	72 - 88	< 100	60
Direct measurement	97.8 - 98.6	> 100.4	64
Direct measurement	95 - 99	> 95	67
Direct measurement	36 - 44	> 30	69
Direct measurement	7.36 - 7.44	> 7.47	74
Direct measurement	33 - 53	> 36	68
C(a-v)O$_2$ = CaO$_2$ - CvO$_2$	4 - 5.5	< 3.5	68
DO$_2$ = CaO$_2$ x CI x 10	520 - 720	> 550	76
VO$_2$ = C(a-v)O$_2$ x CI x 10	100 - 180	> 167	69
O$_2$ ext = (CaO$_2$ - CvO$_2$) • CaO$_2$	22 - 30	< 31	69
RCFR = CI x Hct	0.6 - 1.8	> 1.3	72
BFVR = CI ÷ BV	0.6 - 1.8	> 1.7	75
OTRM = VO$_2$ ÷ RCM	0.06 - .18	> 0.25	79
TOE = avDO$_2$ ÷ RCFR	1.8 - 6.6	> 5.7	75
ETOE = avDO$_2$ ÷ RCM	0.06 - .18	> 1.3	91
OTRF = VO$_2$ ÷ RCFR	1 - 7	< 3	71

This approach was taken to: (a) describe the pattern of nonsurvivors and define criteria for early warning of impending disaster to permit immediate maximal therapeutic effort; (b) describe the pattern of survivors and define objective criteria for therapeutic goals, thus basing therapeutic decisions on empirically derived evidence, rather than on opinion based on anecdotes, philosophy, or a party line; and (c) determine which variables differentiate between survivors and nonsurvivors (Fig. 1). Thus, the capacity of a variable to predict outcome was used as a measure of its relevance and usefulness in making clinical decisions (17-19).

The most commonly monitored variables, BP, PaO_2, CVP, HR and Hct were very poor predictors of outcome, and, therefore, should be of limited value in therapeutic management (18). Cardiac index was slightly better than MAP in predicting outcome; survivors had values which were 50% in excess of normal. PVRI, O_2 delivery ($\dot{D}O_2$) and O_2 consumption ($\dot{V}O_2$) were better predictors; O_2 delivery and $\dot{V}O_2$ were better maintained in survivors. They were reduced in the nonsurvivors and in the case of $\dot{V}O_2$ subsequently increased in compensation. These patterns were remarkably consistent despite the wide variety of illnesses and the even wider variety of operations (Table 2). However, no one variable was completely adequate as a predictor. Since shock is a multifactorial problem, it requires multivariate analysis (16,19,20-22).

Rationale for the Predictive Index

Our approach to prediction is based on the age-old aphorism that if you know everything that is important about a system, you should be able to predict the outcome, and if you can predict outcome, you should be able to modify it. Translated into contemporary scientific terms, adequate description of circulatory events of surviving and nonsurviving emergency patients will provide the basis for a pathophysiologic understanding of the disease. Physiologic studies also help to interpret mechanistically the sequential physiologic events of acute circulatory failure associated with tissue hypoxia. Systematic and objective evaluation of therapy may then be based on these physiologic descriptions and the changes produced by specific therapeutic interventions. Subsequently, organized coherent therapeutic protocols were proposed and tested prospectively (21,22).

Major Premise

The major premise is that death in critical illness follows well defined cardiorespiratory patterns associated with the well known stress response. These physiologic patterns are independent of the specific clinical diagnosis and the specific type of operation. That is, irrespective of the illness or injury, a finite number of physiologic events mark the downhill lethal course and distinguish it from the physiologic pattern of the survivors. Furthermore, complications of life-threatening illness are associated with physiologic derangements that may be described quantitatively and placed in temporal relationship to the primary etiologic event and its compensations.

Several disclaimers should be stated: the predictor and ultimately, the therapy is designed to "optimize" physiologic variables thought to be the major factors in mortality. This is not a panacea; i.e., it will not prevent iatrogenic disaster, misdiagnoses, drug or transfusion reactions, hospital-induced infections, etc.

Hypothesis

The major hypothesis of the clinical studies is that a systematic coherent physiologic approach to management of the life-threatening illness based on clinical and physiologic criteria defined operationally from retrospective analysis of critically ill trauma patients will improve morbidity and mortality. Three essential components of this hypothesis may be examined within this context:

First, the cardiorespiratory patterns of surviving patients are distinctly different from those of nonsurvivors despite the wide spectrum of clinical diagnoses and the even wider spectrum of surgical operations, accidental trauma, hemorrhage, sepsis, etc.

Second, the monitored cardiorespiratory pattern of survivors of life-threatening illness provides objective physiologic criteria that may be used to develop goals of therapy for the critically ill patient.

Finally, these operationally defined goals may also be used to develop a coherent systematic protocol for therapy of acute critical illness. Ideally, a protocol may be expressed in terms of a branch chain decision tree; the branching chain defines (i.e., preselects) clinical groups and sequentially applies therapeutic criteria in a coherent temporal order defined by the survivors' physiologic pattern in order to obtain the most effective and most appropriate clinical decisions.

Assumptions

The underlying assumptions to this hypothesis are:

First, failure of circulatory function is responsible for most postoperative deaths. Critically ill patients more often die of physiologic derangements, rather than the anatomical or structural aspects of their primary disease or the technical features of the disease.

Second, the circulatory system, like other fluid systems, can be characterized by measurements of pressure, flow, volume and physiologic function. These can be measured easily and repetitively by currently available technology and used to characterize physiologic patterns of survivors and nonsurvivors.

Third, functional aspects of the circulation are best assessed by measurements of oxygen transport and metabolism, because oxygen transport is: (a) essential to life, (b) consistently impaired in shock states, and (c) considerably different in survivors and nonsurvivors. This is particularly relevant from the technological standpoint because oxygen has the highest extraction ratio of any blood constituent and, therefore, is the most flow dependent; oxygen cannot be stored, nor can a sizable oxygen debt be accumulated for significant periods of time. These and other experimental studies have suggested that $\dot{V}O_2$ is the controlling or regulating mechanism in the three types of tissue hypoxia (stagnant, anemic, hypoxic) described in Barcroft's classic studies. That is, $\dot{V}O_2$, reflecting the sum of all oxidative metabolism as well as the adequacy the circulatory delivery system, remains normal or somewhat elevated while hemodynamic compensations, such as increased HR, CO, and O_2 extraction, occur to preserve VO_2. When these compensations fail, $\dot{V}O_2$ falls and death rapidly ensues. Measurements of oxygen metabolism are the most sensitive and specific of the monitored cardiorespiratory variables for acute circulatory failure (17,18,20).

Finally, the longer the patient has circulatory deficits, the longer he will be critically ill, and the more likely he will have complications including multiple vital organ failures (renal, respiratory, hepatic and CNS failure), sepsis, and nutritional problems. Post-traumatic deaths most frequently occur after prolonged critical illness which starts with circulatory impairment, but then leads into multiple organ failure.

Formulation of a Predictor

A predictive index based on the probability distributions of each variable was developed using a simple algorithm (16). The relative distance of the value of a given variable from the 90 percentile of nonsurvivors to the 10 percentile of survivors' values was calculated according to an algorithm. The sum of the weighted scores of each variable gives an Overall Severity (Predictive) Index, which serves as a yardstick that tells how far it is to the brink of disaster and how far to safe territory. The sole criterion of this empiric analysis was survival.

Prospective Evaluation of the Predictive Index

Since this Overall Predictive Index was developed retrospectively in a large series of postoperative patients at Cook County Hospital in Chicago and at Mount Sinai Hospital in New York, it was necessary to test the validity of the predictor in a fresh series of critically ill postoperative patients. Table 3 shows the results of this predictive index applied prospectively to a new series of 300 critically ill postoperative patients during the first 5 years of the surgical ICU at Harbor-UCLA Medical Center (20,22). Only about 2% of our surgical patients were monitored; these were critically ill, high-risk, high-mortality patients. As seen from this standard truth table, this index was 93% correct. All 8 incorrectly predicted to die died of late complications or carcinomatosis; the 13 who were predicted to die but who survived, had their catheter removed in less than 18 hours postoperatively. Thus, the Predictive Index was found to be valid and reproducible over a wide range of socioeconomic levels, private vs. public institutions, and in various clinical mixes.

DEVELOPMENT OF PATIENT CARE PROTOCOLS

Definition of Therapeutic Goals

Description of the sequential hemodynamic and O_2 transport patterns also allowed us to define optimal therapeutic goals for each variable as the median value of survivors of life-threatening surgical operations.

TABLE 3

RESULTS OF PREDICTORS AFTER SURGICAL OPERATIONS

		Last Available Predicted Value			
		Survival	Death	Total	% Correct
Actual	Survived	206	13	219	94*
Outcome	Died	8	73	81	90**
	Total	214	86	300	93
	% Correct	96***	85***		

*Sensitivity, percentage of survivors with correctly predicted outcome
**Specificity, percentage of nonsurvivors with correctly predicted outcome
***Predictive accuracy, percentage of survivors among patients predicted to live
****Predictive precision, percentage of nonsurvivors among patients predicted to die

The most important of these optimal values are: (a) BV 500 ml in excess of normal, (b) CI 50% in excess of normal, (c) O_2 delivery and $\dot{V}O_2$ 25% in excess of normal, (d) PVRI less than 225 dyne•sec/cm^5•M^2, and (e) nutritional support (16-20).

Development of a Branch Chain Decision Tree

Therapy of the critically ill trauma patient initially revolves around: (a) volume and choice of fluid therapy and transfusions, (b) vasopressors or vasodilators, cardiotonic agents, and diuretics, (c) correction of hypoxemia, inadequate tissue perfusion, and inadequate tissue oxygenation, (d) correction of acid-base problems, and hyper- or hypo-carbia, and (e) alpha and beta adrenergic agents. It is possible to define indications and contraindications from their known physiologic actions as well as the optimal goals of therapy.

The median values of the survivors were considered a first approximation to optimal goals of therapy. They were placed in their temporal priorities and expressed in a branch chain decision tree or wall-map algorithm (Fig. 1). The criteria for each therapeutic intervention are specified within each diamond decision point according to the priorities derived by the Predictive Index.

EFFECT OF THE DECISION TREE ON OUTCOME

Evaluation of Efficacy

This clinical decision tree was then tested prospectively against concurrent control patients in 223 consecutive postoperative patients.

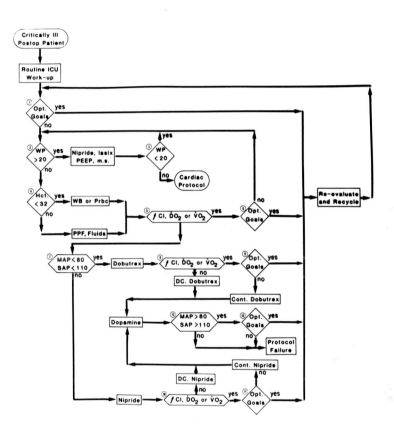

Figure 1

The hypothesis tested was that if physiologic values were brought into the survivors' pattern, they would have a higher survival rate as compared with control patients who had normal values as their therapeutic goals. Table 4 summarizes the results of this clinical trial: 35% of the control patients and 12.5% of the protocol patients died. This was statistically significant at the 2% level of confidence (20,22).

TABLE 4

OUTCOME DATA

	Control	Protocol
Number of patients	143	80
Number of nonsurvivors	50	10
Mortality (%)	35	12.5

Even though the patients were properly allocated to control and protocol groups according to a prearranged schedule worked out in conjunction with our statistician colleagues, it is still necessary to demonstrate that the protocol patients were at least as sick as the control patients (20,22). Table 5, which was developed prior to the onset of the studies, details clinical criteria for identification of preoperative associated severe illnesses. The protocol patients had at least as many associated illnesses as did the control group.

TABLE 5

COMPARISON OF CLINICAL DATA OF THE SERIES

	Control (N=143)	Protocol (N=80)	P-Value
Age (years)	56 ± 20*	51 ± 19*	N.S.**
Males, number (%)	89 (62%)	51 (64%)	N.S.
Lowest MAP (mm Hg)	53 ± 23*	49 ± 19*	N.S.
Time in hypotension (h)	2.2 ± 2.7*	2.4 ± 2.1*	N.S.
MAP < 50 mm Hg, number (%)	48 (34%)	37 (46%)	N.S.
Patients with associated severe illness, number (%)	46 (32%)	50 (62%)	< 0.01
Total number of associated severe illnesses	63	96	< 0.01
Number of associated severe illness/patient	0.45	1.21	< 0.06

*Mean ± SD.
**N.S., not significant.

Table 6 details the major clinical criteria of severe associated illness and demonstrates that the clinical findings of the protocol group were at least as severe as the control group (20).

TABLE 6

ASSOCIATED SEVERE ILLNESS

		Control (N=143)	Protocol (N=80)
1.	MAP < 50 mm Hg with systolic pressure < 75 mm Hg	12 (8%)	17 (21%)
2.	Multiple trauma-injury of > 3 major organs or > 2 organ systems	19 (13%)	14 (18%)
3.	Head injury with coma; i.e., unconscious and unresponsive to verbal or painful stimuli	4 (3%)	3 (4%)
4.	Gunshot or stab wound to major organs (i.e., heart, brain, lungs, liver, spleen, intestinal tract, kidney) with bleeding > 1000 ml	1 (1%)	10 (13%)
5.	Respiratory failure due to chest trauma, head injury, or nonthoracic injury necessitating intubation and mechanical ventilation	5 (3%)	4 (5%)
6.	Massive acute blood loss - loss of > 4000 ml or Hct > 25; slow or chronic blood loss and renal failure not included	7 (5%)	19 (24%)
7.	Septic shock - MAP > 60, temperature < 96°F or > 101°F, and WBC < 4000 or > 12,000	11 (8%)	13 (16%)
8.	Cardiogenic shock - acute MI, CHF or dysrhythmia documented by ECG, laboratory results or autopsy	1 (1%)	5 (6%)
9.	Renal failure	1 (1%)	3 (4%)
10.	Hepatic failure	2 (1%)	7 (9%)
11.	CNS coma (stroke)	--	1 (1%)
	Total number of criteria identified	63	96
	Total number of patients with one or more criteria	43 (30%)	48 (60%)

Postoperative Complications

Table 7 lists the postoperative complications in the protocol and control groups in their order of frequency. The data indicate significantly less complications in the protocol group.

TABLE 7

COMPLICATIONS OF CONTROL AND PROTOCOL GROUPS

Complication	Control (N=143)	Protocol (N=80)	Total (N=223)
Respiratory failure (requiring ventilation)	66	27	93
Sepsis, systemic	44	11	55
Cardiogenic problems, including pulmonary edema, cardiac arrest, arrhythmia	22	9	31
Renal failure (requiring dialysis)	25	5	30
Disseminated intravascular coagulation	8	3	11
Pulmonary embolism	2		2
Hepatic failure, coma	3	1	4
Delirium tremens	1		1
Upper GI hemorrhage	7	1	8
Urinary tract infection	5	1	6
Postoperative bowel obstruction	2		2
Decubitus ulcer	1	1	2
Carcinomatosis		1	1
Pneumothorax		1	1
Bronchopleural fistula	1		1
Pancreatitis	2		2
Metabolic alkalosis	1		1
Allergic reaction	1		1
Total	191	61	253
Average no./patient	1.34	0.76	1.13

SUMMARY

Application of multivariate analysis is particularly appropriate to the multifactorial problems of the severely ill ICU patient. This approach was found to provide a reasonably accurate method to predict outcome in a prospective series of patients (22). The advantage of predictors is that they analyze the complex ICU problems with no preconceptions and an absolute minimum number of assumptions. It is heuristically determined solely by observed values of critically ill trauma and postoperative patients who survived and those who subsequently died.

In conclusion, postoperative deaths are associated with physiologic alterations which can be identified and described. Second, the median cardiorespiratory values of survivors may be used as therapeutic goals in critically ill postoperative patients, as these increased cardio-respiratory values represent compensatory responses that have survival value. Third, there was marked and significant improvement in both morbidity and mortality when these physiologic goals were used in a prospective controlled clinical trial.

We believe, therefore, that the high-risk, intra- and postoperative patients should be treated by titrating therapy to achieve optimal goals empirically defined by the survivors patterns, not the normal values of resting healthy adult volunteers. Cardiorespiratory variables should be monitored prophylactically to maintain these objectively derived goals rather than to wait for physiologic deficits to occur and then to attempt belatedly to correct them.

REFERENCES

1. Cowley RA, Sacco WJ, Gill W, et al: A prognostic index for severe trauma. J Trauma 1971; 14:1029

2. Baker SP, O'Neill B, Haddon W, et al: The injury severity score: a method for describing patients with multiple injuries and evaluating emergency care. J Trauma 1974; 14:187

3. Champion HR, Sacco WJ, Hannon DS, et al: Assessment of injury severity: The Triage Index. Crit Care Med 1980; 8:201

4. Champion HR, Sacco WJ, Carnazzo AJ, et al: The Trauma Score. Crit Care Med 1981; 9:672

5. Teasdale G, Jannett B: Assessment of coma and impaired consciousness: a practical scale. Lancet 1974; 1:81

6. Norris RM, Brandt PWT, Caughey DE, et al: A new coronary prognostic index. Lancet 1969; 1:274

7. Cullen DJ, Civetta JM, Briggs BA, et al: Therapeutic intervention scoring system: a method for quantitative comparison of patient care. Crit Care Med 1974; 2:57

8. Cullen DJ, Ferrara LC, Gilbert J, et al: Indicators of intensive care in critically ill patients. Crit Care Med 1973; 5:173

9. Weil MH, Afifi AA: Experimental and clinical studies on lactate and pyruvate as indicators of severity of acute circulatory failure (shock). Circulation 1970; 41:989

10. Shubin H, Weil MH, Afifi AA, et al: Selection of hemodynamic, respiratory and metabolic variables for evaluation of patients in shock. Crit Care Med 1974; 2:326

11. Siegel J, Goldwin RM, Friedman HP: Pattern in process in the evolution of human septic shock. Surgery 1971; 70:232

12. Knaus WA, Zimmerman JE, Wagner DP, et al: APACHE: Acute physiology and chronic health evaluation: a physiologically based classification system. Crit Care Med 1981; 9:591

13. Synder JV, McGuirk M, Grenvik A, et al: Outcome of intensive care: an application of a predictive model. Crit Care Med 1981; 9:598

14. Shoemaker WC, Elwyn DH, Levin H, et al: Early prediction of death and survival in postoperative patients with circulatory shock by nonparametric analysis of cardiorespiratory variables. Crit Care Med 1974; 2:317

15. Shoemaker WC, Pierchala C, Chang P, et al: Prediction of outcome and severity of illness by analysis of the frequency distributions of cardiorespiratory variables. Crit Care Med 1977; 5:82

16. Shoemaker WC, Chang PC, Czer LSC, et al: Cardiorespiratory monitoring in postoperative patients: I. Prediction of outcome and severity of illness. Crit Care Med 1979; 7:237

17. Bland R, Shoemaker WC, Shabot MM: Physiologic monitoring goals for the critically ill patient. Surg Gynecol Obstet 1978; 147:833

18. Shoemaker WC, Czer LSC: Evaluation of the biologic importance of various hemodynamic and oxygen transport variables. Crit Care Med 1979; 7:424

19. Shoemaker WC, Montgomery ES, Kaplan E, et al: Physiologic patterns in surviving and nonsurviving shock patients. Arch Surg 1973; 106:630

20. Shoemaker WC, Appel PL, Bland R, et al: Clinical trial of an algorithm for outcome prediction in acute circulatory failure. Crit Care Med 1982; 10:390

21. Shoemaker WC, Appel PL, Waxman K, et al: Clinical trial of survivors' cardiorespiratory patterns as therapeutic goals in critically ill postoperative patients. Crit Care Med 1982; 10:398

22. Shoemaker WC, Appel PA, Bland R: Use of physiologic monitoring to predict outcome and to assist in clinical decisions in critically ill postoperative patients. Am J Surg 1983 (in press)

SET UP AND RESULTS ICU DATABASE.

J.A. LEUSINK, M.D., Dept. Anesthesiology,
R. VAN STADEN,
St. Antonius Hospital, Utrecht, The Netherlands.

INTRODUCTION

In recent years many studies have been published to assess the
treatment of patients on intensive care units (ICU). The "Therapeutic
Intervention Scoring System" (TISS) introduced by Cullen et al (1974)
and revised by this group in 1983 (Keene et al 1983) is a well-known
and widely-used method which measures the overall intensity of ICU-
treatment. TISS is used for the classification of ICU-patients in
different ICU's. TISS gives no direct information about the severity
of illness. The therapeutic interventions used in TISS constitute an
indirect measure of the severity of illness. Examples of the therapeutic interventions are given in table 1.
Hypotheses are (1) the same treatment for patients with the same illness from hospital to hospital, (2) all therapeutic interventions described in TISS must be available in all hospitals using this system.
It is arguable whether changes in time e.g. a more frequent use of
pulmonary artery catheters (resulting in higher TISS-points) are an indication of more severe illness.
Knaus et al (1981) recently introduced the "Acute Physiology And Chronic
Health Evaluation" (APACHE). In this system the severity of the acute
illness of a patient is recorded in the first 32 hours after admission
on the ICU, while using 34 criteria which indicate the severity of illness. Examples of the parameters used in APACHE are shown in table 1.
Also the chronic health situation of the patient before the illness
which leads to the ICU-admission is described in terms of daily acti-
vities, a method comparable to the NYHA- or ASA-classificationsystem.
In this system complications occurring after the first 32 hours on the
ICU are not recorded.
In 1980 we started organizing an ICU-database. Lack of data concerning

Table 1.

Comparison TISS[*] and APACHE[**]

	TISS	APACHE
4 pnts	IPPV	heart rate $\geqslant$ 180
	pulmonary art.cath.	PaCO2 $\geqslant$ 70
3 pnts	vasoactive drug infus.	heart rate 141-179
	IMV or CPAP	PaCO2 61- 69
2 pnts	CVP	heart rate 111-140
	stable hemodialysis	PaCO2 50-60
1 pnt.	ECG monitoring	-
	tracheostomy care	-

---

[*] Cullen et al 1974; Keene et al 1983.
[**] Knaus et al 1981.

Table 2.

ICU Admission - Discharge Form.

Name	date of birth
M/F	
Indication for admission	operation
Emergency	perop.complications

Table 3.

Definition "Complications"

Subsystem		Criteria
cerebral		. coma
circulatory	BP	. hypotension > 6 hr $\leqslant$ 80
	i.v. medic.	. catech. > 2 hr
	rhythm	. disturbances
respiratory	IPPV	. > 2 d
renal	diuresis	. oliguria < 400/24 h
		. anuria < 50/24 h
	creatinineconc.	. > 250 mMol/l.
microbiological infections		. severe (sepsis, peritonitis, mediastinitis, multiple infections)
		. pos. culture sputum
	fever, WBC	. > 39°C > 6 hr; WBC > 10
bloodbalance	loss	. > 3000 ml
	transfusions	. > 10 units
	albumine/plasma	. > 10 units

BP = blood pressure
IPPV = intermittent positive pressure ventilation
WBC = white blood count.

many aspects and/or results of the treatment of patients on our ICU
was the main reason.

AIMS.

Aims to set up the ICU database were:

1. the analysis of the composition of the ICU-patient population.
2. the frequency of situations that threaten the patient's life, further
   defined as "complications" (see below).
3. mortality and the relation of "complications" with mortality.
4. (retrospective) investigations concerning ICU-problems.

We defined "complications" as either partial or total lack of normal
function of organ(system)s (e.g. renal function) or as the therapeutic
interventions needed to support or to compensate this lack of function
(c.q. dialysis, administration of catecholamines, IPPV).
The "St. Antonius Ziekenhuis" in Utrecht, The Netherlands is a general
hospital with 633 beds, specialized in cardiopulmonary and vascular
surgery. The hospital has an ICU of 25 beds. The treatment of patients
is multidisciplinary. The department of anesthesiology is in charge
of the daily management of the ICU.

METHODS.

At admission of the patient on the ICU, descriptive data are filled
in on the so-called "Admission and discharge form-ICU" (table 2).
At the patient's discharge from the ICU the occurrence of "complications" during the whole ICU-period is tested with the help of defined
criteria. These criteria (table 3) are compared with the possible
life-threatening situations of the patient's subsystems (cerebral, circulatory, respiratory, renal, microbiological, blood-balance deviations). For each patient 74 items could be described. The time spent on
writing in the forms was usually 2 - 5 minutes, for patients after a
long and protracted stay on the ICU it sometimes took more than 10
minutes.

INPUT OF DATA AND MANIPULATION OF THE ICU-DATABASE.

For input and retrieval of the data a database-program called
"ADAMO" was used. This program was developed at the Department of Medical Informations (Free University, Amsterdam, The Netherlands) and

published by Hasman et al (1982). This database program can easily
be used for all kinds of research applications. Special programs have
been written for the editing and monthly reports of all inserted data.
Of each patient 74 items could be described. Items could be free text
(a maximum of 30 characters e.g. description of complications), numbers (e.g. units of bloodtransfusions) or code (0 to 9, e.g. 0 = normal
spontaneous respiration; 1 = insufficient spontaneous respiration;
2 = mechanical ventilation $\leqslant$ 48 hours; 3 = mechanical ventilation
$>$ 2 days).
Via the ICU-terminal all data were inserted; the terminal was connected
with a PDP 11/34 computer. Passwords were used to secure the database
and the programs. Weekly copies were made of all inserted data and
programs.

RESULTS.
   The results of our investigation during 1982 are shown below.
1. Composition ICU patient population.
   The number of admissions on the ICU was 2197, 83% men, 27% women;
16% emergency admissions. Of the 2197 patients, 91% were postoperative.
The mean age was 57 years, $<$ 20 years 3%, 20 to 40 years 8%, 40 to 60
years 40%, 60 to 70 years 35% and $\geqslant$ 70 years 15%. The admission categories and the mean duration of the ICU-period are shown in table 4.
Of the 2197 patients 3% remained on the ICU for more than 14 days.
2. Mortality.
   Overall mortality was 5.1%. Mortality for postoperative patients
was 3%, for non-postoperative patients 27%. The mortality rates for
the different patient-categories are shown in table 5. The mortality
for emergency admissions was 22%. A clear relation exists between age
and mortality. Below 60 years 3% mortality, 60 to 70 years 5%, 70 to
80 years 12% and $\geqslant$ 80 years 16%. The mortality of patients staying for
more than 10 days was 26%.
3. Mortality and "complications".
   In table 6 the mortality rates in patients with "complications" are
shown. The highest mortality rate was found in patients with anuria
(81%), followed by coma (72%). A mortality rate of about 50% was found
in patients with hypotension, oliguria, severe infections or after many
bloodtransfusions or many albumin or plasma-infusions. A mortality rate

82

Table 4.

Composition ICU patient population and mean duration of the
ICU-period

	%	days
postoperative		
cardiac surgery	62	4.54
pulmonary surgery	11	4.27
vascular surgery	12	5.27
general surgery/trauma	7	4.14
non-postoperative		
pulmonary and/or cardial	5.5	7.28
internal and/or neurological	3.5	4.91

Table 5.

Mortality rate

Postoperative: ✝

cardial surgery	2%
pulmonary surgery	3%
vascular surgery	6%
general surgery	13%

Non-postoperative:

pulmonary/cardial	32%
internal/neurological	17%

Table 6.

Occurrence of "complications" in all ICU-patients and the
mortality rate in patients with these complications.

Criteria	occurrence % of 2197	mortality %
coma	4 %	72%
hypotension	5 %	54%
catecholamines	11 %	35%
rhythmdisturbances	30 %	10%
IPPV > 2d	7 %	37%
oliguria	2.5%	45%
anuria	2 %	81%
creat.conc. > 250	5 %	48%
dialysis	2 %	49%
severe infections	1.5%	52%
pos.cult.sputum	6 %	18%
fever + WBC > 10	6 %	30%
bloosloss > 3 l	2 %	39%
bloodtrans. > 10 units	1 %	50%
alb./plasma > 10 units	1.5%	51%

Table 7.

Mortality rates in patients with combinations of "complications"
of two different subsystems.

Subsystem	* 1	2	3	4	5	6
* 1. cerebral	72%					
2. circulatory	83%	35%				
3. respiratory	68%	54%	37%			
4. renal	79%	68%	65%	48%		
5. microbiol.	73%	51%	51%	75%	30%	
6. bloodtransf.	74%	36%	46%	57%	45%	18%

* 1 = coma, 2 = catech. > 2 hr., 3 = IPPV > 2 d, 4 = creat. >250
5 = fever + WBC > 10, 6 = transf. > 5 units.

Table 8.

Mortality rates in ICU-studies

	composition		mortality
	postop.(%)	non-postop.(%)	%
Phillips et al (1979)	43%	57%	8%
Pybus et al (1982)	60%	40%	11%
Snyder et al (1981)	88%	12%	19%
Teres et al (1982)	-	-	17%
St. Antonius (1983)	91%	9%	5%

Table 9.

Comparison of criteria for "complications" and the mortality rates
in patients with these complications (Teres et al 1982; our study).

criteria		mortality (%)	
Teres	St. Antonius	Teres	St. Antonius
coma > 48 hr	coma	77%	72%
BP ≤ 90 + catech.	BP ≤ 80 > 6 hr	55%	54%
IPPV > 4 d	IPPV > 2 d	51%	37%
creat.conc. > 330	> 250 mMol/l.	57%	48%
hemodialysis	dialysis	41%	49%
1 infection	pos.cult.sputum	18%	18%
2 or > infections	severe or multiple	47%	52%
temp ≥ 40°C	≥ 39°C + WBC > 10	61%	30%
bloodtrans. 5-9 Un.	5-10 Units	14%	12%
id. ≥ 10	> 10 Units	30%	50%

of about 30% was found in patients treated with catecholamines, mechanically ventilated longer than 2 days or with fever and leucocytosis.
In table 7 the mortality rates in patients with combinations of two
"complications" of different subsystems are shown. In these calculations we used one complication of each subsystem that occurred frequently ($\geq$ 4%). The highest mortality rates were found in patients
with coma and circulatory insufficiency (83%), or coma and renal insufficiency (79%). The mortality rate in patients with renal insufficiency and a microbiological problem was high (75%). Also high mortality rates were found in patients with circulatory insufficiency and renal (68%) or respiratory (65%) insufficiency.

DISCUSSION.

The ICU-database has supplied us with many data about the patient
population, complications and intensity of treatment. In our opinion
the severity of illness can be discribed in the way shown.
The overall mortality of 5.1% is low when compared to the results of
many other authors (table 8). The composition of the ICU-patient population strongly influences the mortality rate. In all studies the mortality of postoperative patients is lower than that of non-postoperative
patients. Also mortality in ICU-patients after complicated general surgery is higher than after cardiac surgery. Also the definition of mortality: ICU-mortality versus hospital-mortality can explain different results.
The relation between "complications" and mortality is clearly shown. The
high mortality rate after acute renal insufficiency is reported by many
authors (Sweet et al 1981, Teres et al 1982, Pybus et al 1982).
A comparison of mortality in relation to complications in ICU-patients
is possible with the data of Teres et al (1982) (table 9).
Although the composition of the patient population in the study of
Teres is not exactly known, the mortality rates in patients with coma,
hypotension, dialysis, moderate and severe infections, multiple bloodtransfusions are exactly the same. The differences in the mortality
rates for IPPV, creatinine-concentration and fever can be explained by
differences in the definition of "complications".
The cumulative effect of coma and renal insufficiency was also shown in
a study of Pybus et al (1982). Sweet et al (1981) showed a synergistic
effect of renal and respiratory failure on mortality.

Also in our study the mortality rate in patients with respiratory insufficiency (37%) increased after addition of renal insufficiency (65%).

REFERENCES.

1. Cullen DJ, Civetta JM, Briggs BA et al. 1974. Therapeutic Intervention Scoring System; A method for quantitative comparison of patient
   care. Crit.Care Med. 2:57.
2. Keene AR, Cullen DJ. 1983. Therapeutic Intervention Scoring System:
   up date 1983. Crit.Care Med. 11:1.
3. Knaus WA, Zimmerman JE, Wagner DP, Draper EA, Lawrence DE. 1981.
   APACHE-acute physiology and chronic health evaluation: a physiologically based classification system. Crit.Care Med. 9:591.
4. Hasman A, Chang, SC. 1982. Adamo, a data storage and retrieval system for clinical research. Comput. and Biom.Res. 15:145.
5. Pybus DA, Gatt S, Torda TA. 1982. Clinical audit of an intensive care
   unit. Anaesth.Intens.Care. 10:233.
6. Teres D, Brown RB, Lemenshow S. 1982. Predicting mortality of intensive care unit patients. The importance of coma. Crit.Care Med.
   10:86.
7. Sweet SJ, Glenney CU, Fitzgibbons JP, Friedman P, Teres D. 1981.
   Synergistic effect of acute renal failure and respiratory failure in
   the surgical intensive care unit. Am.J.Surg. 141:492.

AN INTERACTIVE INFORMATION SYSTEM FOR ANAESTHESIA

G. L. OLSSON

1. INTRODUCTION

In the midsixties a computeraided anaesthetic record-keeping system was designed at the Karolinska Hospital (1). The goals of this system was presented at the Forth World Congress of Anaesthesiologists in London 1968: "The medical goal is to create possibilities for a systemic follow up of the routine anaesthetic activities..... The administrative goal is to create a sound basis for rational planning and use of the available resources" (2).

This system today contains information from approximately 220.000 anaesthetics and it has been widely used for description of anaesthetic work, clinical follow up and research, in education and for administrative tasks such as planning of rebuildings, on-duty work etc. During the elapsed 16 years the development of computer technique has been fast, and a revision of the system became desireble to overcome some drawbacks of the originally designed system.

Therefore, a new system was designed during 1982 at the department of paediatric anaesthesia St Görans Hospital, Stockholm. This new system will soon be introduced within the County of Stockholm including 13 hospitals and approximately 100.000 anaesthetics per year.

2. METHODS

2. 1. The computer system

The County Council in Stockholm has built up an extensive ADB system within the field of medical services. The basis of this information system is a data bank drawn from several different registers. One includes all residents of the county, approximately one and a half million, and contains both details of their registered addresses and the most important medical information about the hundreds of thousands of persons who have recieved treatment at any of the county council hospitals since

1968. Another is a register of patients presently admitted to hospitals while another contains various kinds of medical data. The system is also used for a number of laboratory analyses. The display terminals connect the hospitals to the computer system which is gradually being expanded to link more and more units to the ADB system and thus make full use of its many possibilities. In many cases the computer is part of the daily routine. Within a few seconds details of a blood group, any previous examinations and the result of laboratory tests can be produced. One data service bureau is responsible for the ADB-activities in the County Council, which is called L-DATA.

2. 1. 1. Equipment. The central machine configuration is composed of two computers IBM 3031 with 5 and 6 MB memory. One is a 3031 AP. To the computers are connected disc drives 3350 and 3380. They are accessible from both computers via control units 3830. There are two high speed printers 3211, one laser printer 3800, two 3203 and two card readers. The data communication is controlled by four 3705 communication controllers. Besides these two IBM 3031 there is also one 360/168. The 360/168 is among many other things used during the designing of new applications.

At the department of paediatric anaesthesia at St Görans Hospital we use a display terminal for registration and communication with the 360/168. This is an IBM 3276 connected through a modem and the telephone net to the computer located at L-DATA 8 km away. Reports are printed on the laser printer 3800.

2. 1. 2. Program products. L-DATA uses the operation system MVS with JES2 (IBM). The user communicates with the operation system with the aid of TSO (Time Sharing Option). For database/datacommunication L-DATA uses IMS and DL/1.

2. 2. The anaesthetic system

2. 2. 1. Registration. Selection of data: Our system is to be used by many departments and we preferred to start with a limited amount of information pieces in order not to force a heavy, timeconsuming system upon collegues that possibly do not have our own interest in and knowledge of information technique. Table 1 shows the data that were selected in collaboration with all anaesthetic departments in the area.

TABEL 1. Information pieces that are to be registered.

      patients personal registration number
      name
      date of operation
      clinic/department
      inpatient/outpatient
      elective/emergency
      risk classifikation (ASA)
      time for start of anaesthesia
      time for termination of anaesthesia
      performed operation (code)
      anaesthetic technique (code)
      locality of the performance
      results, complications, comments

Coding systems for anaesthetic technique and performed surgical operations are produced by the national Board of Health and Welfare and are widely used in Sweden (3, 4). A new code-list for anaesthetic consultations i. e. cannulation of vessels, cardiopulmonary resuscitations, etc has been constructed. This will cover interventions performed by anaesthetists not including anaesthesia. In addition to these data a free information field will be available where an anaesthetic department can registrate any information of interest. It is also a great advantage if the system is flexible and easily permits the introduction of additional information fields when the users recongnize new relevant data.

Programs for registration: During the designing of the system at St Görans hospital a program tool called APE (APL Prototyping Environment) was used. This system facilitates easy construction of terminal screens for registration.

Personel: Our opinion is that the registration should be done by personel belonging to the staff of the anaesthetic department. This will minimize misinterpretations when transfering data from the source to the system. At St Görans hosptial anaesthetic nurses make the registration when spare time is available. The time required for the registration is approximately 45 seconds per record. The display terminal is located inside the operating ward. The items to be registered are read from a copy of the anaesthetic chart and no additional form is used to transfer data from where it was created to the information system.

Controls: The system checks the values of registered data according to preset limits e. g. in the field for clinic/department only existing departments are accepted, the operation cannot take place before

date of birth etc. The personal registration number is also checked
against a central register by means of the system. An anaesthetic nurse
checks with the operating list that no anaesthetic record is missing.

2. 2. 2. <u>Retrieval</u>. The reports constitutes the results of the information system. This is the aim of the projekt and we must start with
planning the presentation of all the measures that will become available
when the system is running. It is a great advantage for the staff to
be able to use the system interactively whenever needed and to be able
to execute those retrievals that currently are of interest. This is
especially important during the early phase of implementing the primarily designed system. At St Görans hospital this has been achieved with
the aid of the general purpose inquiry facility ADI (APL Data Interface)
that operates under VS APL in the TSO environment. This system is designed for users who require ready access to information stored in APL
Data Interface files. After registration the information is stored in a
sequential file which with a simple command is converted to an APL Data
Interface file. This transposed file concept is used to increase the
speed of file access. With standard sequential or keyed files, all data
from one record are processed before any of the next are processed.
This processing is wasteful when you wish to access only a few fields
in many records. A transposed file has the elements from a single field
from many records grouped into one logical record. The advantage of this
organisation is that only the fields of interest are read, ignoring all
other fields.

The functions of ADI provide a relatively simple way to interactively
access, analyse, manipulate, and report on information stored in on-
line files. The functions allow you to select data using "and/or" logic,
relational terms such as "less than" or "equal to" and computed values.
Combining these functions can significantly reduce the need for application programming. Besides providing powerful selection capability,
there are many functions that operate upon the data extracted from the
files. You can summarise, count, obtain frequency distributions, accu-
mulate statistics, sort, cross tabulate, rank and subtotal. Knowledge
of APL is not necessary, although the full power of APL is available.
At St Görans hospital three of the anaesthetic nurses, without any previous knowledge of computer technique has learned to use ADI and to
produce reports. Already after a couple of hours training retrievals

of reports were possible. ADI is used in full screen mode and the active
workspace size is approximately 3 MB.

2. 2. 3. Presentation. It is essential to present results in an
attractive and readable mode. No sign or letter should be presented
that an anaesthetist could not interpret and the paper should not be
striped as a pyjamas. Therefore a word/text-processing system, DCF
(Documentation Composition Facility, IBM) was used for the presentations.
Figures 1 - 6 are photos of tables from the various reports.

2. 2. 4. The future. When the system will be introduced in all the
other anaesthetic departments in Stockholm County the system will be
incorporated in the general medical systems and the information will
be stored together with medical data from other medical fields. This
database is working in the IMS environment and the use of ADI will not
routinely be possible. On the other hand all the reports then are
settled and there will also be possibilities to interactively retrieve
stored information on the display terminal at the anaesthetic departments. It will also be possible to combine anaesthetic information
with other medical information such as outcome (total hospital mortality), staytime, diagnoses, complications etc. The registration will be
performed by a secretary at the anaesthetic clinic and she will also
take care of the correction of missing or erroneous data. Progress is
also achived in using microcomputers as display terminals in order
combine the field of applications of a micro with the power of a big
computer.

3. RESULTS

3. 1. Annual report

During 1982 6140 records were registered in the system. This corre-
sponds to 4474 patients. There were 4486 anaesthetics performed, not
including local infiltration anaesthesia. 4978 surgical operations and
1021 anaesthesia consultations were recorded. Information on these interventions are presented in the annual report in 71 tables. Figure 1 shows
the first part of the table of content of the annual report. The table
presents information from all clinics together and first are all kinds
of interventions presented together. After this the anaesthetics are
presented in 7 tables. Figure 2 constitutes an example (table Aa7,
complications and risk classification).

FIGURE 1. First part of the table of content of the annual report.

Aa7. Results and complications / riskclassification

This classification is similar to the ASA classification. Group 5 is included in group 4.

RESULT/COMPLIKATION	RISK 1	RISK 2	RISK 3	RISK 4	NOT REG.	TOT
no comment	3336	608	88	26	16	4074
tooth injury	1	0	0	0	0	1
hypersensitiv. react.	9	3	1	0	0	12
insufficient anaesth	29	8	2	0	0	39
remaining drugeffect	66	20	2	0	0	88
difficult intubation	20	12	5	2	0	39
bronchospasm	1	4	1	0	0	6
laryngospasm	26	10	1	0	0	37
aspiration	3	1	1	0	0	5
hypotension	0	1	0	3	0	4
serious arrythmia	2	6	3	2	0	13
bloodloss 20 %	2	4	4	3	0	13
cardiac arrest	0	0	2	1	0	3
devicefailure	2	1	0	1	0	4
insuff premedication	12	4	1	0	1	18
vomiting	16	3	0	0	0	19
other comment	85	37	8	3	0	133
reg missing	16	4	2	0	2	24
total	3611	705	117	34	19	4486

FIGURE 2. Anaesthetics. Tables from the annual report 1982. Complications and risk classification.

92

Consultations are presented in 5 tables and figure 3. (table Ak2 and Ak3) presents emergency/elective, inpatient/outpatient and an age and sex distribution. The anaesthetic consultations are mostly venous cannulations, performed by anaesthetic nurses on children in a ward needing i.v. infusions. Finally, performed surgical operations are presented in 7 tables. Figure 4 presents time consumption of common surgical interventions (first page of table Ao7).

FIGURE 3. Anaesthetic consultations. Tables from the annual report 1982. Emergency/elective and inpatient/outpatient, age and sex distribution.

Dept. Paed. Anaesth.
ST GÖRANS HOSPITAL   14
Box 12500 S-11281 Stockholm
1983-04-25

Annual report 1982
Gunnar L. Olsson

Ak2. Consultations emergency/planned , outpatients/inpatients

EMERG / PLANNED	OUT-PAT	IN-PAT	TOTAL
emerg	40	880	920
planned	12	89	101
total	52	969	1021

Ak3. Consultations, age and sex

AGE-GROUP	MALE	FE-MALE	TOT
0-6 d	19	14	33
7-30 d	16	17	33
1-2 m	112	47	159
3-5 m	52	22	74
6-11 m	96	40	136
1 year	128	75	203
2 years	45	35	80
3-4 y	45	47	92
5-9 y	59	43	102
10-14 y	45	43	88
≥15 y	3	18	21
total	620	401	1021

After these tables the annual report presents each clinic separately with the same tables. This makes the annual report a comprehensive document but the logical disposition will facilitate the search for demanded information.

FIGURE 4. Surgical operations. Table
from the annual report 1982.
Numbers of operations and time consumption.

CODE	NUM-BERS	MEAN TIME MIN	CODE-TRANSLATION
4206	526	61	hernia ing. repair
8200	500	40	fract. rep + plaster
4510	395	74	appendicectomy
8228	243	18	fracture - plaster
8910	238	44	extirp(skin, tum, scars)
6901	232	59	phimosis plast. surg.
6790	210	98	ectopia testis
8070	98	64	extrac osteosynt mat
4899	86	25	anal pressuremeas.
6999	64	36	phimosis
8215	64	130	fract - open rep
8900	63	40	skin - inc. drain.
4200	58	75	hern ing radicalop
6840	57	49	ext of hydatid
8320	55	31	artrocentesis
8201	51	68	extension, thread
7499	48	14	gyn examination
9013	47	36	rectoscopy
8902	45	54	rev wound , sutur
9006	43	79	cystoscopy

3. 2. Monthly report

A monthly report is produced as soon as possible after a turn of the
month. This is important in order to avoid lag in registration. The report consists of 4 tables and permits a continous follow up of the
daily work.

There used to be two paediatric surgery clinics in Stockholm but in
April 1982 the clinic at the Karolinska Hospital moved to St Görans hospital. The number of surgical operations in the clinic of
paediatric surgery, as represented in the monthly reports
of January 1982-March 1983, was expected to increase by 50%
after the move. A certain increase was seen already in April
1982 but not until February 1983 the full effect of the move
was seen.

3. 3. Personal report to the surgeons

The codes for performed operation are delivered by the surgeon to the
anaesthetist who record it on the anaesthetic chart. Quarterly the surgeons get a report on the interventions they have participated in as
first surgeon or as assistent. Figure 6 shows the first page of such a
report. This report includes anaesthetic time consumption.

3. 4. Clinical follow up

The surgeons often use the system to find a special patient or groups of patients. Such a retrieval is accomplished in a couple of minutes. The system also facilitates a more accurate follow up of various techniques used i. e. the yearly report tells us that 82 cases of arterial cannulation were performed during the year and a study of complications is readily performed.

3. 5. Clinical follow up - education

The system is continously used at the staffmeetings to retrieve information on recently occurred complications during anaesthesia. Interesting cases are easy to find. Students, residents and nurses thus are taught with a close reality as a basis.

4. DISCUSSION

Essential for the maintaining of a high reliability of an information system is that a fast feedback of information to the personel that creates and records data is obtained. The reports to the surgeons, the monthly report and the continous use of the system at the weekly staffmeetings are examples of our solution of this issue. ADI has facilitated the designing of a system that will be used by many other hopitals. With the experience from the system used at the Karolinska Hospital as a basis we think we have designed a system that creates possibilities for a systematic follow up of the routine anaesthetic activities and creates a sound basis for rational planning and use of the available resources.

REFERENCES

1. Hallen B. 1973. Computerized anaesthetic record-keeping. Acta Anaesth Scand: Suppl. 52.
2. Hallen B, Eklund J, Gordh T, Hall P, Selander H. 1968. Computer application in clinical anaesthesia. A report on two years experience. Exerpta Medica International Congress series. No 200, p 618-622.
3. Socialstyrelsen 1979. Klassifikation av operationer, 4th Ed. Stockholm, Liber.
4. Socialstyrelsen 1970. Anestesiklassifikation, 2nd Ed. Stockholm, Socialstyrelsen.

FIGURE 5. Personal report to the surgeons.

GUNNAR L OLSSON
Dept. Paed. Anaesth.
St Görans hospital

SURGEON/ASSISTENT
performed operations
1983-04-24

REPORT ON PERFORMED OPERATIONS.

This report is intended to present those surgical operations
that a surgeon has performed (first surgeon) or assisted.

Period: Jan - march 1983
Surgeon: Paul Tordal

Intervention as first surgeon

Numbers of operation codes	83
numbers of interventionoccasions	77
numbers of patients	77
anaesthetic time consumption, hours	83.9
anaesthetic time consumption, average	1.1

INTERVENTION	N
hernia ing. repair	21
fracture, reposition	14
appendicectomy	7
extirp skin (tumour, scar)	7
phimosis	5
fract., repos. + plaster	4
pyloromytomy	3
nerv suture	2
orchidectomy	2
ectopia testis	2
gyn examination	2
extraction osteosynt. material	2
inc. tendon sheet	2
app.ect. en passant	1
neurolysis	1
extirp in pharynx	1
extirp of hydatid	1

AUTOMATED ANALYSIS OF THE ESOPHAGEAL ACCELEROGRAM AS A MINIMALLY INVASIVE MONITOR OF MANIFEST CONTRACTILE STATE

RALPH S. WILEY, M.S., LEE S. SHEPARD, M.D., AND LEWIS B. WOLFENSON, Ph.D.

Departments of Anesthesiology and Biometry
Cuyahoga County Hospital and Case Western Reserve University School of Medicine
Cleveland, Ohio

ABSTRACT

Automated real-time monitoring of the heart's relative contractile state was achieved simply and cost effectively through automated analysis of the esophageal accelerogram (EA) and electrocardiogram (ECG). Previous work showed that the first major complex of the EA contains information which is a sensitive indicator of the left ventricle's mechanical activity. An automated system was developed around a small, inexpensive, personal computer through the application of current software engineering design and implementation techniques. The resulting system has freed the physician from tedious, time consuming data analysis in the operating room. The ECG and EA analog signals are obtained from conventional physiologic monitors and processed by the system to yield an index of the relative contractile state every five seconds. This discrete index is trended along with heart rate (HR) by plotting the last twenty minutes of data. In addition, the most current numeric values of HR and the contractile index are presented. The system is contained on a single cart, and therefore, is easily rolled into the operating room (OR). Operation of the system was designed to be simple and unoccupying in the sometimes hectic environment of the operating room. System performance was tested and found to be accurate when supplied with correct analog signals. Electrocautery device generated electromagnetic interference of the ECG or EA caused the system to produce an appropriate error message and "hold" until an acceptable signal was obtained. Due to the minimally invasive nature of the esophageal probe, monitoring of the heart's relative contractile state is performed on a routine basis with minimal risk to the patient.

1. INTRODUCTION

The ability to routinely monitor the contractile state of the anesthetized patient's heart remains a difficult task. Through invasive means we are able to monitor contractile indices such as left ventricular dp/dt max[1,2], mean electromechanical $\Delta P/\Delta t$[3,4], the collection of force-velocity-length indicators[5], and pressure-volume-stress relationships to name a few.[6,7] These indices provide useful information, but owing to their invasiveness are inappropriate for routine monitoring. There is also a variety of indices which can be obtained noninvasively; primarily, systolic time intervals (STI)[8] and the echocardiography techniques.[9] Of these noninvasive techniques only the STIs have been automated[10,11] to produce a real-time monitor for the operating room. Even STI monitoring is limited in application due to the rather critical transducer positioning.

Recently there has been some work done[12,13,14] with a variety of transducers placed in proximity to the heart via the esophagus. There exists a great potential for producing a simple, automated system from these techniques. Several important features are 1) minimal invasiveness, 2) simple transducer electronics, and 3) analog signals which are appropriate for straightforward computer analysis. Pinchak et al[15] first placed a miniature accelerometer in an esophageal stethoscope and demonstrated that high quality signals produced by the mechanical activity of the heart and great vessels could be obtained with relative ease. Further work by this laboratory has established very strong relationships between the indices derived from the esophageal accelerogram (EA) and more conventional cardiovascular parameters, e.g., dp/dt max, mean electromechanical$\Delta p/\Delta t$, and STI.

Our goal, however, is not to establish merely a correlate with a variety of "indices of contractility." Our intention is to produce a clinically useful tool for the anesthesiologist by providing an automated system for monitoring the relative manifest contractile state of the heart. In this paper we will present the development of such an automated system. The automated system receives ECG and EA waveforms as inputs, and outputs three myocardial contractile indices (MCI).

2. SYSTEM DESCRIPTION

It is our design philosophy to configure systems from commercially available and supported components which are truly pin-for-pin compatible. Our intent is to produce a simple and inexpensive system requiring a minimum of user integration and virtually no modification. This philosophy, we feel, makes the system readily available to a variety of institutions and interested users. It provides a flexible environment in which a system can evolve. There is also the advantage of being able to use a competitive pricing structure for the various components to keep costs down. We have therefore constrained the system to be:

1. inexpensive,
2. simple to operate,

3. easy to maintain, and

4. portable.

2.1. Hardware Configuration

The hardware system consists of three parts: 1) an esophageal accelerometer, 2) two physiologic amplifiers, and 3) a microcomputer system. Below are detailed descriptions of each of these.

2.1.1. Esophageal Accelerometer. The principal transducer of the system is an accelerometer positioned in the distal end of a conventional esophageal stethescope. See Figure 1. The original acoustical properties of the stethescope

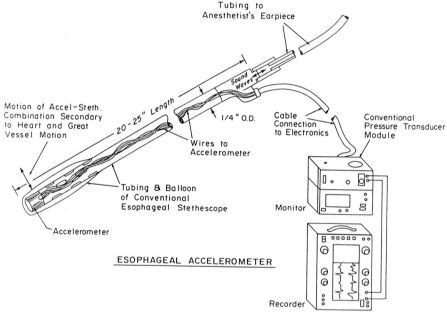

FIGURE 1. Esophageal accelerometer recording system.

are retained and aid in properly positioning the accelerometer. The accelerometer used is manufactured by Entran Devices, Inc. (Model No. EGAXT2-R-50-D). This device is a biaxial piezoresistive accelerometer which employs a fully active semiconductor Wheatstone bridge. A less expensive single axis version can be used to keep costs to a minimum. The semiconductor circuitry is fully compensated for temperature changes in the environment. The high output from this device allows readily available OR physiologic amplifier systems to be used with excellent signal-to-noise ratios. The accelerometers are internally damped and have a flat frequency response of greater than 600 Hz. The accelerometer has overrange protection to 10,000 g.

2.1.2. Physiologic Amplifiers. Two separate amplifiers are used by the system. One is for obtaining the ECG analog signal, and the other is a standard bridge amplifier to drive the accelerometer. Most commercialy available pressure transducer amplifiers are of this type. Both amplifier systems are available as a single physiologic monitor with one ECG channel and one pressure channel. In the operating room we use the Datascope 870 with the P3 module. For our animal work we use Gould #13-4615 series amplifiers. Any amplifier may be used if an analog output between ± 2.5 volts is available. In addition the bridge amplifier must produce an excitation voltage between ± 7.5 volts. We have purposefully chosen commercially available units which most, if not all, anesthesia departments possess. An additional advantage is that all such devices have already passed the electrical tests for patient contact.

2.1.3. Microcomputer System. Again in adherance to our design philosophy, we configured the computer portion of the system from commercially available hardware. We selected an Apple II-plus with a monitor and two 5¼ inch disk drives.

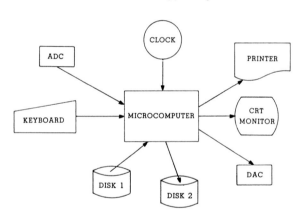

To this basic system we added a 16K RAM card, a printer with interface, a real time clock, and an analog-to-digital converter (ADC). For testing purposes we temporarily incorporated a digital-to-analog converter (DAC) to facilitate synchronization of data acquisition with our Gould 2600 strip chart recorder. Figure 2 shows a block diagram of the system.

FIGURE 2. Block diagram of the hardware system configuration.

2.2. Software Configuration

Like the constraints imposed upon the hardware system, the software portion of the monitoring system must be:

1. easy to maintain and modify,
2. simple to operate, and
3. resistant to user error.

Much time and energy was spent designing and implementing a similar system with identical constraints.[11] It was decided to test the flexibility of this previous design by modifying it to meet our current application. The modified system's physical structure chart is shown in Figure 3. Those modules requiring modification are denoted by an asterisk under the name. One module, GETDIST, is a completely new module which was added. This approach saved much time by minimizing new design efforts and unnecessary implementation cycles. We also experienced the advantage of building upon a clinically tried and tested system.

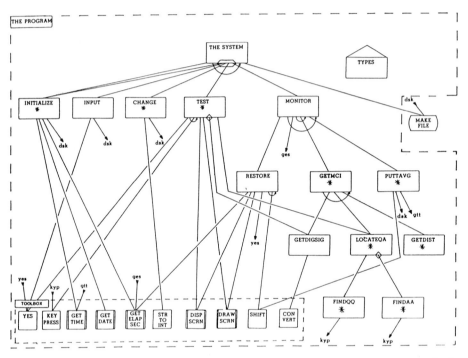

FIGURE 3. The MCI system physical structure chart. Notation follows Myers (16).

The software system was designed, implemented, and tested according to the principles and methodologies of structured design[16] and top-down implementation.[17] The software environment for development and operation was the Apple Pascal system. Only a few speed-critical modules were written not in Pascal, but in the 6502 assembly language.

The resulting single-user system is composed of an executive module (THE SYSTEM) which receives commands from the keyboard and then executes the appropriate functional module. The seven functions implemented were:

1. INITIALIZE. . .sets to initial state,

2. INPUT. . .receives patient identification information,

3. CHANGE. . .modifies operating parameters (display rate, printer on/off, initial ADC conversion rate),

4. TEST. . .verifies quality of ADC and identification algorithms,

5. MONITOR. . .acquires and displays HR and MCIs,

6. HELP. . .lists valid system commands,

7. QUIT. . .exits system.

All modules are highly independent in that they perform only single functions. This allows the system to be configured as a collection of functional modules. By controlling intermodule communication through strictly defined interfaces we reduced any ripple effect that might be introduced from modifying or adding modules.

TEST allows the user to decide if the analog-to-digital converter and the landmark identification algorithms are performing correctly. This is accomplished by plotting the raw digitized signal and the landmarks selected on the video monitor.

MONITOR continuously cycles through the acquisition and display of HR and the myocardial contractile indices. It is fully automated and does not require user interaction.

2.2.1. <u>Signal Analysis.</u> Both the QRS detection and EA landmark detection algorithms use multiple stage, slope analysis techniques. In short, each waveform is represented as a one dimensional array of integer values. By comparing the value at index i in the array with the value at index i plus some look ahead offset it is possible to detect the presence, magnitude, and direction of a slope. See Figure 4a.

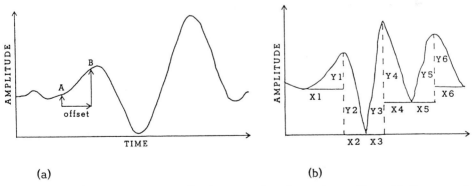

(a)   (b)

FIGURE 4. a) Depiction of amplitude comparison for a given offset. b) Decomposition of EA into sequence of right triangles.

By basing processing control decisions on polarity and magnitude of this slope one may determine the location and value of the waveform peaks and valleys. The characteristics of this algorithm are tuned by changing the look ahead offset and the slope response.

2.2.2. <u>QRS</u> <u>Detection</u> <u>Algorithm</u>. For the purpose of monitoring we typically use lead II or lead V. The algorithm takes advantage of this fact by being less general than many diagnostic algorithms. The result is increased execution speed and smaller size; both being important considerations for an eight-bit microcomputer. The module FINDQQ (see Figure 3) receives as input the array which contains the digitized ECG waveform. This array is processed to determine a cardiac cycle denoted QQ'. To accomplish this it must find two consecutive Q waves. This is done by the following algorithm:

1.   Search and skip until a preset positive threshhold value is exceeded.

2.   Back up and crudely search for upstroke of R wave.

3.   If R wave is found, back up and finely search for onset of Q.

    3.1   If first Q is found then search for second:

        3.1.1 Skip over first QRS.

        3.1.2 Search for second Q in same manner as for first.

    3.2   Else write error message and exit.

2.2.3. <u>EA</u> <u>Analysis</u> <u>Algorithm</u>. The myocardial contractile indices produced by the system are designated as M1 through M3. Given the series of triangles formed in Figure 4b, M1 equals the sum of the ratios Y:X for each triangle. M2 and M3 are the average acceleration and the root mean square average acceleration, respectively. M2 and M3 are calculated directly from the raw digitized waveforms and require no sophisticated waveform analysis. Since M1 requires interpretation of the waveform as a series of triangles it is necessary to detect the corresponding peaks and valleys. This is accomplished by:

1.   Search and skip within a specific window begining with the Q wave until a crude slope value is found.

 .2.   If the slope found is positive then

    2.1   Search for value and index where the slope turns negative

    2.2   Record value and index in vector as a peak.

3.   Else (slope is negative)

    3.1   Search for value and index where the slope turns positive

    3.2   Record values and index in vector as a valley.

4.   Repeat until not in window.

At this point in time the system serves mainly as a research tool to aid us in the characterization of the various EA indices. For this reason we calculate and display all indices. In the purely clinical version we will calculate and present only the most useful indices.

3. RESULTS

3.1. System Hardware

We are satisfied that the hardware system has met our computing needs while being constrained to be inexpensive, simple, and portable. All the components of the hardware system are engineered for the "personal" computer market. The result is an inherently simple system. It is easy to connect, operate, and maintain the components. The operation manuals are reasonably well written and do not require special technical knowledge to understand. Our main concern was durability in the equipment-hostile environments of critical care medicine and animal research laboratories. To date we have experienced no serious environmental effects. Hardware reliability has been excellent. The only hardware failure was the early demise of a single integrated circuit on the Apple Language Card. This was remedied the same day. The system tolerates the continual moving from room to room.

Another concern was the extreme interference generated by the operation of electrocautery devices during surgery. The older spark-gap devices are not tolerated but hardware damage was not observed. The newer, solid state devices do not adversely affect the computer system's operation. They do, however, induce much noise in the ECG analog signal.

The primary hardware limitation is the slow access time of the floppy disk drives. This, however, did not significantly impact our software design. The 5¼-in. diskette format is useful since it is desirable for each user to keep the resulting patient data diskette.

3.2 System Software

Our decision to use the Apple Pascal language for the development and operation of our MCI monitoring system has produced no major regrets. Pascal, being a strongly typed and structured language, facilitated adherence to the principles of software engineering. Its block structure and flexible control structures made the desired high modularity simple to achieve. Clearly defined module interfaces were forced by excluding global variables and passing all information (whether control or data) as parameters. This approach is fully supported by Pascal. We encountered no major operating system bugs. The constraints imposed by the operating system were in keeping with our philosophy of structured design and top-down implementation and thus were accepted. The clock routines supplied by the manufacturer, however, reflected inflexible design and unmaintainable coding.

3.3 MCI Monitoring System

To obtain a preliminary evaluation of the system's performance six patients were selected at random for evaluation from our OR schedule. The cases selected included abdominal and extremity procedures, but no thoracic procedures. The esophageal accelerometer was positioned in accordance with our Human Investigation Committee approved protocol #7914-A-79. The ECG and EA analog signals were recorded on a Teac R-71 FM recorder. These recordings were used later to evaluate the system's performance by comparison with manual data reduction. Using the digital-to-analog converter, a Gould 2400 strip chart recorder was synchronized to the data acquisition cycle of the MCI system. This allowed a direct comparison between manually derived MCI and system calculated MCI. The manual processing of the strip chart recording was accomplished using a Houston Instruments Digitizer driven by an Apple II-plus. (Maximum resolution for this system is .001 in.) Twelve determinations of each MCI were made from each patient by both methods. The data from each patient were then correlated using a simple linear model. The resulting r^2 statistics ranged from .89 - .96 for M1, .92 - .98 for M2, and .91 - .98 for M3.

The behavior of the system was tested with extremes of inputs. The system's response to high amplitude noise was either a message correctly detecting no ECG, or a false reading. These false readings are easily distinguished from valid physiologic readings by their generally absurd values. Low amplitude noise (i.e. below threshold value) produced a message stating that no complexes were found. Grounding of inputs gave the same response. The system is highly resistant to erroneous input and will not crash due to bad analog signals. The worst case is an erroneous "MCI value."

4. CONCLUSION

In contrast to the difficulty of noninvasively monitoring contractile indices the system has performed very well. Our evaluation was based upon three criteria: 1) ease of use, 2) clinical utility, and 3) ease of configuration. Ease of use was established by simple observation and user comments. Out of six users none found the system confusing or intimidating. All were able to operate the system from either the manual alone or 10 minutes of verbal instructions. Clinical utility was confirmed by the value of the indices themselves and the minimally invasive nature of the esophageal probe. Our work in animals indicate that MCI will be extremely useful in the management of patients that require a sensitive balance between positive inotropic state and afterload control. Finally, the system can be configured without an engineer. By far the most complex part is the packaging of the accelerometer since prepackaged devices are not yet available. The amplifier systems are already widely used by most clinicians. The vast and rapid acceptance of the personal computer speaks for itself. The minimal requirement on the user is that the cables necessary to connect these three subsystems be provided.

Such a system will allow us to quickly and extensively evaluate the clinical utility in the EA contractile indices in a broad spectrum of patients and surgical procedures.

REFERENCES

1.   Broughton, A. and Korner, P.I.   Estimation of maximum left ventricular inotropic response from changes in isovolumic indices of contractility in dogs. Cardio. Res., 15, pp. 382-389, 1981.

2.   Diamond, G., et al. Mean electromechanical $\Delta p/\Delta t$ - An indirect index of the peak rate of rise of left ventricular pressure. Amer. J. Cardiol., 30, pp. 338-342, 1972.

3.   Brubakk, O. and Folling, M. Mean electromechanical $\Delta p/\Delta t$ and systolic time intervals in coronary artery disease. Europ. J. Cardiol., 7/5-6, pp. 367-377, 1978.

4.   Van den Bos, G.C., et al. Problems in the use of indices of myocardial contractility. Cardio. Res., 7, pp. 834-848, 1973.

5.   Weber, K.T., and Janicki, J.S. Instantaneous Force-Velocity-Length relations: Experimental findings and clinical correlates. Amer. J. Cardiol., 40, pp. 740-747, 1977.

6.   Grossman, W., et al. Contractile State of the left ventricle in man as evaluated from end-systolic pressure-volume relations. Circulation, 56:5, pp. 845-852, 1977.

7.   Lewis, R.P., et al. A Critical review of the systolic time intervals. Circulation, 56:2, pp. 146-158, 1977.

8.   Folland, E.D., et al. Assessment of left ventricular ejection fraction and volumes by real-time, two dimensional echocardiography. Circulation, 60:4, pp. 760-766, 1979.

9. Pouleur, H., et al. Assesment of left ventricular contractility from late systolic stress - volume relations. Circulation, 65:6, pp. 1204-1212, 1982.

10. Divers, R.T., et al. Continuous real-time computation and display of systolic time intervals from surgical patients. Comput. Biomed. Res., 10, pp. 45, 1977.

11. Wiley, R.S., et al. A computerized system for monitoring systolic time intervals from esophageal accelerograms. Comput. Biomed. Res., 16, pp. 44-58, 1983.

12. Cahalan, M.K., et al. Intraoperative myocardial ischemia detected by transesopohageal 2-dimensional echocardiography - prognostic implications. In Proceedings of 5th annual meeting of Society of Cardiovascular Anesthesiologists., pp. 122, 1983.

13. Dauchot, P.J., et al. Detection of ischemia-induced left ventricular dyskinesia by the esophageal cardiokymogram in dogs. In Proceedings of 5th annual meeting of Society of Cardiovascular Anesthesiologists., pp. 126, 1983.

14. Wiley, R.S. and Shepard, L.S. Noninvasive monitoring of left ventricular contractile dynamics from esophageal accelerograms. In Proceedings of 5th annual meeting of Society of Cardiovascular Anesthesiologists., pp. 128, 1983.

15. Pinchak, A.C., et al. Esophageal accelerometer-Indicator of cardiovascular function. J. Biomech. Eng., Trans. ASME 103, pp. 160-167, 1981.

16. Myers, G.J. "Composite/Structured Design." Van Nostrand-Reinhold, New York, 1978.

17. Hughes, J.K. and Michtom, J.I. "A Structured Approach to Programming." Prentice-Hall, Englewood Cliffs, N.J., 1977.

INFORMATION TRANSFER FROM OPERATING ROOM TO ICU

RICHARD M. PETERS, M.D.

The period from the termination of anesthesia until completion of
transfer to the ICU is one of high risk. Not only is the patient emerging
from the stress of surgery and anesthesia and being moved, but management
is also being transferred to a new professional team. A safe and effective
patient management system requires appropriate monitoring of patient state
and transfer of information. Unfortunately, under usual conditions the
information transfer is often incomplete and even haphazard, as is the
monitoring. Automation has the potential of improving the quantity and
quality of information transfer.

Information about patient state with its variance during the operative
procedure is essential to management of the postoperative period. The
patient is acutely ill during operation. Postoperatively the operative
record is an important information set for appropriate care. The present
system creates an anesthesia record in an obtuse code, often not available
and more often difficult if not impossible to interpret.

Some of you may think this information is relatively irrelevant or,
if available, would not be used. Reed Gardner and his colleagues at
Latter Day Saints Hospital in Salt Lake City, Utah, have shown the fallacy
of this conclusion. During cardiopulmonary bypass, intraoperative
information is entered into the computer and is available to the ICU
nurses while the case is proceeding. When the nurses discovered this
information was available without prompting, they began to monitor this
information to evaluate how soon and in what state the patient will be
on arrival in the cardiac surgery ICU.

What information can we make available in a usable format, and how
can this be done in 1983, or perhaps in the year of George Orwell, 1984?
I believe we have passed the day when such services were available only
to rich developers of such systems. The microprocessor has radically

changed this situation. Change has occurred both in cost of systems hardware and software, and, most important, in user attitude. The nurses and physicians whose 10-year-old children are programming and playing with computers can no longer admit to being threatened by them. Their children's greater aptitude is a constant reminder of their inadequacy. They want effective systems. We have only to make information useful and operation facile.

Over the past year we have been transferring programs formerly available only on our Hewlett-Packard patient monitoring system to the IBM PC computer. The cost at present of such a computer with color video graphics printer is around $5000. We anticipate this will fall by 20 to 30 percent over the next 12 to 18 months. Now we have modular computer hardware that can be at each bedside or each operating table. Our job is to catch up with the available resource hardware and the fast developing software. We must learn how to use the information that will be available.

Table I illustrates the information that may be needed during anesthesia for a complex patient. The starred information is that needed for all operations. To speed development and maintain flexibility, we have had rules for the development of our PC system. (1) No systems program would be written if one could be purchased. (2) Program transfer would start with direct patient monitoring and testing, supplemented by keyboard-entered information.

The following is a list of the presently available programs:

Blood gases

Cardiac output

Lung water

Hemodynamics

Ventilation and work

Pulmonary wedge pressure

Figures 1 and 2 are examples of some of the reports.

We must decide how to include another vital piece of information, the intake and output. I propose that each information acquisition start on the PC in the operating room, and that the disc accompany the patient to the ICU, where collection and interpretation will continue.

With computer cost and capability removed as a barrier, the next issue is what front end hardware should be used for data collection. We can reach our goal in steps starting relatively simply and adding modules for

Fig. 1 ICU Patient Testing & Information System

Hemodynamic Calculations

ID # 12345   Name Doe   John
Date 05-11-83   Time 00:00

```
                    Cardiac Output (L/min)   8.5
                        Heart rate (/min)    80      ( 60- 90)
      Systemic Arterial Pressure (mm Hg)   120/ 80
             Mean Arterial Pressure (mm Hg)  95      ( 70-105)
            Central Venous Pressure (mm Hg)   4      (  0-  4)
         Pulmonary Artery Pressure (mm Hg)  45/ 22
    Mean Pulmonary Artery Pressure (mm Hg)  30      (  9- 19)              ***
           Pulmonary Artery Wedge (mm Hg)   10      (  5- 13)
```

```
                                          Value                 Index
                    Cardiac Output (L/M)    8.5                  4.2 (2.5-4.3)
                       Stroke Volume (ml)   106                  52  ( 35- 45)***
    Total Periph Resist (dyne sec cm^-5)    856    (800-1500)
    Pulm Vascular Resist (dyne sec cm^-5)   188    (105-165)                 ***
        Left Ventricular Stroke Work (g M)  123                  61  ( 40- 55)***
       Right Ventricular Stroke Work (g M)   37                  18  (  7- 10)***
```

Normal values in parentheses.
*** = value outside normal range.

Fig. 2 ICU Patient Testing & Information System

BLOOD GAS CORRECTIONS & CALCULATIONS

```
           ID #  12345              NAME  Doe            John
           DATE  05-11-83           TIME  14:36
                                    INPUT
   Temp(C)    38.0 (36.5-37.5)           Hcta    35  (35-48)
      pHa    7.45 (7.37-7.43)            Hgba        (12-16)
      PaO2    75   (80-100)              SaO2(%)     (95-100)
     PaCO2    34   (35-45)               CaO2(vol%)  (15.5-22)
      pHv    7.44 (7.35-7.41)            Hctv        (35-48)
      PvO2    35   (35-40)               Hgbv        (12-16)
     PvCO2    36   (41-51)               SvO2(%)     (71-79)
    FiO2(%)   21   (20-100)              CvO2(vol%)  (13-17)
                                         (A-V)DO2    (3.5-5)
                         CORRECTIONS & CALCULATIONS
  pHa   7.44          pHv   7.43              (A-V)DO2    4.2
  PaO2  80            PvO2  38         Base Excess(mEq/l)  -0.0  (-2-+2)
  PaCO2 36            PvCO2 38            Bicarb(mEq/l)    23    (22-27)
  SaO2  96            SvO2  70             Shunt[QsQt]     0.10  (<.05)
  CaO2  15.2          CvO2  11.1        (A-a)DO2(torr)    25    (0-30)
```

new information. We can start by having the anesthesiologist enter data using the keyboard instead of a pen at the frequency of the anesthesia record, q 5 min, blood pressure, pulse, respiration, drugs, fluids and events. This will be displayed on the CRT in color distinctive for each parameter and stored on a disc. If the patient is a candidate for a Swan-Ganz catheter, PWP and PAP should be entered with blood pressure. When cardiac output is done q 15-30 min, all hemodynamic parameters will be calculated and displayed with the abnormal values highlighted (Fig. 1: Hemodynamic Report). In the future, with further development for patient with arterial lines, respirator monitors, and automatic infusers, much of this information would be automatically acquired and edited to give information on significant change in state. For example, windows could be set around blood pressure values and, if they fall out of the window, an automatic display made. The time, type, and amount of fluid infusion, blood loss and urine output for each half-hour period should be associated with a simple event record -- incision, chest opened, etc.

My concepts of how the functional state of respiration should be monitored depart most from present concepts. More morbidity and mortality occurs intraoperatively and in the ICU due to accidents of ventilation management than is acceptable. Such tragedies can be avoided by better testing. The nasogastric tube with a balloon catheter provides an additional sensor, without extra invasion. This simple modification of nasogastric tube permits patients undergoing major procedures to have both airway and intrapleural pressure monitored. (In the supine posture, the suggestions of Baydur and colleagues for positioning the balloon above the heart should be followed.) The pressures alone will give a great deal of information. During assisted ventilation, what is the concordance of airway and esophageal pressure? For example, a rise in airway pressures without an equivalent rise in esophageal pressure suggests a misplaced endotracheal tube. A concordant rise in both pressures may indicate pneumothorax or that the surgeons are leaning on the patient, both poor for the patient. A change in transpulmonary pressure, airway pressure minus esophageal pressure, indicates fall in compliance of the lung, airway obstruction or lung congestion.

Respiratory monitor values should be recorded at least q 5 min and graphed to show the time course of change. A pneumotachograph to record flow allows calculation of tidal volume, respiratory rate, lung mechanics.

Esophageal pressure provides other important information about the true filling pressure, preload, of the heart and true afterload. Since the heart is in the chest, the preload is equal to pulmonary wedge pressure minus pleural pressure, and afterload, mean arterial pressure minus pleural pressure.

The use of monitors of expired gases -- CO_2, O_2 -- will enhance anesthetic safety by preventing accidents. If blood gases are determined, the calculation of the A-A CO_2 difference to correct end-tidal PCO_2 will permit estimation of arterial PCO_2. However, in my opinion the most important function of CO_2 monitor is to prevent anesthetic accidents. This requires a continuous monitor to determine that CO_2 goes to zero at mid-inspiration and rises during expiration to near arterial levels. The transfer of the information about CO_2 cycling will have little importance to subsequent care since it primarily indicates the skill or somnolence of the anesthesiologist. Blood gases and hematocrit when done should be entered to permit calculation of shunt, etc., as illustrated in blood gas report.

Let me illustrate how such a system could work using as an illustration the subject of a talk I gave the last time I was in Rotterdam. A vigorous 50-year-old man with good pulmonary function and exercise tolerance is to have a pneumonectomy using a double lumen endotracheal tube. A nasogastric tube with a balloon, central venous pressure, and radial artery catheter are inserted. Let us consider how a computer system in which transferred information as described above might forewarn the ICU team of the risk of pulmonary edema. First review would be of intraoperative events.

A review of the anesthetic record is given in Table II. On first glance it again seems to portray a benign course, an easy operation with small blood loss. However, there are predictors of trouble. A right pneumonectomy for a patient who received fluids in excess of amounts required for resuscitation had a high intraoperative urine output with a net positive balance at end of operation of over 2000 cc. The pleural pressure, i.e., transpulmonary pressure, is modestly elevated. The patient requires careful monitoring of his respiratory and fluid balance state. A more subatmospheric mean, end-inspiratory, and end-expiratory pleural pressure would indicate fall in lung compliance due to pulmonary congestion. In this patient, high fluid intake, high urine output, greater transpulmonary pressure indicate high risk for postpneumonectomy pulmonary edema. The patient needs continued monitoring with insertion of Swan-Ganz catheter, not discharge from the ICU.

Another area requiring new interpretation is the traditional measure of adequacy of cardiac function, the blood pressure. It has proven to be an inadequate and, on occasion, dangerous indicator of cardiac function. If drugs which alter blood pressure are administered, then blood pressure becomes at best a controller of the drug infusion rate. Without any drugs being given, excitation of the sympathetic adrenal system can maintain blood pressure despite dangerously low cardiac output.

How should blood pressure be interpreted in 1983? As in use of all monitoring information, the importance is determined by physiology, not by signal. The level of blood pressure determines both the afterload on the heart and the perfusion force for various organs. However, a high blood pressure does not guarantee adequate organ perfusion.

The question of critical importance to patient management in 1983 is when should afterload, peripheral resistance, be manipulated? Afterload is a major determinant of cardiac output and the ratio of oxygen consumed by the heart to mechanical work done by the heart. Lowering afterload will increase cardiac output for the same preload. If afterload is to be manipulated, then information requirement goes up. We must know cardiac output and cardiac filling pressures.

There are many instances when therapy degrades signals so knowledge of drugs given colors interpretation. All such information must be transferred. By using the same information format from the intraoperative to the postoperative period, the intraoperative risk factors will guide those responsible for postoperative care. For this stage of our development of automated data acquisition and information system, a common OR-ICU system is needed. Rather than transferring illegible sheets of paper with incomplete information, we can transfer plastic discs that permit facile and fast review of all the information together with interpretations. This type of information collection and transfer with increasingly sophisticated forms of interpretation must be our new standard in 1984.

REFERENCES

1.   Brimm JE, Shelton RE, Zeldin RA. An adaptable system for respiratory
     analysis. Presented at fifth annual international symposium,
     Computers in Critical Care and Pulmonary Medicine, Salt Lake City,
     Utah, U.S.A., June 1983.
2.   Zeldin RA, Shelton RE, Brimm JE. A microcomputer-based ICU patient
     testing and information system. Ibid.
3.   Baydur A, Behrakis PK, Zin WA, Jaeger M.,Milic-Emili J. A simple
     method for assessing the validity of the esophageal balloon technique.
     Am Rev Respir Dis 126:788-791, 1982.

Table I
Parameters to be Monitored

1) Intake and Output
   a) Fluid infused type and amount*
   b) Blood loss*
      Other losses*
   c) Urine output
      Urine osmolality
   d) Net fluid intake*
   e) Fluid interpretation*
   f) Hematocrit*

2) Cardiovascular State
   a) Blood pressure*
   b) Pulse*
   c) Cardiac output
   d) Peripheral resistance
   e) P-A pressure
   f) PWP
   g) A-V DO_2

3) Gas Exchange
   a) Tidal volume, spontaneous and ventilator*
   b) Respiratory rate, spontaneous and ventilator*
   c) Tidal CO_2 and O_2 interpretation*
   d) pH, PCO_2 and interpretation+
   e) PO_2, SaO_2, SVO_2, Q_s/Q_t
   f) Muscle force, fatigue

4) Kidney Function
   Urine output, rate and volume
   Urine osmolality

5) Cerebral function
   State awareness

*Required on all patients

+A safety device that could prevent anesthetic accidents

Table II

Review of Anesthetic Record

	7:45	8:00	8:15	8:30	8:45	9:00	9:15	9:30	9:45	10:00	10:15	10:30	10:45	11:00
Pulse	100	80	80	80	95	95	95	100	95	90	90	100	100	100
Sys/Dia	120/80	90/50	90/50	90/50	120/80	110/75	110/75	110/75	110/75	110/75	110/75	130/90	130/90	130/90
Fluids	750 RL	750 RL	500 RL	250 RL	250 RL	250 RL	250 RL	250 RL	250 RL	250 RL	250 RL	250 RL	300 RL	100 RL
Total intake		1500	2000	2250	2500	2750	3000	3250	3500	3750	4000	4250	4650	4650
PaH		7.40				7.37	7.38		7.42				7.35	
$PaCO_2$		40				35	38		30				45	
PaO_2		300				55	50		350				200	
Tidal volume			1000	1000	1000	1000	700	650	650	650	650	550	400	400
Resp. rate			8	8	8	8	11	12	12	12	12	16	20	24
Airway pressure			20	20	20	35	30	25	25	25	25	0	0	0
Esophageal pressure		-10	6	6	6	0	0	0	0			-10	-15	-15
Blood loss								250					350	
Urine						1000				1750			2000	
Event	1		2	3	4	5	6	7	8	9	10	11		12

Events:

1. Insertion of catheters
2. Intubation
3. Turned, prepped
4. Incision
5. R chest opened
6. R lung deflated
7. Pulmonary artery tied
8. Superior vein
9. Inferior vein
10. Bronchus stapled, lung removed
11. Chest closed
12. Skin closed

ENERGY METABOLISM

BURSZTEIN S., M.D., BSHOUTY Z., M.D.
Intensive Care Department Rambam Medical Center,
and Technion School of Medicine, Haifa (Israel).

Without going through the details of the biochemical and thermodynamical
basics and principles of energy production in man, for the matter of
simplicity and understanding, it can be stated that the energy expenditure in man (energy metabolism), presented in the form of calories, is
being constantly produced by the oxidation of the different nutritional
elements. This calories can be liberated in the form of heat, or
coupled with other reactions at the cellular level to drive such vital
processes as synthetic reactions, muscular contraction, nerve conduction
and active transport, or can be stored in the form of A.T.P.

MECHANISM OF ENERGY PRODUCTION

The nutritional elements producing energy are essentially presented to
the body in the form of charbohydrates (CH), proteins (P) and lipids (F).
Assuming a complete oxidation, 1gram of (CH) requiering 0.829 liters of
O_2 (STPD) will produce 0.829 liters of CO_2 and 0.6 milliliters of water
and will liberate 4.1 calories. Therefore, the following equations can
be written:

$$1g(CH) + 0.829 \text{ L. } O_2 \longrightarrow 0.829 \text{ L. } CO_2 + 0.6 \text{ ml } H_2O + 4.1 \text{ Cal} \qquad (1)$$

Imagining a situation where the only nutritional element metabolized is
(CH), the amount of CO_2 produced per unit time ($\dot{V}CO_2$) will be equal to
the amount of O_2 consumed ($\dot{V}O_2$). The Respiratory Quotient ($RQ = \dot{V}CO_2/\dot{V}O_2$)
will then be equal to one.
Similar equations can be written for the metabolism of proteins and lipids respectively:

$$1g(P) + 0.966 \text{ L. } O_2 \longrightarrow 0.782 \text{ L. } CO_2 + 0.41 \text{ ml } H_2O + 4.1 \text{ Cal} \qquad (2)$$

$$RQ = 0.809$$

$$1g(F) + 2.019 \text{ L. } O_2 \longrightarrow 1.426 \text{ L. } CO_2 + 1.06 \text{ ml } H_2O + 9.3 \text{ Cal} \qquad (3)$$

$$RQ = 0.71$$

QUANTITATIVE EVALUATION

There are basically two methods to evaluate the energy metabolism:
1. Direct Calorimetry
2. Indirect Calorimetry
In general, the direct calorimetry measures heat loss while the indirect
calorimetry measures heat production. Both measurements are equivalent
if there is no change neither in the core body temperature nor in the
body energy reserves during the time interval between both measurements.

1. DIRECT CALORIMETRY

In the direct calorimetry the subject is placed in an isolated chamber, his heat loss is measured directly by recording the total amount of heat transferred to a weighed quantity of water circulating through the calorimeter. The oxygen intake, the CO_2 output and the nitrogen excretion in the urine and feces are also measured during the entire period of observation (1).

2. INDIRECT CALORIMETRY

In the indirect calorimetry, the amount of heat produced, carbohydrate, protein and lipid metabolized and the amount of endogenous water produced are calculated by measuring:
O_2 consumption ($\dot{V}O_2$), CO_2 production ($\dot{V}CO_2$) and nitrogen excretion (NM), and by the resolution of the following equations (2):

a) in the fasting state:

$$ME \quad = 4.1 \quad dP + 4.1 \quad dCH + 9.3 \quad dF$$
$$\dot{V}O_2 \quad = 0.966 \ dP + 0.829 \ dCH + 2.019 \ dF$$
$$\dot{V}CO_2 = 0.782 \ dP + 0.829 \ dCH + 1.427 \ dF$$
$$H_2O_m = 0.41 \quad dP + 0.60 \quad dCH + 1.06 \quad dF$$
$$dP = 6.25 \quad NM$$

b) in the postabsorptive state:

$$ME \quad = 4.1 \quad dP + 4.1 \quad dCH + 9.3 \quad dF$$
$$\dot{V}O_2 \quad = 0.829 \ dP + 0.829 \ dCH + 1.865 \ dF$$
$$\dot{V}CO_2 = 0.860 \ dP + 0.829 \ dCH + 1.311 \ dF$$
$$H_2O_m = 4.1 \quad dP + 0.6 \quad dCH + 1.06 \quad dF$$
$$dP = 6.25 \quad NM$$

The difference in the numerical factors, between both states, being attributed to the specific dynamic action (SDA) of each foodstuff (3,4, 5,6).

dP, dCH, dF = grams of totally metabolized protein, carbohydrate and fat per minute.
ME = energy metabolism in Kcal/min.
$\dot{V}O_2$ = oxygen consumption in liters/min.
$\dot{V}CO_2$ = carbon dioxide production in liters/min.
NM = nitrogen excretion, in grams/min., in the urine.

The resolution of these equations enables us to obtain the values of ME, dP, dCH, dF and H_2O_m. A special computer program has been written to obtain these data rapidly. $\dot{V}O_2$ and $\dot{V}CO_2$ being obtained by analysis of inspired and expired O_2 and CO_2 concentrations and by measuring the expired gas volumes, all constructed into the apparatus shown in Figure 1 (7).

118

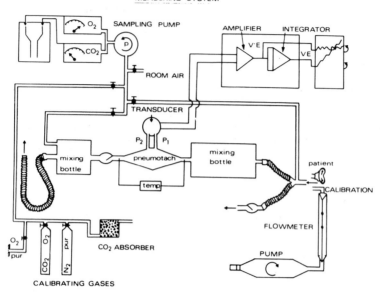

FIGURE 1

PROCESSES OF ENERGY PRODUCTION

In order to be able to understand the processes of energy production in
the acute and hypercatabolic patient, it is important to understand the
processes of energy production and metabolic adaptation to starvation in
the normal subject. A sudden, brief deficit of fuel is handled metaboli-
cally by appropriating for energy some nutrients that would normally be
used for other purposes. These sources are carbohydrates, lipids and
proteins being converted in the intestine to monosaccharides, fatty acids
and amino acids. To provide immediate fuel, more monosaccharides are
converted directly to glucose; fewer are compounded to glycogen and none
are converted to fatty acids. More fatty acids are processed in the
liver for oxidation, fewer or none are stored as fat. More amino acids
are stripped of nitrogen and converted for oxidation. If the emergency
is brief, no harm is done.

In starvation however, no further ingested nutrients are available and
the reserve must be used. Carbohydrates provide a small but significant
component of the body's fuel for only the first few days. Thereafter,
protein and fat are the sole sources of fuel, the former contributing
20% of the calories and the latter the balance (8).

A limited amount of glycogen is stored in the liver and in the muscle for quick depolymerization to glucose. Of roughly 500 grams of glycogen in a typical 70Kg adult male (< 1% of body weight), 200 grams are stored in the liver and are available for systemic use. The rest are in muscles and are essentially burned there. This total glycogen reserve can maintain an individual for about only 24 hours.

After the first day or two, free fatty acids become the primary source of fuel for the body, most of which flow to the heart, kidneys and other organs, where they are oxidized directly. About 25% are partially oxydized in the liver to produce ketone bodies, which are burned in the peripheral tissues. The typical adult male has 15% of his body weight as protein, a third of which is available for energy. In the first several days of starvation, muscle protein is utilized fairly rapidly. The protein is split into amino acids, most of which are passed to the liver for gluconeogenesis to supply energy, especially to the central nervous system, glycolytic tissues and erythrocytes. Some amino acids are burned directly and others are reassembled as protein to maintain vital organs. If the process of starvation is prolonged further, the central nervous system is adapted to utilize the ketone bodies as a source of energy in an attempt to reduce the catabolism of protein to minimum (9).

In the state of starvation, because of the fact that almost no glucose is being metabolized, the RQ will essentially be less than one (RQ of fat = 0.706). In the postabsorptive state, as carbohydrates are being fed, glucose is being shifted towards the production of energy, glycogen and fat synthesis. In the production of glycogen there is neither consumption of O_2 nor production of CO_2, while in the synthesis of fat from glucose there is a release of O_2, a process that will reduce the O_2 consumption relative to the CO_2 production and the RQ will essentially rise to values obve one (2).

In extreme starvation, the body becomes drained of readily available protein. Certain organs are depleted first, and their amino acids are utilized both for energy and for protein repair in more vital organs. Muscle tissue atrophies early. Among the next organs to lose significant protein are the liver and the spleen, followed by the kidneys and by albumin and other blood proteins. Eventually, skeletal muscle is severely atrophied, and where this wasting is associated with total weight loss of more than 20 or 30%,an increased mortality has been observed (10). The organs protected to the last include the heart, adrenals and the central nervous system.

In order to be able to administer enough energy and in the right combination to critically ill patients, it is essential to first be able to measure it in an attempt to reduce their catabolic state to minimum or even reverse it to an anabolic state.

In injury or disease, as has been shown by several investigators, the metabolic rate is frequently increased (11,12,13,14), causing an increased demand for energy. This in turn causes an increase in O_2 consumption and accelerates the use of adipose tissue reserves and speeds the wasting of protein. This increased demand of O_2 is provided by an increase in ventilation and/or cardiac output. In a critically ill patient where these two systems are affected, such an increase can lead the patient into a state of decompensation and inevitable death. Connecting these patients to assisted ventilation has been proved to reduce the O_2 consumption (12).

The protein wasting is caracterized by an increase in nitrogen excretion and by negative nitrogen balance. One sign of these combined effects is loss of body weight. Typically 4 to 8 % after elective surgery and not infrequently reaching 10 to 20% after major fractures, multiple injuries or septicemia. An increased weight loss of over 30% has been shown to be quite often fatal (10).

An attempt to reduce the severity of this weight loss can be done by trying to achieve a zero or positive nitrogen balance.

REFERENCES

1. Atwater WO, and Rosa EB. A New Respiratory Calorimeter. Bulletin no. 63, Washington D.C., U.S. Department of Agriculture, 1899.

2. Bursztein S, Glaser P, Trichet B, Taitelman U, Nedey R. Utilisation of protein carbohydrate and fat in fasting and postabsorptive subjects. Am.J.Clin.Nutr. 33: 998-1001, 1980 .

3. Peters JP, and Van Slyke DD. in: Quantitative Clinical Chemistry Interpretation, Vol.1, pp. 3-93. The William and Wilkins Company, Baltimore, 1946.

4. Forebs EB,and Swift RW. Associative dynamic effects of protein carbohydrate and fat. J. Nutrition, 29: 253-468, 1943.

5. Glickman N, Mitchell HH, Lambert EH, and Keeton RW. The total specific dynamic action of high protein and high carbohydrate diets on human subjects. J. Nutrition, 36:41 -48, 1948.

6. Hunt LM. An analytic formula to instantenously determine total metabolic rate. J. Appl. Physiol., 27: 731 - 734, 1969.

7. Bursztein S, Glaser P,Taitelman U, De Myttenaere S, Nedey R. Determination of energy metabolism by respiratory function alone. J. Appl. Physiol., 42: 117 - 119, 1977.

8. Duke JHJr, Jorgensen SB, Broell JR, Long CL,Kinney JM. Contribution of protein to caloric expenditue following injury. Surgery, 68: 168-175, 1970.

9. Cahill GF Jr. Starvation in man. New Engl.J.Med. 282: 668-675, 1970.

10. Kinney JM. Energy requirements in injury and sepsis. Acta Scan. Suppl. 55: 15 - 20, 1974.

11. Benedict FG, and Higgins HL. The influence of the respiratory exchange of varying amounts of carbohydrate in the diet. Am.J.Physiol., 30:217-229, 1912.

12. Bursztein S, et Al. Reduced oxygen consumption in catabolic states with mechanical ventilation. Crit.Care Med.6(2):162-164,1978.

13. Cairnie AB,Campbell RM, Pullar JD, Cubertson DP. The heat production consequent on injury. Brit.Exp.Pathol.38: 504 - 511, 1957.

14. Zarem HA,Kinney JM, Nichols S. Energy expenditure during early and late convalescence from multiple fractures. Surg. Forum. 11: 450-463, 1960.

Gas Distribution and Ventilation-Perfusion Relationships during Anaesthesia and in Acute Respiratory Failure. Clinical Implications.

G. Hedenstierna and S. Baehrendtz

Department of Clinical Physiology, Huddinge Hospital and Department of Medicine I, South Hospital, Stockholm, Sweden.

Hypoxemia is a recurrent complication during anaesthesia and in intensive care. In a review from 1975, Rehder et al., concluded that hypoxemia during anaesthesia may be caused by alveolar hypoventilation, reduced cardiac output, true shunt (perfusion of non ventilated regions) and mismatching between ventilation and perfusion ($\dot{V}/\dot{Q}$ mismatch). Since the time of that review additional information has been gained and today a sharper picture of lungfunction in anaesthetized man has emerged. Our deeper insight mainly concerns the regional differences in lung function that occur in the vertical plane. The "physiological" inequality of ventilation and perfusion distributions that is seen during anaesthesia may also occur in patients with acute severe pulmonary insufficiency and add to that caused by their pulmonary disease, leading to severe hypoxemia. In the following, the "physiological" mismatching is analyzed in more detail and possible messures to counteract it are discussed.

Regional ventilation and perfusion in awake man

In the healthy subject, ventilation increases down the lung from top to bottom. This is a consequence of the sigmoid shape of the pressure-volume curve of the lung and the vertical plural pressure gradient (Milic-Emili et al., 1966). Dependent lung units are located on the lower, steeper part of the pressure-volume curve, and non-dependent units on the upper, flatter part. For a given increase in transpulmonary pressure, the lower lung regions expand more than the upper ones. However, in older subjects ventilation may be reduced in dependent lung regions, this being attributed to airway closure (Milic-Emili et al., 1966). Closure of the airway may occur when the peribronchial pressure exceeds that in the airway. Since the intrathoracic, and thus peribronchial pressure is higher in dependent than in non-dependent regions, airway closure begins at the bottom of the lung. Intrathoracic pressure increases during expiration, and this causes airway closure to spread up the lung during a sustained exhalation. In young subjects, airways close only during a deep expiration, below the functional residual capacity (FRC). Under such circumstances the distribution of ventilation will remain unaffected during normal breathing. In older subjects, airway closure occurs at a higher lung volume, within or even above the tidal volume. The distribution of ventilation to dependent regions will thereby be affected, i.e. either reduced or abolished.

A change from the upright to the supine position reduces the resting lung volume, i.e. FRC, by 0.5-1 litre (Briscoe, 1964), while the lung volume at which airways begin to close, the closing capacity, remains essentially unaltered (Le Blanc et al., 1970; Craig et al., 1971). Airway closure within or above the tidal volume may thus occur more easily in the supine than in the upright position. Taking into consideration both age and body position, it can be predicted that in the upright position airways will close above FRC in subjets aged 65 years or older, whereas in the supine position such closure will occur above FRC already in 45 years old subjects (Le Blanc et al., 1970; Craig et al., 1971).

The distribution of inspired gas will also depend on the regional lung resistance. This is a function of regional volume and inspiratory flow rate (Jonson, 1970; Bake et al., 1974). It increases with decreasing lung volume and increasing inspiratory gas flow. The smaller regional volume in dependent than non-dependent lung regions will thus increase the airway reistance, impeding the ventilation of dependent units. However, regional differences in airway resistance appear to have minor influence on gas distribution during quiet breathing (Rehder et al., 1981).

In the healthy subject, perfusion also increases from top to bottom of the lung, this being due to hydrostatic forces (West et al., 1964). A small reduction in regional perfusion may be seen in the lowermost region of the lung (Ueda et al., 1964). This minor reduction in dependent lung perfusion may be due to compression of extraalveolor vessels by interstitial oedema and, in case of airway closure, to hypoxic vasoconstriction - diverting the blood flow to better ventilated regions (von Euler and Liljenstrand, 1946; West, 1977). The uppermost region may be poorly or not at all perfused if the pulmonary arterial pressure is low (so called zone I).

Thus, both ventilation and perfusion increase down the lung, although there is a greater difference in perfusion than in ventilation between topmost and lowermost lung regions. But, if there is no preponderant airway closure in the dependent lung regions and no zone I (unperfused lung units) in non-dependent regions, a good "matching" between ventilation ($\dot{V}$) and perfusion ($\dot{Q}$) ensues, the $\dot{V}/\dot{Q}$ ratio being close to ideal (0.5-5) at all vertical levels of the lung (Fig. 1). This matching ensures an optimum gas exchange.

Regional ventilation and perfusion during anaesthesia and mechanical ventilation

The distribution of ventilation is altered during anaesthesia, during spontaneous breathing as well as during mechanical ventilation. Thus, Rehder and Sessler (1973) showed that during spontaneous breathing under general anaesthesia,

124

more of the tidal breath was distributed to the non-dependent than to the dependent lung with the subject in the lateral position. The results were obtained by using a double lumen bronchial catheter and measuring the ventilation of each lung separately. Mechanical ventilation during anaesthesia, with or without muscle paralysis, resulted in much the same gas distribution as during spontaneous

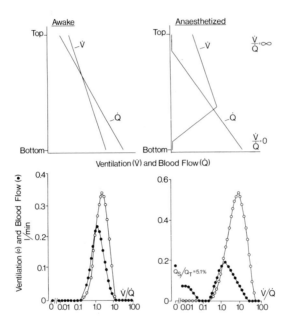

Fig. 1.
Schematic drawing of the vertical distribution of ventilation ($\dot{V}$) and perfusion ($\dot{Q}$) of the lung in the awake and the anaesthetized subject (left and right upper panels), and the corresponding ventilation-perfusion distributions recovered by the multiple inert-gas elimination technique (Wagner et al., 1974), (lower panels). Note the increase in $\dot{V}$ and $\dot{Q}$ down the lung and the unimodal distribution of $\dot{V}/\dot{Q}$ in the awake subject, indicating a good match between ventilation and perfusion. During anaesthesia, dependent and non-dependent perfusion are reduced or abolished increasing the scatter of $\dot{V}/\dot{Q}$, from zero (shunt, $\dot{Q}S/\dot{Q}T$) and "low" $\dot{V}/\dot{Q}$-regions to "high" $\dot{V}/\dot{Q}$.

breathing in the anaesthetized subject. Thus 60 % of the ventilation was distributed to the non-dependent lung in the lateral position (Rehder et al., 1973; Bindslev et al., 1981 a). Moreover, during an end inspiratory pause, gas was redistributed from the less ventilated dependent to the better ventilated non-dependent lung, resulting in 68 % being delivered to the upper lung (Bindslev et al., 1981 a). A similar preference for non-dependent lung ventilation has also been shown for anaesthetized humans in the supine position, using radio-active Xenon (Rehder et al., 1977). Finally, with the application of positive end expiratory pressure (PEEP) of approximately 10 cm $H2O$, a uniform distribution between the upper and lower lung was observed in the lateral position (Rehder et al., 1973; Bindslev et al., 1981 a). How can this altered distribution of inspired gas during anaesthesia be explained? It was observed by Froese and Bryan (1974) that in the supine awake, spontaneously breathing subject the dependent part of the diaphragm made the largest excursions during ventilation. On the other hand, in the anaesthetized mechanically ventilated subject the uppermost part of diaphragm was moving most during the ventilation. This observation has often been interpreted as demonstrating better ventilation of dependent regions during spontaneous breathing and of non-dependent regions during mechanical ventilation. However, there are several reasons why this can not be true. Firstly, in the anaesthetized spontaneously breathing subject, the dependent part of the diaphragm makes the largest excursions (Froese and Bryan, 1974), but the ventilation is preferentially distributed to non-dependent lung regions (see above). Secondly, the more homogeneous ventilation with PEEP will not fit in with regional differences in diaphragmatic motion. Thirdly, it has been suggested that the lung behaves as an isotropic tissue, i.e. a tissue that expands in the same fashion irrespective of where the forces are applied (Mead et al., 1970). Support for an isotropic behaviour is the observation that predominantly rib cage or predominantly diaphragmatic breathing results in much the same distribution of the inspired gas, as assessed by isotope technique (Bake et al., 1976).

Froese and Bryan (1974) also observed a cranial shift of the diaphragm during anaesthesia. This suggests reduced functional residual capacity (FRC) which has also been demonstrated with gas dilution techniques (Laws, 1968; Don et al., 1970) as well as with body pletysmography (Westbrook et al., 1973; Hedenstierna et al., 1981 c). The fall in FRC amounts to 0.4-0.7 litres and causes the lung to slide down its pressure-volume curve so that dependent lung regions locate on the lower, flatter part of the curve while non dependent regions are positioned on the steeper part of it. This would explain the altered ventilation distribution during anaesthesia (Rehder et al.,1973; Bindslev et al., 1981 a). But what elastic properties of the lung cause the flattening of the pressure volume curve when approaching smaller lung volumes? Not only does the lung slide down its pressure volume curve during anaesthesia, the curve itself is also altered. Thus, several studies have shown that the lungs are stiffer during anaesthesia with a right shift and a flatter slope of the pressure-volume curve (e.g. Butler and Smith, 1957; Westbrook et al., 1973). Why the lung is less compliant during anaesthesia is not fully understod and is also beyond the scope of this presentation. The inflection point, i.e. the point where the pressure volume curve begins to flatten when approaching smaller volumes, is easier to explain and coincides with the onset of airway closure. With continuing expiration more and more of the dependent lung regions are closed off and the lung behaves as if it is stiffer (Demedts et al., 1975; Ingram et al., 1974). The majority of studies have also shown that while FRC is reduced with anaesthesia, closing capacity remains unaltered (Gilmour et al., 1976; Hedenstierna et al., 1976; Hedenstierna and Santesson, 1979), and that airway closure may occur within a greater part of dependent lung regions, as measured in each lung separately, with the subject in the lateral position (Hedenstierna et al., 1981 b). This implies that airway closure will be more common during anaesthesia. Indeed, assuming that the fall in FRC with anaesthesia is similar at all ages, it may be anticipated that airway closure will occur above FRC in subjects as young as 30 years, and with an increasing distribution of airway closure with increasing age. The authors thus consider airway closure to be the most likely explanation to impeded dependent ventilation during anaesthesia. However, different findings of a decrease in closing capacity in parallel with the decrease in FRC have been presented by Juno et al. (1978), so the question what causes the altered gas distribution during anaesthesia has not yet been definitely answered. An objection to unaltered closing capacity with anaesthesia has been the simultaneously stiffer lung creating greater transmural airway pressure which should act to reduce closing capacity. However, this objection postulates unaltered airway tone with anaesthesia, but there is evidence that the airways are more compliant under this condition (Hedenstierna and Lundberg, 1975).

During general anaesthesia, the pulmonary arterial and systemic pressures may be reduced. The decrease in the former will impede perfusion of the uppermost, non dependent lung regions. Institution of mechanical ventilation will increase alveolar pressure, which will further interfere with the perfusion of the non dependent regions (West et al., 1964). The anaesthetic agent may reduce or abolish the hypoxic vasoconstrictor response which favours perfusion of poorly ventilated, mainly dependent lung regions (Benumof and Wahrenbrock, 1976; Sykes et al., 1973). Thus, during anaesthesia and mechanical ventilation these factors act in common to force perfusion down the lung, creating an increased preference for dependent perfusion, in opposition to the preference for the non-dependent ventilation. Moreover, the increased intrathoracic pressure may impede venous return (Werkö, 1947) and the anaesthetic agent may have a cardiodepressant effect (Merin ,1975), both of which may reduce the cardiac output.

Ventilation perfusion relationships during anaesthesia

The impaired ventilation in dependent lung regions and, in per cent of total perfusion, augmented blood flow during anaesthesia would be expected to cause low ventilation- perfusion ($\dot{V}/\dot{Q}$) ratios ($\dot{V}/\dot{Q}<0.1$) and even true shunt ($\dot{V}/\dot{Q}=0$). Upper lung units may be poorly or not at all perfused but still ventilated and this would be expected to create high $\dot{V}/\dot{Q}$ ratio and dead space. Thus, $\dot{V}/\dot{Q}$ may vary from zero to infinity (Fig. 1). Evidence has also accumulated during the last years that this is the case. Thus, using a multiple inert gas elimination technique (Wagner et al., 1974), a virtually "continuous" distribution of $\dot{V}/\dot{Q}$ ratios can be recovered. Assuming a 50 compartment lung model, each compartment being defined by a certain $\dot{V}/\dot{Q}$ ratio, evenly distributed on a log axis from below 0.005 (true shunt) to above 100 (dead space), the distribution of ventilation and perfusion to each of these compartments can be calculated. Using this technique, Dueck et al. (1980) could demonstrate greatly increased dispersion of $\dot{V}/\dot{Q}$ ratios in elderly subjects with chronic lung disease on induction of anaesthesia. True shunt could exceed 20 % of cardiac output and large regions of low $\dot{V}/\dot{Q}$ developed. Similar although less marked changes in the $\dot{V}/\dot{Q}$ distribution were observed in middle-aged clinically lung-healthy patients during anaesthesia. True shunt averaged 8 % (Bindslev et al., 1981 b). In young subjects below 30 years of age, moderate increases in the dispersion of $\dot{V}/\dot{Q}$ and almost no shunt appeared on induction of anaesthesia (Rehder et al., 1979). This age dependence would fit well with the idea that airway closure has a major impact on gas exchange, young subjects suffering no or little airway closure during anaesthesia, in contrast to those above 30 years of age. A separate mode within high $\dot{V}/\dot{Q}$ regions was sometimes observed during mechanical ventilation and was consistently the finding after the application of PEEP (Bindslev et al., 1981 b). Moreover, the ventilation to high $\dot{V}/\dot{Q}$ regions increased with increase in PEEP. A similar high $\dot{V}/\dot{Q}$ mode had previously been observed in PEEP ventilated dogs (Dueck et al., 1979). By using radioactive microspheres to assess the perfusion distribution in conjunction with microscopy of lung tissue samples it could be demonstrated that the high $\dot{V}/\dot{Q}$ mode corresponded to zone I, i.e. non-dependent lung regions with no capillary blood flow (zone I) but maintained corner-vessel blood flow (Hedenstierna et al., 1979). The patent corner-vessels, located in the junctions of interalveolar septa create a certain gas exchange, signified by high $\dot{V}/\dot{Q}$ ratios. It can thus be concluded that the expected range of $\dot{V}/\dot{Q}$ ratios from zero to infinity can be recovered in the anaesthetized subject, with the notion that (alveolar) dead space did not increase as much as might be expected with the development of zone I, but rather that a distinct high $\dot{V}/\dot{Q}$ mode appeared.

Gas distribution and $\dot{V}/\dot{Q}$ in acute respiratory failure

A more marked fall in FRC than in normal subjects during anaesthesia can be seen in patients with acute respiratory failure. Thus, Katz et al. (1981) reported a fall in FRC to 55 % of the predicted value in the supine position, corresponding to a 1.3 litre reduction, in patients suffering from acute respiratory failure after massive trauma, major surgery, or metabolic or infectious disease. Pontoppidan and co-workers (1973) proposed that such a fall in FRC promotes airway closure. Although no studies seem to have been reported on this subject, it appears that in acute respiratory failure the vertical distribution of ventilation may be similar to that seen in anaesthetized subjects, and possibly the decrease in ventilation of the dependent lung is even more marked than during anaesthesia. High airway and alveolar pressures are often required for adequate ventilation, which will force perfusion further down the lung. $\dot{V}/\dot{Q}$ inaquality similar to, or more advanced than that in the anaesthetized subject may thus ensue. This mismatching, which is "physiological" in the sense that it mimics that seen in healthy, elderly, anaesthetized subjects, adds to the $\dot{V}/\dot{Q}$ inequality caused by the lung disease through other mechanisms, creating the well known severe and sometimes life threatening hypoxemia.

General positive end-expiratory pressure

The reduction in FRC can be counteracted by the application of positive end-expiratory pressure (PEEP), which may thus serve as a tool for improving oxygenation of the blood (Ashbaugh et al., 1969; Kumar et al., 1970). However valuable, PEEP has not become an indispensable method in intensive care and has shown no clearcut advantage in routine anaesthesia (Hewlett et al., 1974; McCarthy and Hedenstierna, 1978). There may be at least two explanations for the lack of a beneficial effect. Firstly, the increased intrathoracic pressure reduces cardiac output by impeding venous return (Colgan and Marocco, 1972), and a concomitant increase in alveolar pressure forces lung blood flow to dependent regions (West et al., 1964). Secondly, the effect of PEEP on the regional lung volume is unfavourably distributed, dependent lung tissue being less expanded than non-dependent tissue. This has been demonstrated by constructing pressure-volume curves for each lung separately with the human subject in the lateral position (Bindslev et al., 1980). Certain assumptions are necessary here, such as a linear pleural pressure gradient, but the value assigned to this will not interfere with the analysis (Hedenstierna et al., 1981 a). The crucial reason for the unfavourable effect of PEEP is the sigmoid shape of the pressure-volume curve of the lung, in conjunction with the different locations of each lung on these curves - a consequence of the pleural pressure gradient (Fig. 2).

The dependent lung is positioned on the lower, flatter part of its pressure- volume curve, while the non-dependent lung lies higher up on the steep portion of its pressure-volume curve. During inspiration or mechanical inflation, the airway and alveolar pressures increase equally in the two lungs. Application of a certain PEEP will then increase the dependent less than the non-dependent lung volume. Application of a PEEP of 10-12 cm H2O should suffice to raise the dependent lung volume above its closing capacity in most subjects with normal lungs (Bindslev et al., 1980). This amount of PEEP raises the dependent lung volume by the 0.2-0.3 1 necessary to counteract airway closure. Simultaneously, however, the non-dependent lung volume increases by 0.8-1.0 1 and approaches the maximum expansion. Not only does this entail unnecessary impedance to cardiac output, but it also increases the danger of barotrauma (Kumar et al., 1973). It may thus be concluded that PEEP does not provide the physiological basis for an optimum match between ventilation and perfusion, and it may cause lung damage.

Differential ventilation with selective PEEP

Ideally, ventilation should be distributed in proportion to regional lung blood flow. The supine posture does not permit a perfustion matched distribution of ventilation. However, with the subject in the lateral position, the anatomical configuration of the human broncial tree enables a subdivision of ventilation to two vertically different lungcompartments, i.e. the dependent and the non-dependent lung. Ventilation may then be vertically distributed in proportion to the assumed distribution of perfusion (differential ventilation), more gas being delivered to the

132

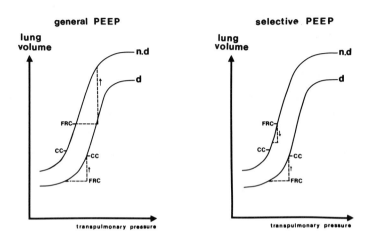

Fig. 2.
Separate pressure-volume curves of the non-dependent (n.d.) and the dependent (d) lung in the lateral decubital posture during anaesthesia and mechanical ventilation. Left panel: General PEEP is applied unitarily for the two lungs of such a magnitude that FRC of the dependent lung is raised to its closing capacity (CC). Note the considerably larger increase in the non-dependent than in the dependent lung volume (revised from Bindslev et al., 1980).
Right panel: Selective PEEP is applied solely to the dependent lung. Note the concomitant reduction of the non-dependent lung volume. The net increase in lung volume (FRC) is thus considerably larger during general PEEP than during selective PEEP.

dependent and less to the non-dependent lung than would have been the case with conventional ventilation. By applying PEEP only to the dependent lung, distribution of inspired gas to lower regions within that lung can be ensured (selective PEEP). Because of less overall intrathoracic pressure and lung expansion, interference with the total lung blood flow and the danger of barotrauma should be less than with general PEEP. But most important, an improved ventilation-perfusion ratio within separately ventilated units can be achieved. Since differential ventilation and selective PEEP will affect the intrathoracic pressure and regional lung inflation, this ventilation concept will also have an impact on the distribution of perfusion. In anaesthetized, lung-healthy subjects an "optimum" match between ventilation and perfusion was obtained when half of the tidal volume was distributed to each lung, and a selective PEEP of 10 cm H2O was applied to the dependent lung (Baehrendtz et al., 1982). This resulted in an equal distribution of perfusion between the two lungs, as assessed by injecting radio-active boli of Xenon 133. Cardiac output was reduced less than with general PEEP and arterial oxygen tension increased by 20-40% (Baehrendtz and Klingstedt, 1983).

In the operating theatre the lateral position has limited use. However it is a frequently used position during upper urinary tract and esophageal surgery. The lateral position is also accompanied by a higher incidence of atelectasis in the dependent lung (Lambert et al., 1955). A ventilation method that may reduce the demand for a high fraction of inspired oxygen and which allows the selective inflation of dependent lung regions (i.e. differential ventilation with selective PEEP) may be an efficient tool against atelectasis. Moreover, the high concentrations of nitrous oxide sometimes required for analgesia, limits the space for oxygen administration and increases the demand for an efficient utalization of the alveolar oxygen. Thus, in selected patients with extensive airway closure, e.g. elderly, extremely obese and heavily smoking patients, differential ventilation with selective PEEP may be valuable. Accidental or intentional hypotension during surgery may make the use of general PEEP dangerous whereas selective PEEP might be a better tool for reducing the venous admixture without causing further deterioration of central hemodynamics.

A more important application of differential ventilation with selective PEEP is presumably during intensive care of patients treated with mechanical ventilation due to acute severe respiratory failure. These patients are frequently suffering from hypoxemia in spite of high and potentially toxic concentrations of oxygen in the inspired gas. The lateral position is commonly used in the intensive care unit and rotating scheme with the patient alternatively on his right and left side is used to counter bedsores and to improve the elimination of airway secretions. In a number of patiens with severe acute respiratory failure due to a diffuse, bilateral lung disease (bronchopneumonia, aspiration-pneumonia and near drowning) differential ventilation and selective PEEP have been tested, so far during short periods of time only. Using differential ventilation with equal distribution of the tidal volume between the lungs and a selective PEEP of 12 cm H2O to the dependent lung as "a rule of thumb", arterial oxygen tension could be improved by an average of 40% and with no impedement of cardiac output in comparison with that during conventional ventilation (Baehrendtz, 1982), (Fig. 3). It thus appears that differential ventilation with selective PEEP can offer a considerable improvement of the gas exchange in acute bilateral lung disease, but long term studies are required for a final evaluation.

Changing the perfusion-distribution

So far the discussion has dealt with healthy lungs or bilateral lung disease. In diseases affecting only one lung, differential ventilation can be used, and uni-lateral lung disease has indeed been the major indication for such ventilator treatment (Carlon et al., 1978). However, there are also other means in order to improve gas exchange in uni-lateral lung disease. Placing the patient in the lateral position with the sick lung up reduces the perfusion of

that lung in which the gas exchange is impaired. If the
sick lung is stiffer than normal one may expect an increased

Fig. 3.
Cardiac output ($\dot{Q}T$), venous
admixture($\dot{Q}S/\dot{Q}T$) and arterial
oxygen tension (PaO2) from
seven patients in acute respiratory failure, illustrating
the effects of the different
ventilator settings:
A) conventional ventilation
   with ZEEP in the supine
   posture.
B) conventional ventilation
   with general PEEP in the
   supine posture.
C) conventional ventilation
   with ZEEP in the lateral
   decubital posture.
D) differential ventilation
   with even tidal volume distribution and ZEEP in the
   lateral decubital posture.
E) differential ventilation
   with even tidal volume distribution and selective
   PEEP to the dependent lung
   in the lateral decubital
   posture.
Mean value + SEM; x =
P<0.05, xx = P<0.01.

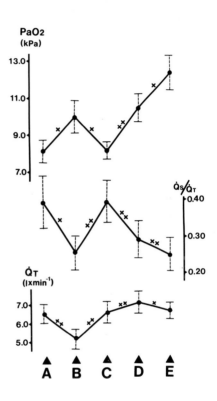

ventilation of the healthier lung, even with a conventional
single lumen tracheal tube. The possibility of gravitation-
al distribution of infectious secretions down to the healthier lung is under debate.
Another measure to direct the perfusion from the sick lung
is to enter a balloon catheter to the main pulmonary artery
of the sick lung where the balloon is inflated to occlude
the vessel (Alfery et al., 1981). This might be a valuable
treatment in desolate cases, but the experience is very limited.

Conclusion

The mismatching of ventilation and perfusion regularly observed during anaesthesia and acute respiratory failure im-
pedes gas exchange and may lead to severe hypoxemia.
General PEEP can improve matching of ventilation and perfusion but can not restore it to normal. However, this can be
achieved by placing the subject in the lateral position,
ventilating each lung in proportion to its blood flow (differential ventilation) and applying PEEP solely to the dependent lung to ensure an even distribution of inspired gas
within that lung (selective PEEP). Another approach, of
possible value in unilateral lung disease, is to divert perfusion away from the sick lung. This can be accomplished by
positioning the patient in the lateral posture with the sick
lung up (gravitation causing a preferential blood flow of
the dependent healthy lung), or by occluding the main pulmonary artery in the sick lung by a balloon-catheter.

REFERENCES

Alfery, D.D., Zamost, B.G., Benumof, J.L. Unilateral lung lavage: Blood flow manipulation by ipsilateral pulmonary artery balloon inflation in dogs. Anesthesiology 55, 376-380 (1981).

Ashbaugh, D.G., Petty, T.L., Bigelow, D.B., Harris, T.M. Continuous positive pressure breathing in adult respiratory distress syndrom. J. Thorac Cardiovasc. Surg. 57, 31-41 (1969).

Baehrendtz, S. Differential ventilation and selective positive end-expiratory measure. Effects on patients during anaesthesia and intensive care. Opuscula Medica (1983), suppl. 61.

Baehrendtz, S. and Klingstedt C. Differential ventilation and selective PEEP during anaesthesia in the lateral decubital position. Acta Anaesth. Scand. (1983).

Baehrendtz, S., Hedenstierna, G., Santesson, J., Bindslev, L., Klingstedt, C., Dalbom, M., Söderberg, B., Norlander, O. Perfusion of each lung during differential ventilation with selective PEEP. Anesthesiology 57, A458, ASA Abstracts suppl. 3A (1982).

Bake, B., Wood, L., Murphy, B., Macklem, P.T., Milic-Emili, J. Effect of inspiratory flow rate on regional distribution of inspired gas. J. Appl. Physiol. 34, 8 (1974).

Bake, B., Dempsey, J., Grimby, G. Effects of shape changes of the chest wall on distribution of inspired gas. American review of respiratory disease 114, 1113-1120 (1976).

Benumof, J.L., and Wahrenbrock, E.A. Local effects of anesthetics on regional hypoxic pulmonary vasoconstriction. Anesthesiology 43: 525 (1976).

Bindslev, L., Hedenstierna, G., Santesson, J., Norlander, O., Gram, I. Airway closure during anaesthesia and its prevention by positive end-expiratory pressure. Acta Anaesth. Scand. 24, 199 (1980).

Bindslev, L., Santesson, J., Hedenstierna, G. Distribution of inspired gas to each lung in anaesthetized human subjects. Acta Anaesth. Scand. 25, 297 (1981a).

Bindslev, L., Hedenstierna, G., Santesson, J., Gottlieb, I., Carvallhas, A. Ventilation-perfusion distribution during inhalation anaesthesia. Effects of spontaneous breathing, mechanical ventilation and positive end-expiratory pressure. Acta Anaesth. Scand. 25, 360 (1981b).

Briscoe, W.A. Lung volumes. Handbook of physiology, vol. III. Section 3: Respiration. American Physiolgical Society, Washington, p. 1363 (1964).

Butler, J. and Smith, B. H. Pressure-volume relationships of the chest in the completely relaxed anaesthetized patient. Clin. Sci. 16, 125-146 (1957).

Carlon, G.C., Cole Jr., R., Klein, R., Goldiner, P.L., Miodownik, S. Criteria for selective positive end-expiratory pressure and independent synchronized ventilation of each lung. Chest 74, 501-507 (1978).

Colgan, F.J., Marocco, P.P. The cardiorespiratory effect of constant and intermittent positive pressure breathing. Anesthesiology 36, 444 (1972).

138

Craig, D.B., Wahba, W.M., Don, H.F., Contare, J.G., Becklake, M.R. "Closing volume" and its relationship to gas exchange in seated and supine positions. J. Appl. Physiol. 31, 717 (1971).

Demedts, M., Clement, J., Stanescu, D.C., van de Woestijne, K.P. Inflection point on transpulmonary pressure-volume curves and closing volume. J. of applied physiology 38, 228-235 (1975).

Don, H.F., Wahba, M., Cuadrado, L., Kelkar, K. The effects of anesthesia and 100 per cent oxygen on the functional residual capacity of the lungs. Anesthesiology 32, 521 (1970).

Dueck, R., Wagner, P.D., West, J.B. Effects of positive end-expiratory pressure on gas exchange in dogs with normal and edematous lungs. Anesthesiology 47, 359-366 (1977).

Dueck, R., Young, I., Clausen, J., Wagner, P.D. Altered distribution of pulmonary ventilation and blood flow following induction of inhalational anesthesia. Anesthesiology 52, 113 (1980).

Euler, U.S. von and Liljenstrand, G. Observations on the pulmonary arterial blood pressure in the cat. Acta Physiol. Scand. 12, 301-320 (1946).

Froese, A.B. and Bryan, C. Effects of anesthesia and paralysis on diaphragmatic mechanics in man. Anesthesiology 41, 242-255 (1974).

Gilmour, I., Burnham, M., Craig, D.B. Closing capacity measurement during general anesthesia. Anesthesiology 45, 477 (1976).

Hedenstierna, G. and Lundberg, S. Airway compliance during artificial ventilation. Br. J. Anaesth. 47, 1277-1281 (1975).

Hedenstierna, G., Santesson, J. Airway closure during anesthesia: a comparison between resident-gas and argon-bolus techniques. J. Appl. Physiol. 47, 874 (1979).

Hedenstierna, G., McCarthy, G., Bergström, M. Airway closure during mechanical ventilation. Anesthesiology 44, 114 (1976).

Hedenstierna, G., White, F.C., Mazzone, R., Wagner, P.D. Redistribution of pulmonary blood flow in the dog with PEEP ventilation. American Physiological Society 278-287 (1979).

Hedenstierna, G., Bindslev, L., Santesson, J. Pressure-volume and airway closure relationships in each lung in anaesthetized man. Clin. Physiol. 1, 479 (1981a).

Hedenstierna, G., Bindslev, L., Santesson, J., Norlander, O.P. Airway closure in each lung of anesthetized human subjects. J. Appl. Physiol. 50, 55 (1981b).

Hedenstierna, G., Löfström, B., Lundh, R. Thoracic gas volume and chest-abdomen dimensions during anesthesia and muscle paralysis. Anesthesiology 55, 499 (1981c).

Hewlett, A.M., Hulands, G.H., Nunn, J.F., Milledge, J.S. Functional residual capacity during anaesthesia. III: Artificial ventilation. Br. J. Anaesth. 46, 495 (1974).

Ingram Jr., R.H., O'Cain, C.F., Fridy Jr., W.W. Simultaneous quasi-static lung pressure-volume curves and "closing volume" measurements. J. of Applied Physiology 36, 135-141 (1974).

Jonson, B. Pulmonary mechanics in normal men, studied with
the flow regulator method. Scand. J. clin. Lab. Invest.
25, 363-373 (1970).
Juno, P., Marsh, H.M., Knopp, T.J., Rehder, K. Closing ca-
pacity in awake and anesthetized-paralyzed man. J. Appl.
Physiol. 44, 238 (1978).
Katz, J.A., Ozanne, G.M., Zinn, S.E., Fairly, H.B. Time
course and mechanism of lung-volume increase with PEEP in
acute pulmonary failure. Anesthesiology 54, 9 (1981).
Kumar, A., Falke, K.J., Geffin, B., Aldredge, C.F., Laver,
M.B., Löwenstein, E., Pontoppidan, H. Continuous
positive-pressure ventilation in acute respiratory failure.
New Engl. J. Med. 238, 1430 (1970).
Kumar, A., Pontoppidan, H., Falke, K., Wilson, R., Laver,
M.B. Pulmonary barotrauma during mechanical ventilation.
Crit. Care Med. 1, 181 (1973).
Laws, A.K. Effects of induction of anesthesia and muscle
paralysis on functional residual capacity of the lungs.
Canad. Anaesth. Soc. J. 15, 325 (1968).
LeBlanc, P., Ruff, F., Milic-Emili, J. Effects of age and
body position on "airway closure" in man. J. Appl.
Physiol. 28, 448 (1970).
McCarthy, G.S., Hedenstierna, G. Arterial oxygenation dur-
ing artificial ventilation. The effect of airway closure
and of its prevention by positive end-expiratory pressure.
Acta Anaesth. Scand. 22, 563 (1978).
Mead, J., Takishima, T., Leith, D. Stress distribution in
lungs: a model of pulmonary elasticity. J. Appl. Physiol
28, 596-608 (1970).
Merin, R.G. Effects of anesthetics on the heart. Surg.
Clin. N. Amer. 55, 759 (1975).
Milic-Emili, J., Henderson, J.A., Dolovich, M.B., Trop, D.,
Kaneko, K. Regional distribution of inspired gas in the
lung. J. Appl. Physiol. 21, 749 (1966).
Pontoppidan, H., Geffin, B., Lowenstein, E. Acute respira-
tory failure in the adult. N. Engl. J. Med. medical
progress series. Little, Brown and Company, Boston 1973, p.
9-16.
Rehder, K., Sessler, A.D. Function of each lung in spontaneously breathing man anesthetized with
Thiopental-Meperidine. Anesthesiology 38, 320-327 (1973).
Rehder, K., Wenthe, F.M., Sessler, A.D. Function of each
lung during mechanical ventilation with ZEEP and with PEEP
in man anesthetized with Thiopental-Meperidine.
Anesthesiology 39, 597-606 (1973).
Rehder, K., Sessler, A.D., Marsh, M. General anesthesia and
the lung. American review of respiratory disease 112,
541-563 (1975).
Rehder, K., Sessler, A.D., Rodarte, J.R. Regional intrapulmonary gas distribution in awake and anaesthetized-paralyzed
man. J. Appl. Physiol Respirat. Environ Exercise Physiol. 42, 391 (1977).
Rehder, K., Knopp, T.J., Sessler, A.D., Didier, E.P.
Ventilation-perfusion relationship in young healthy awake
and anesthetized man. J. Appl. Physiol. 47, 745 (1979).
Rehder, K., Knopp, T.J., Brusasco, V., Didier, P.

140

Inspiratory flow and intrapulmonary gas distribution. Am. rev. respir. dis. 124, 392–396 (1981).

Sykes, M.K., Loh, L., Seed, R.F., Kafer, E.R., Cahkrabarti, M.K. The effect of inhalational anaesthetics on hypoxic pulmonary vasoconstriction and pulmonary vascular resistance in the perfused lugns of the dog and cat. Brit. J. Anaest. 44, 776 (1973).

Ueda, H., Iio, M., Kaihara, S. Determination of regional pulmonary blood flow in various cardiopulmonary disorders. Jpn Heart J. 5, 431 (1964).

Wagner, P.D., Salzman, H.A., West, J.B. Measurement of continuous distributions of ventilation-perfusion ratios: theory. J. Appl. Physiol 36, 588 (1974).

Werkö, L. The influence of positive pressure breathing on the circulation in man. Acta Med. Scand. suppl. 193 (1947).

West,J.B., Dollery, C.T., Naimark, A. Distribution of blood flow in isolated lung; relation to vascular and alveolar pressures. J. Appl. Physiol 19, 713 (1964).

West, J.B. Regional differences in the lung. Academic Press, New York, pp 281 (1977).

Westbrook, P.R., Stubbs, S.E., Sessler, A.D. Effects of anaesthesia and muscle paralysis on respiratory mechanics in normal man. J. Appl. Physiol 34, 81 (1973).

CONTINUOUS MONITORING OF INTRATHORACIC FLUID

KORSTEN, H.H.M. [*†], MEIJER, J.H. [□], HENGEVELD, S.J. [††],
DELEMARRE, J.B.V.M. [†††], LEUSINK, J.A. [†], SCHURINK, G.A. [†], SCHNEIDER, H. [□]

ABSTRACT

A computerized system is presented to measure the mean specific thoracic
impedance as an index for intrathoracic fluid content, according to the
method of differential impedance plethysmography. Preliminary results,
obtained from patients after cardiac surgery, are found to be in
agreement with data obtained from chest X-ray photography, pulmonary
arterial pressure measurements and urine production. Measurement of the
basic impedance Z_o according to Kubicek is found to be an unreliable
parameter in monitoring intrathoracic fluid content. Some typical
examples of registrations are shown.

KEYWORDS

Intrathoracic fluid, continuous monitoring, mean specific impedance,
basic impedance, cardiac surgery

I. INTRODUCTION

The homeostasis of body fluid during anaesthesia and in the intensive
care unit is of paramount importance. However, (sub-)clinical lung edema
of different etiology is a complicating factor frequently met in the
critically ill patient. A good method for detection of changes in
intrathoracic fluid content will lead to: a) early detection and
therefore early treatment; b) adequate evaluation and therefore adequate
adjustment of individual as well as general therapies; and c) extension of
knowledge about the different pathophysiological mechanisms and therefore
possibilities for general prevention.

[□]   Department of Medical Physics, Free University, Amsterdam, Netherlands
[†]   Department of Anaesthesiology, St.Antonius Hospital, Utrecht, Netherlands
[††] Department of Instrumentation and Automation, St.Antonius Hospital

Though the importance of the subject is well recognized, no satisfactory method is available [1]. The ideal method should be: a) *reliable*, i.e. produce no false positive or negative results; b) *specific* to the detection of intrathoracic fluid; c) *sensitive* to a degree that clinically relevant amounts of fluid can be detected; d) *non-invasive*; and e) *suitable to serve as a monitor*, which means in practice that the detecting signal should be available in the form of an electrical signal, which can be processed electronically, e.g. to detect a trend in the amount of fluid.

Transthoracic electrical impedance measurements potentially possess the ability to fulfil these requirements. A large number of investigators have studied in particular the monitoring of chest fluid using the non-invasive bioelectrical impedance technique both in clinical situations and animal experiments [2,3,4,5,6,7,8,9,10,11]. Those investigators found a significant correlation between the variation of the basic impedance, and the amount of fluid overload or fluid withdrawal. However, values varied greatly from one patient to another and from one investigator to another. Variation in the basic impedance, as measured by Kubicek's electrode arrangement [12] appeared to be dependent on the individual. Furthermore, the distance between the electrodes, and the posture of the patient were of critical importance. The electrical field distribution appeared to be inhomogeneous in the upper thoracic and neck region, a fact which introduced an uncontrollable error into the measurements [13,14].

The purpose of the present study is: a) to show the origin of these defects of Kubicek's basic impedance measurement, resulting in reduced reliability, loss of sensitivity, position- and subject-dependency; b) to propose a method for measuring thoracic impedances designed to avoid those defects; and c) to present a computerized measurement device and show some typical examples of registrations.

II. BASIC IMPEDANCE MEASUREMENT ACCORDING TO KUBICEK

Fig. 1 shows the electrode arrangement according to Kubicek's method [12]. A constant, alternating electrical current of 2 mA r.m.s., with frequency 100 kHz, is applied to the thorax by means of two circum-ferential electrodes: electrode 1 around the neck, and electrode 2 around the abdomen. The consequent voltage-difference is measured

between electrode 2 around the neck, and electrode 3 around the thorax.
According to Kubicek the ratio of voltage-difference to electrical current:
the thoracic basic impedance Z_o, is supposed to be a reliable measure of
intrathoracic fluid content.

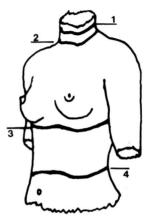

*Figure 1. Electrode configuration
according to Kubicek
et al. [12].*

This method is subjected to fundamental criticism: a) *loss of sensitivity*
due to inhomogeneities in the electrical field distribution; b) *loss of
reliability* caused by changes in body position or relocation of the
electrodes; and c) *lack of comparability*, since different subjects have
different physical dimensions.

In order to demonstrate the influence of the electrode configuration, we
measured the basic impedance Z_o at different electrode positions, in a
healthy, male volunteer: Electrode 2 around the neck was duplicated at a
distance of 2 cm, distal to the original electrode 2. The measuring
electrode 3 was applied to the trunk 8-fold. Three electrode configurations
were studied:

a) Basic impedances Z_o were measured between the cranial electrode 2 and the
   successive trunk electrodes;

b) Basic impedances Z_o were measured between the distal electrode 2 and the
   successive trunk electrodes;

c) Two upper electrodes around the trunk served as cranial current and
   measuring electrodes 1 and 2.

The results of the three experiments are presented in figure 2.

144

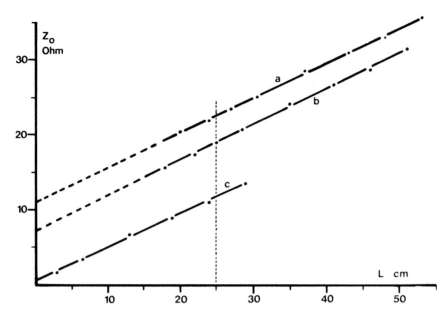

Figure 2. Relationship between Z_o and the distance L between the measuring electrodes, using Kubicek's method, in three electrode configurations a,b,c (see text). Note the difference in measured Z_o in the three configurations at the same distance (dotted vertical line).

From these results four important conclusions can be drawn:

a) The relationship between Z_o and electrode-distance L is linear to a high degree of significance (all coefficients of linear correlation r > 0.999; all p < 0.005);

b) At equal distances between the measuring electrodes 2 and 3 substantially different basic impedances are measured;

c) The slopes of the three lines are essentially the same;

d) Extrapolation to zero distance between the measuring electrodes results in a Z_o identical to zero, in experiment c only.

The difference in zero-shift between the experiments a and b is due to the inhomogeneity of the electrical field close to the upper current electrode. The difference in zero-shift between the experiments a and b on one hand, electrical field in the region of the neck and shoulders. The differences in Z_o measured at equal distances in the three experiments are caused by the different zero-shifts as a consequence of the inhomogeneities in the electrical field.

III. DIFFERENTIAL THORACIC IMPEDANCE MEASUREMENT

A method was designed to eliminate these zero-shifts [14].This method is expected to increase the sensitivity and reliability of the impedance measurements. This measurement is based upon computation of the mean impedance per unit length: dZ/dL. This figure is multiplied by the thoracic axes perpendicular to the vertical body axis. In this way a measure analogeous to the mean specific impedance is obtained. The thus calculated mean specific thoracic impedance Rho can be expected to be inter-individually comparable.

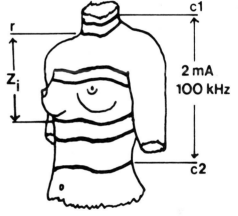

Figure 3. Electrode configuration used for the differential method according to Meijer et al. [14].

Four measurement electrodes are applied to the thorax (see fig. 3). In female subjects two of these electrodes are applied above, and two are applied below the mammae. Electrode 2 in the neck serves as a reference (r). The basic impedances Z_i are measured between the thoracic electrodes i= 1,.....,4 (distance to the reference electrode: L_i) and the reference around the neck. By means of coupled linear regression the additional shift in the $Z_i \leftrightarrow L_i$ relationship in female subjects at the level of the mammae is eliminated (see figure 4).

146

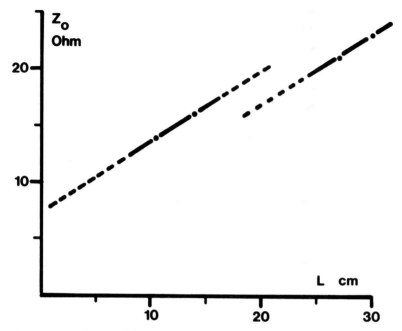

*Figure 4. Relationship between the basic impedance Z_o and
the distance L between the measuring electrodes
in a healthy female volunteer. Note the shift
in the linear relationship at the level of the
mammae.*

Two straight lines with the same slopes dZ/dL are calculated for the two
assemblies of two points (Z_i, L_i), measured from the upper and lower group
of two electrodes, according to [14]:

$$\frac{dZ}{dL} = \frac{\Sigma L_i Z_i - N_u \overline{L}_u \overline{Z}_u - N_1 \overline{L}_1 \overline{Z}_1}{\Sigma L_i^2 - N_u \overline{L}_u^2 - N_1 \overline{L}_1^2} \qquad \text{Ohm.cm}^{-1} \qquad (1)$$

In which u and l indicate the upper and lower point assemblies, N the
number of points per assembly (in this configuration: 2), and i the
measuring electrodes. The bar denotes the mean. For instance $\overline{Z}_1 = (Z_3 + Z_4)/N_1$,
i.e. the mean of the basic impedances measured at the measuring
electrodes 3 and 4.

In general, the mean impedance per unit length dZ/dL depends upon the dimensions of the conductor, i.e. the thorax, which is subjected to interindividual differences. To obtain comparable results between subjects, the mean specific impedance of the thorax is computed as follows [*] :
The main thoracic axes f and g are measured at the level of the manubrium sterni. The product f.g.dZ/dL is identified with the mean specific thoracic impedance Rho:

$$\text{Rho} = f.g.\frac{dZ}{dL} \quad \text{Ohm.cm} \tag{2}$$

IV. COMPUTERIZED DATA PROCESSING

Figure 5 shows a schematic drawing of the computerized impedance measurement system. The system consists of a standard impedance cardiograph (IFM model 403A), a 64kRAM microcomputer based on a Z80 microprocessor (Sinclair ZX-81), an A/D converter and a one-shot timer. By means of a mechanical switch, controlled by the microprocessor, successive thoracic measurement electrodes are linked to the cardiograph, which is in turn connected to the computer. The measurement frequency of the system is controlled by the programmable one-shot timer. The microprocessor computes the mean specific impedance Rho. An on-line trend-analysis in time of Rho and Z_o is performed by means of least-square linear curve-fitting.

*) As an example the following data are processed:

i	L_i, cm	Z_i, Ohm	
1	10.5	13.9	$N_u = 2$
2	14.0	16.0	
3	27.0	21.0	$N_l = 2$
4	30.0	23.0	

Thoracic axes f×g = 26×19 cm²

$$\frac{dZ}{dL} = \frac{1626.95 - 2\times12.25\times14.95 - 2\times28.5\times22}{1935.25 - 2\times150.0625 - 2\times812.25} = 0.628 \quad Ohm.cm^{-1}$$

coefficient of correlation: r = 0.9995
Rho = 0.628×26×19 = 310 Ohm.cm

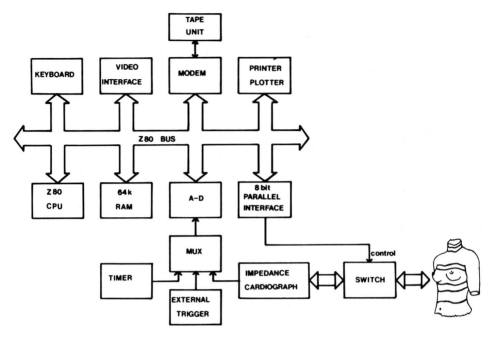

Figure 5. Data registration/processing system.
Modem = modulator/demodulator; CPU = central processor unit; RAM = random
acces memory; A-D = analog to digital converter; MUX = multiplexer.

V. PRELIMINARY RESULTS

During 36 hours after cardiac surgery the changes in basic impedance Z_o and
mean specific impedance Rho were studied in 16 patients. Trends in time in Z_o
and Rho were compared with changes in intrathoracic fluid content as
concluded by a radiologist from serial chest X-ray photographs. The results
are listed in table I.

TABLE I. Comparison of the two impedance methods with chest X-ray diagnostics.
Numbers of patients in which the impedance method agreed (+), disagreed (-),
or in which no agreement or disagreement could be formulated (o),
compared with the observations from serial chest X-ray photographs.

	+	o	-
Rho method	14	2	0
Z_o method	6	6	4

There appeared to be no correlation at all between the basic thoracic impedance Z_o and the chest X-ray diagnostics (χ^2-test; $p < 0.005$). The correlation between the latter and the mean specific impedance Rho was fairly good (χ^2-test; $p > 0.5$).

VI. TYPICAL EXAMPLES

Three typical examples of measuring results are shown in fig. 6,7,and 8. Fig. 6 shows recordings from a patient during the first 56 hours following mitral- and tricus pid-valve replacement. A period of low cardiac output, as concluded from the low urine production, resulted in a sharp rise of the pulmonary artery pressure about 23 hours post-operative. The mean specific impedance Rho showed a marked decrease at this instant, whereas the basic impedance Z_o showed no significant change. After therapy, e.a. digitalis, sodium nitroprusside and furosemide, the urine production increased, pulmonary artery pressure decreased and the specific impedance Rho increased.

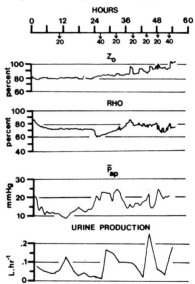

Figure 6. Registration from a patient after cardiac surgery. Basic impedance Z_o and mean specific impedance Rho are plotted as a percentage of the pre-operative values. $\overline{P}_{ap}$ denotes the mean pulmonary arterial pressure. Also the hourly urine production is shown. On top of the figure the amounts and moments of furosemide injections are given. See text for discussion.

In fig. 7 registrations are shown from a patient during the first 46 hours following aortic valve replacement. The steady decrease in Rho of about 20% during the first 26 hours post-operative was accompanied by a steady increase in mean pulmonary arterial pressure and low urine production, indicating diminished left ventricular function. No significant change in Z_o was observed. Both in figure 6 and 7 the post-operative values of both impedances were 20% lower than the pre-operative values, indicating a

150

significant increase in intrathoracic fluid content. This is in
agreement with ultrastructural changes in lung tissue immediately after
cardiac surgery [15].

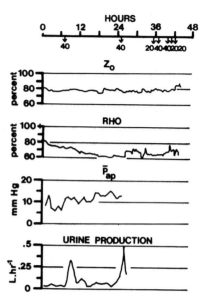

*Figure 7. Registration from a patient
after cardiac surgery. Basic impedance
Z_o and mean specific impedance Rho
are plotted as a percentage of the
pre-operative values. $\overline{P}_{ap}$ denotes the
mean pulmonary arterial pressure. Also
the hourly urine production is shown.
On top of the figure the amounts and
moments of furosemide injections are
given. See text for discussion.*

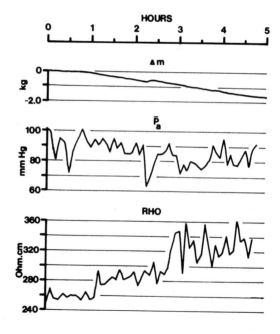

*Figure 8. Course of the
mean specific impedance
Rho in a patient during
5 hours of heamodialysis.
Δ m is the loss of weight
caused by ultrafiltration
$\overline{P}_a$ denotes the mean
arterial pressure. See
text for discussion.*

Figure 8 shows the mean specific impedance Rho, mean arterial pressure $\bar{P}_a$ and weight loss Δm during a 5 hours period of haemodialysis. The specific impedance is very low at the onset of haemodialysis, indicating significant fluid overload (normal value in subjects below 35 years of age: 316 $\pm$ 26 Ohm.cm, [14], mean $\pm$ s.d.). At the end of the heamodialysis session, in which 1.6 l of fluid was withdrawn, the Rho was returned to a normal value of about 330 Ohm.cm.

VII. CONCLUSIONS

It can be concluded that measurement of the mean specific impedance Rho is a usefull tool in monitoring the critically ill patient during surgery and in the intensive care unit. The relationship between the basic impedance Z_o and the intrathoracic fluid content appears to be predominantly stochastic, so the measurement of Z_o is unreliable as a guide to intrathoracic fluid content.

REFERENCES

1. Staub, N.C., and Hogg, J.C.
   Conference report of a workshop on the measurement of lungwater
   Crit. Care Med.,8: 752 - 759 (1980)
2. Hill, D.W., Mohapatra, S.N., Welham, K.C., and Stevenson, M.L.
   The effect of a progressive decrease in circulating blood volume
   of the dog on the transthoracic impedance
   Europ. J. Intens. Care Med.,2: 119 - 124 (1976)
3. Hull, E.T., Heemstra, H.,and Wildevuur, Ch.R.H.
   De transthoracale impedantiemethode ter bepaling van de graad van
   verandering van het extravasculaire water
   Acta Pneumolog. Belg.,68: 369 - 377 (1979)
4. Keller, G.,and Blumberg, A.
   Monitoring of pulmonary fluid volume and stroke volume by impedance
   cardiography in patients on haemodialysis
   Chest,72: 56 - 62 (1977)
5. Luepker, R.V., Michael, J.R., and Warbasse, J.R.
   Transthoracic electrical impedance: quantitative evaluation of a
   non-invasive measure of thoracic fluid volume
   Am. Heart J.,85: 83 - 95 (1973)

152

6. Pomerantz, M., Baumgartner, R., Lauridson, J., and Eiseman, B.
    Transthoracic electrical impedance for the early detection of
    pulmonary edema
    Surgery,66: 260 - 268 (1969)

7. Pomerantz, M., Delgado, F., and Eiseman, B.
    Clinical evaluation of transthoracic electrical impedance as a
    guide to intrathoracic fluid volumes
    Ann. Surg.,171: 686 - 694 (1970)

8. Spence, J.A., Baliga, R., Nyboer, J.,Seftick, J., and Fleischmann, L.
    Changes during haemodialysis in total body water, cardiac output and
    chest fluid as detected by bioelectrical impedance analysis
    Trans. Am. Soc. Artif. Intern. Organs,XXV: 51 - 55 (1979)

9. Van de Water, J.M., Philips, P.A., Thouin, L.G., Watanabe, L.S., and
    Lappen, R.S.
    Bioelectrical impedance: new developments and clinical application
    Arch. Surg.,102: 541 - 547 (1971)

10. Van de Water, J.M., Mount, B.E., Barela, J.R., Schuster, R., and
    Leacock, F.S.
    Monitoring the chest with impedance
    Chest,64: 597 - 603 (1973)

11. Baker, L.E., and Denniston, J.C.
    Noninvasive measurement of intrathoracic fluids
    Chest,65: 35s - 37s (1974)

12. Kubicek, W.G., Karnegis, J.N., Patterson, R.P., Witsoe, D.A., and
    Mattson, R.H.
    Development and evaluation of an impedance cardiac output system
    Aerosp. Med.,37: 1208 - 1212 (1966)

13. Sakamoto, K., Muto, K., Kanai, H., and Lizuka, M.
    Problems of impedance cardiography
    Med. & Biol. Eng. & Comput.,17: 697 - 709 (1979)

14. Meijer, J.H., Reulen, J.P.H., Oe, P.L., Allon, W., Thijs, L.G., and
    Schneider, H.
    Differential impedance plethysmography for measuring thoracic impedances
    Med. & Biol. Eng. & Comput.,20: 187 - 194 (1982)

15. Anyanwe, E., Dittrich, H., Gieseking, R., and Enders, H-J.
    Ultrastructrural changes in the human lung following
    cardiopulmonary bypass
    Basic Res. Cardiol.,77: 309 - 322 (1982)

THE POTENTIAL OF COMPUTER MODELLING TECHNIQUES IN INTENSIVE CARE MEDICINE

C J HINDS, C J DICKINSON

Mathematical modelling and systems simulation using digital computers has become an established technique in a wide variety of disciplines ranging from economics[1] to the control of industrial processes.[2] Computer models can be used, for example, to verify hypotheses or suggest new avenues for research, while the response of the model to specific manipulations may predict the likely effects of the same intervention on the real system. Computer simulation can also be useful as a teaching aid and has been used successfully for training skilled personnel, such as airline pilots, without endangering either people's lives or expensive machinery.

Applications of computer modelling relevant to medicine include the investigation of normal physiological mechanisms, such as the control of breathing,[3] as well as pathological states, such as the respiratory dysfunction associated with sepsis[4] or cardiopulmonary bypass.[5] Computer simulation has also been used to study gas exchange during anaesthesia[6] and for teaching medicine to both undergraduates and postgraduates.[7,8]

Since a large proportion of intensive care medicine is concerned with applied physiology and pharmacology, and because it is often possible to produce mathematical descriptions of many of the relevant components of these systems, it is a specialty in which computer modelling techniques might be expected to be of value.

Using a previously described computer model of human respiration[9] we set out to determine firstly whether accurate computer simulation of intensive care patients was clinically feasible and secondly whether it could be of assistance in the management of such patients. We have also used this, and other, computer models for training both graduates and undergraduates in aspects of intensive care, applied physiology and pharmacology.

154

The computer model of human respiration (Fig 1)

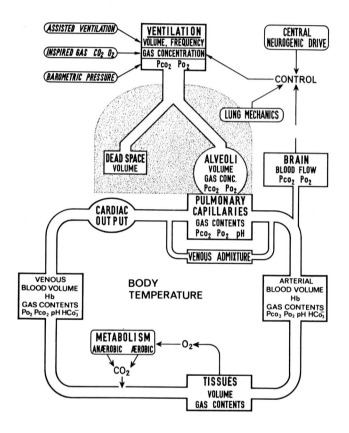

U.C.H.M.S. 2921/271-74. V.K.A.

The model used in these studies[9] was originally designed as a self-instructional device and is of intermediate complexity. It is written in FORTRAN and consists essentially of a model of lung function and gas exchange linked to a single tissue compartment by a circulation. At present the model contains a simple three compartment representation of pulmonary function consisting of dead space (V_D) venous admixture ($\dot{Q}_s/\dot{Q}_t$) and perfectly matched ventilation/perfusion ($\dot{V}/\dot{Q}$). The lungs and airways are represented in terms of their volumes and mechanical properties, while alveolar ventilation is described dynamically. Empirically derived functions, fully described by Dickinson,[9] allow effective dead space and venous admixture to change dynamically with tidal volume, cardiac output, positive end-expiratory pressure (when used) and alveolar gas tensions. Blood circulates, at a rate determined by the cardiac output, through the lung model and into a 1 litre arterial pool. From here it passes to the tissues and thence into a 3 litre venous pool. The tissues are treated as a single compartment containing reasonable descriptions of the likely oxygen and carbon dioxide dissociation curves. Here oxygen is consumed and carbon dioxide produced in amounts dependent on the metabolic rate and tissue respiratory quotient respectively. In each blood pool contents of O_2, CO_2 and bicarbonate are determined by mass balance equations. The partial pressures of oxygen and carbon dioxide are calculated using the equations described by Kelman[10,11] as approximating their known dissociation curves. The acid-base state of each blood pool is established by considering total CO_2 content and standard bicarbonate content. The whole model also incorporates many other aspects of human respiration, including a complex description of the control of ventilation by central and peripheral neural mechanisms.

It was felt that, although originally designed for teaching, this model also had potential for clinical use since it is comprehensive and yet contains sufficient simplifications to make it economical both in terms of storage space and computer time. It is also capable of describing dynamic changes. Furthermore the user can easily interact with the model and adjust any of a large number of changeable values. The equations of the model are then solved repeatedly at intervals of ten seconds of simulated time (or less) until a new 'steady state' is reached.

CLINICAL APPLICATIONS OF COMPUTER MODELLING

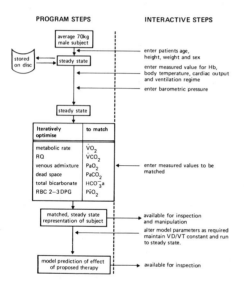

Procedure for creating a computer simulation

In order to use this model to assist in the management of individual patients, an accurate simulation of the patient had first to be produced. Our initial attempts to match the model to values obtained from patients were made using manual adjustments of model parameters. However, because of interactions within the model, this proved both difficult and time consuming. A technique for producing an accurate simulation of the patient had therefore to be developed which could be used easily in the clinical situation. Because of the complexities involved in analysing spontaneously breathing subjects, we have so far confined our clinical studies to artificially ventilated patients.

Fig 2 illustrates the procedure which has been developed for producing a steady-state representation of a patient undergoing intermittent positive pressure ventilation (IPPV). The model always starts with a representation of a normal, 70 kg male subject. The first step is therefore to enter the age, height, weight and sex of the patient being studied. Expected values for resting cardiac output, oxygen consumption, lung volume and anatomical dead space are then automatically computed within the model and a new steady-state description is produced. Next the actual ventilation regime and the patient's measured cardiac output, haemoglobin concentration and body temperature are entered, together with the barometric pressure. These values are 'fixed' within the model which is again run until a new steady state is achieved. At this stage the model contains a simulation of a subject with normal metabolism, lung function and acid-base status undergoing IPPV. In most cases, therefore, the model values for arterial partial pressure of oxygen (PaO_2) will be considerably higher and those for the arterial partial pressure of carbon dioxide ($PaCO_2$) lower than those measured in the patient and the acid-base state will not be appropriately 'matched'. Therefore, measured values to be 'matched' are entered into an algorithm which iteratively optimises metabolic rate to match oxygen consumption ($\dot{V}O_2$), tissue respiratory quotient to match carbon dioxide production ($\dot{V}CO_2$), venous admixture ($\dot{Q}_s/\dot{Q}_t$) to match PaO_2, dead space (V_D) to match $PaCO_2$ and the total mass of bicarbonate to match actual arterial bicarbonate concentration. Optimisation of $\dot{Q}_s/\dot{Q}_t$ and V_D is performed using a combination of linear search and quadratic interpolation to match PaO_2 and $PaCO_2$ to within $\pm$ 1.5 mmHg, while the arterial bicarbonate was matched to within $\pm$ 0.5 mmol using a calibration procedure. It was not necessary to set tolerance limits for $\dot{V}O_2$ and $\dot{V}CO_2$ since these were always closely matched. Finally the model red cell 2-3 diphosphoglycerate concentration is optimised to achieve matching for $P\bar{v}O_2$. The equations used in this last step are so designed that they do not artifically correct for small discrepancies between the model and measured values for $P\bar{v}O_2$ caused by the slight mismatching of venous pH. Following this last adjustment further iterations of the matching algorithm are required.

Evaluation of accuracy of simulation

In order to evaluate the accuracy of the simulation produced in this this we studied 12 patients being artificially ventilated following cardiac bypass surgery.[12]

DATA COLLECTED

	Information required for simulation	Additional information obtained to check accuracy
General patient details	Age, Ht, Wt, Sex	
Ventilation regime	F_{IO_2}, V_T, f, PEEP	
Metabolism	$\dot{V}O_2$, $\dot{V}CO_2$	
Blood gas analysis	PaO_2, $PaCO_2$ HCO_3^- art $P\bar{v}O_2$	pHa, CaO_2 pH$\bar{v}$, $P\bar{v}CO_2$ $HCO_3^-\bar{v}$, $C\bar{v}O_2$
Others	Hb, Body temp, cardiac output barometric pressure	$\dot{Q}s/\dot{Q}T$, VD

The data required to produce the simulation, together with additional information obtained in order to check its accuracy, is shown in Table 1. Briefly, the methodology was as follows: the inspired oxygen fraction (FIO2) was measured using a paramagnetic oxygen analyser. Simultaneous collection and analysis of expired gas over a timed period allowed calculation of tidal volume and carbon dioxide production. Cardiac output was determined using the thermodilution technique with a modified Swan-Ganz catheter which also allowed sampling of mixed venous blood. Oxygen consumption was calculated from the cardiac output and the arterio-venous content difference. A total of 58 sets of data were obtained in this way. Matching of PaO_2, $PaCO_2$ and arterial bicarbonate was always within the preset tolerance limits as defined above. $\dot{V}O_2$ and $\dot{V}CO_2$ were also invariably closely matched. Furthermore the values for venous admixture and dead space generated within the model by the matching algorithm correlated closely with those derived from values measured in the patients (r>0.99). The most crucial test of the correctness of the model's steady-state description is clearly on the venous side of the systemic circulation and not surprisingly here the correlations were less close. However, even for venous blood, the simulation was within clinically acceptable limits with correlation coefficients always greater than 0.91. Thus it is now possible to produce a steady-state simulation of an artificially ventilated patient which is sufficiently accurate to have clinical potential. It was felt that interaction with this simulation should provide additional insight into the patient's pathophysiology and that it might, therefore, prove to be useful both for teaching and to facilitate the physician's assessment of the patient. It also seemed possible that the simulation could be used to predict the patient's response to alternative proposed treatment regimes so that the optimal therapy for each patient could be discovered without recourse to the usual 'trial and error' procedure.

Farrell and Siegel have adopted a very similar approach.[4,5] They have used CSMP (Continuous System Modelling Program) programming techniques, together with their previously described model,[13] to generate simulations of patients being artifically ventilated following coronary artery bypass surgery. The simulations enabled them to assess the nature and severity of the cardiorespiratory dysfunction in these patients and they presented illustrative cases in which the simulation was used to predict the effects of alternative therapy (altering minute volume and/or $\dot{Q}_t$). Although their impression was that these predictions were qualitatively correct, they did not make any formal assessment of the accuracy achieved.

Evaluation of the accuracy of model predictions

The ability of the model simulation to predict an individual patient's response to alterations in the ventilation regime has therefore been evaluated.[14]

A simulation of the patient was first created using the method outlined above. Next the patient's minute volume and/or FIO2 were altered. The same adjustments were made to the ventilation regime of the simulated patient and this was then used to predict the cardiorespiratory consequences of these alterations. The actual changes produced in the patient were then measured and compared with the model's prediction.

Although the correlation between measured and predicted values for PaO_2 was reasonable (r=0.94) there was an appreciable random inaccuracy (SEE = $\pm$ 17.3 mmHg). This was caused by errors in shunt prediction and compounded by fluctuations in $\dot{V}O_2$ and $\dot{Q}_t$ which were largely unpredictable. There was a consistent tendency to overestimate when predicting $PaCO_2$ and for this reason, values for arterial pH were generally too low. There were small, random fluctuations in arterial bicarbonate between each set of measurements and these were responsible for minor, random inaccuracies in arterial pH. The random errors in $PaCO_2$ prediction were probably largely attributable to small errors in predicted V_D as well as alterations in $\dot{V}CO_2$. However these were insufficient to explain all of the random error and could not account for the consistent tendency to overestimate $PaCO_2$. It is possible that either the model or the patient, or both, had not reached a steady state at the time of measurement and that the time course of CO_2 uptake, storage or excretion in the model requres modification.

The errors in $PaCO_2$ and pHa were reflected in the predictions for $P\bar{v}CO_2$ and $pH\bar{v}$. As anticipated, the least accurate predictions were those for $P\bar{v}O_2$ since this is influenced by many factors, including PaO_2, $\dot{Q}_t$, $\dot{V}O_2$ and alterations in the position of the oxyhaemoglobin dissociation curve.

Failure to predict arterial and venous blood gas/acid-base state sufficiently accurately can therefore be attributed to deficiencies in the model/simulation (mainly errors in prediction of shunt, dead space and, possibly, CO_2 exchange), compounded by unpredictable alterations in the patient's physiology (most importantly $\dot{V}O_2$, $\dot{V}CO_2$ and $\dot{Q}_t$). Finally the limitations and inaccuracies of the measurement techniques at our disposal have also to be considered.

Modifications to improve the accuracy of simulation and prediction

Perhaps the most important limitation of the model as described is the use of a three compartment lung. A more realistic simulation could be achieved by using a sophisticated lung model, such as the ten compartment representation described by Farrell and Siegel,[13] which would be capable of accurately simulating ventilation/perfusion $(\dot{V}/\dot{Q})$ mismatch. However, the difficulties associated with routine measurements of $\dot{V}/\dot{Q}$ distributions in the clinical situation remain. On the other hand, Farrell and Siegel claim[5] that when matching blood gas tensions using their model there were sufficient constraints to allow detailed and accurate characterisation of a patient's respiratory dysfunction in terms of $\dot{V}/\dot{Q}$ disparity, diffusion gradient, venous-arterial pulmonary shunt and respiratory dead space. At present our intention is to develop a lung model using continuous $\dot{V}/\dot{Q}$ distributions[15] in order to achieve more accurate simulation and prediction.

As discussed, the modelling of CO_2 uptake, storage and excretion may not be sufficiently accurate and possibly the time course of slow CO_2 changes requires modification. Furthermore it is important to ensure that both the patient and the simulation have reached a steady state at the time comparisons are made.

Farrell and Siegel[5] derived $\dot{V}O_2$ and $\dot{V}CO_2$ from the product of $\dot{Q}_t$ and the arterio-venous O_2 and CO_2 content differences (calculated using the same Kelman's equations as are incorporated in the models), whereas we derived $\dot{V}CO_2$ from an analysis of mixed expired gas and measured oxygen contents directly with a fuel cell analyser. By adopting Farrell and Siegel's procedure the discrepancy between model and patient values could certainly be reduced, although to a certain extent this would be an artificial improvement.

Further developments to facilitate creation of a simulation

The generation of 'physiological profiles'[16] is now a routine clinical procedure in many intensive therapy units. Although it requires invasive monitoring, including insertion of a thermodilution Swan-Ganz catheter, as well as accurate determination of blood gas tensions, oxygen saturation, acid-base state and haemoglobin concentration, the required data can be obtained fairly easily in the clinical situation. Using a small computer program, many important derived values are then rapidly produced.

In order to simplify the modelling process, a 'physiological profile' program was written which not only collates, derives and displays relevant cardiorespiratory data, but also automatically provides the matching algorithm with the information required to generate a simulation.

The clinical potential of computer simulation

Further development of this technique is limited not by computer technology (either hardware or software), but rather by our incomplete understanding of the physiological mechanisms involved and an inability to measure rapidly, reliably and accurately all the data required to generate a correct simulation. For example, accurate modelling of the patient's probable response to the application of a positive end-expiratory pressure (PEEP) could be of considerable assistance clinically. Although a complex algorithm describing the effects of PEEP on altered cardiorespiratory function could theoretically be designed, additional measurements such as functional residual capacity, compliance and myocardial performance, would be required in order to achieve a reasonable simulation. Similarly prediction of the patient's response to a period of spontaneous respiration could help the clinician to decide when to discontinue artificial ventilation. Unfortunately the modelling of spontaneous respiration is complex and influenced by many unquantifiable factors such as the effect of sedation on the respiratory centre, the adequacy of neuromuscular function and the influence of psychological factors. Whether it will prove possible to develop models capable of dealing with other complex situations, such as intermittent mandatory ventilation or high frequency ventilation, remains to be established.

Even if an infinitely complex and accurate model could be constructed the applicability of this approach suffers because such a model still deals with only one aspect of the patient's physiology; in reality cardiovascular function, fluid and electrolyte balance and drug administration, to name only a few, are closely interrelated. Models of these other systems are already available and could theoretically be appropriately modified and linked together to form a comprehensive patient model for use in the critically ill.

COMPUTER MODELLING FOR SELF-INSTRUCTION AND ASSESSMENT

Computer assisted learning (CAL) techniques are becoming a widely accepted method of teaching in many fields, including medical education. As well as overcoming certain practical difficulties, such as limited availability of teachers, CAL is a versatile and stimulating means of acquiring knowledge, forming a useful adjunct to traditional teaching methods. Because CAL is interactive, providing frequent questions and immediate feedback, the students interest and attention is maintained, while repeated attempts at solving the same problem reinforce the information acquired.

Those trainees who find formal teaching, in which mistakes are exposed to both teachers and peers, a daunting experience, may find CAL particularly helpful because only the computer discovers their ignorance. Furthermore, when groups of students run through an exercise together a more vigorous discussion may ensue if they are not inhibited by the presence of a teacher. However, CAL should only be used to supplement traditional teaching methods, not as a substitute. This is particularly important in medical education because CAL, by its very nature, tends to provide information in an unqualified, factual form, which is often remote from the realities of clinical practice.

At present CAL usually involves the use of case studies to teach clinical decision making. For example, programs have been developed which are concerned with the management of conditions likely to be encountered in general practice[17] as well as in anaesthesia and intensive care.[18] A more sophisticated program has also been produced which presents problems concerned with the clinical management of emergency cases and includes a representation of changes in the patient's vital functions with time and in response to prescribed treatment.[19] Others have concentrated on problem-solving behaviour in association with history taking,[20] while the 'CASE' system allows the student to interrogate the patient and obtain the results of investigations before proceeding to diagnosis and treatment.[21] Some of these exercises are linked to projectors which display relevant information such as X-rays and ECGs,[22] and they may be supplemented by written texts.

The use of computer models adds a new dimension to CAL since it provides a degree of realism not possible with other methods. The user need not be constrained in his choice of therapy by a pre-determined list of options since the model will always respond realistically to the chosen treatment and the student is able to explore the effects of various therapeutic options quite safely. A number of computer models designed for teaching the principles of fluid and electrolyte balance,[23,24] applied cardiorespiratory physiology[25] and drug administration[26] have been developed, including the model of human respiration described above.[9] De Land[23] has described an extensive and accurate model which has been used for teaching the management of fluid and electrolyte disturbances. However, in order to represent the clinical situation more accurately it is necessary not only to have dynamic models, which can simulate the passage of real time and take account of renal excretory function, but also to integrate correctly the relevant aspects of circulation and respiration. One of the authors (C J D) has attempted to produce a teaching model specifically designed to examine these interrelationships.[24] Unfortunately current uncertainties about some of the physiological parameters and functions (eg interstitial compliance and dynamics) mean that the model is not sufficiently accurate for clinical use. Nonetheless it can be used effectively for teaching many of the basic principles of fluid and electrolyte balance. A comprehensive model has been published by Guyton,[27] and although there are still certain limitations, this is probably the best available. Coleman[28] has been working on an even more comprehensive model which, like MacPuf,[9] cuts as many corners as possible to speed operation. A comprehensive and accurate model for teaching pharmacokinetics is also available[26] and has been tried out in teaching situations.[29] At present this model is being equipped with a pharmacodynamic limb to make it easier to translate drug level predictions to actual clinical effects.

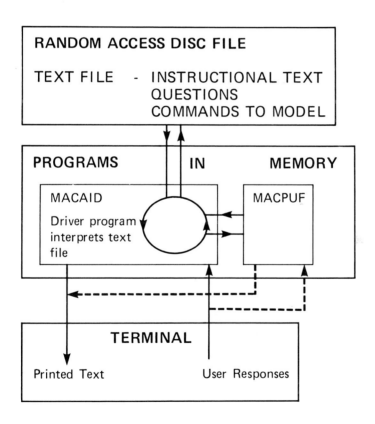

These models can, of course, be used interactively on their own as originally intended. However, a more entertaining and thorough teaching program can be offered by linking the model to a computer-assisted instructional driver[30] in the manner illustrated in Fig 3. The teaching exercises are written into text files which consist of a series of labelled 'frames'. Each frame may contain instructional text, questions (single or multiple choice, together with answers and scores) or a 'string' of commands to a model. The texts are contained in a direct access disc file and are designed to allow a tutor to write, add to or edit exercises easily via a computer terminal. The instructional driver is a general purpose software tool with facilities for the creation of many types of interrogative sequences. It reads and processes the text file and is situated, together with the free-standing model program, in main memory (Fig 3). The driver program transmits instructional text and questions to the visual display unit and interacts with the student, moving through the frames of the text file in a sequence determined by his responses, while at the same time scoring his answers. It can also relay commands to a model to create and control simulations. Facilities are included to allow such a set of commands to be interrupted, permitting the user to interact with the model directly, following which control returns to the instructional driver.

Unlike any comparable system, the instructional driver program has been written in FORTRAN to ensure portability on to a wide range of computer systems and is capable of running virtually any CAL exercise. It has proved easy to adapt and has been used in a MUMPS program to teach cardiopulmonary resuscitation[31] and in BASIC programs on intensive care.[18] Using the computer model of human respiration described above,[9] together with the instructional driver, we have so far written two exercises dealing with the respiratory management of intensive care patients,[7] as well as others dealing with respiratory physiology.

The development of such a universal 'text interpreter' means that, provided that the teaching material is written in a suitable form, the necessity to write basic interactive software, which is a time-consuming task, can be eliminated and dissemination of teaching exercises may be promoted.

In conclusion, it is likely to be some time before computer simulations are sufficiently sophisticated to make a significant contribution to patient care, although they can enhance our understanding of pathophysiological mechanisms. The use of computer models for teaching, on the other hand, is already proving to be a valuable technique.

REFERENCES

1. Tintner G (1968): Methodology of mathematical economics and econometrics. University of Chicago Press

2. Westcott J H (1969): Application of optimal methods to control of industrial processes. Computers in Simulation, IBM Symposium Proceedings

3. Yamamoto W, Hori T (1971): Phasic air movement model of respiratory regulation of carbon dioxide balance. Computers and Biomedical Research 3: 699-717

4. Siegel J H, Farrell E J (1973): A computer simulation model to study the clinical observability of ventilation and perfusion abnormalities in human shock states. Surgery 73: 898-912

5. Farrell E J, Siegel J H (1981): Cardiorespiratory simulation for the evaluation of recovery following coronary artery bypass surgery. Comput Biol Med 11: 105-128

6. Scrimshire D A, Tomlin P J (1973): Gas exchange during initial stages of N_2O uptake and elimination in a lung model. J Appl Physiol 34: 775-789

7. Hinds C J, Ingram D, Dickinson C J (1982): Self-instruction and assessment in techniques of intensive care using a computer model of the respiratory system. Intensive Care Medicine 8: 115-123

8. Skinner J B, Knowles G, Armstrong R F, Ingram D (1983): The use of computerised learning in intensive care: an evaluation of a new teaching program. J Med Educ (in press)

9. Dickinson C J (1977): A computer model of human respiration. Lancaster, England- MTP Press Ltd

10. Kelman G R (1966): Digital computer subroutine for the conversion of oxygen tension into saturation. J Appl Physiol 21: 1375-1376

11. Kelman G R (1967): Digital computer procedure for the conversion of PCO_2 into blood CO_2 content. Respiration Physiology 3: 111-115

168

12. Hinds C J, Ingram D, Adams L et al (1980): An evaluation of the clinical potential of a comprehensive model of human respiration in artificially ventilated patients. Clinical Science 58: 83-91

13. Farrell E J, Siegel J H (1973): Investigation of cardiorespiratory abnormalities through computer simulation. Computers and Biomedical Research 5: 161-186

14. Hinds C J, Roberts M J, Ingram D, Dickinson C J: Computer simulation to predict patient responses to alterations in the ventilation regime. Intensive Care Medicine (in press)

15. Butter J P, Mohler J G (1970): The alveolar-arterial difference for O_2 and CO_2 in an infinite alveolus lung model. Mathematical Biosciences 9: 195-203

16. Shabot M M, Shoemaker W C, State D (1977): Rapid bedside computation of cardiorespiratory variables with a programmable calculator. Crit Care Med 5: 105-111

17. Murray T S, Cupples R W, Barber J H et al (1977): Teaching decision making to medical undergraduates by computer-assisted learning. Med Educ 11: 262-264

18. Kenny G C, Schmubian C (1979): Computer-assisted learning in the teaching of anaesthesia. Anaesthesia 34: 159-162

19. Murray T S (1977): Developing methods of evaluation appropriate to the undergraduate teaching of general practice of Glasgow University. PhD Thesis, University of Glasgow

20. Warner H R, Woolley F R, Kane R L (1974): Computer-assisted instruction for teaching clinical decision making. Comp Biomed Res 7: 564-574

21. Harless W G, Orennon G G, Marxer J J et al (1971): CASE: A computer-aided simulation of the clinical encounter. J Med Educ 46: 443-448

22. Aida K, Minamikawa T, Takai Y et al (1977): A simulation oriented CAI system for diagnosis and treatment in cardiology. In: Shires, Wolf (eds) IFIP Medinfo 77. Amsterdam, Oxford, New York, North Holland Publishing Company, pp 841-845

23. De Land E C, Dell R B, Ramakrishnan R (1977): On-line patient simulation for trial fluid therapy. MEDCOMP 77, Proceedings, Berlin

24. Dickinson, C J Shephard E P (1971): A digital computer model of the systemic circulation and kidney, for studying renal and circulatory interactions involving electrolytes and body fluid compartments. J Physiol (Lond) 216: 11P

25. Dickinson C J, Sackett D L, Goldsmith C H (1973): MacMan: A digital computer model for teaching some basic principles of haemodynamics. J Clin Comput 2: 42-50

26. Bloch R, Ingram D, Sweeney G D et al (1980): MacDope: A simulation of drug disposition in the human body. Mathematical considerations. J Theor Biol 87: 211-236

27. Guyton A C, Coleman T G, Granger H J (1972): Circulation: Overall regulation. Ann Rev Physiol 34: 13-32

28. Coleman T G (1978): A mathematical model of the human body in health, disease and during treatment. Proceedings of the Joint Automatic Control Conference 4: 77-86

29. Ingram D, Dickinson C J, Saunders L et al (1979): Application of a pharmacokinetic simulation program in pharmacy courses. Computers in Education 3: 335-345

30. Ahmed K, Ingram D, Dickinson C J (1980): Software for educational computing: a general purpose driver for computer-assisted instruction, interrogation and system simulation (MACAID). Lancaster, England, MTP Press Ltd

31. Hoffer E P, Barnett G O, Farquar BB (1972): Computer simulation model for teaching cardiopulmonary resuscitation. J Med Educ 47: 343-348

AN INTERACTIVE PROGRAM FOR INTRAVENOUS DRUG INFUSION MANAGEMENT

Michael N. Skaredoff, M.D. and Paul J. Poppers, M.D.

Department of Anesthesiology, Health Sciences Center

State University of New York

Stony Brook, New York   USA

INTRODUCTION

In critical care medicine, the rational use of drugs with rapid and powerful effects on the cardiovascular and other vital systems has become ever more important. Vasodilators, inotropic agents, antiarrhythmic drugs and even some tocolytic compounds are often administered by intravenous infusion.

The safe and effective administration by this route of such medications demands sophisticated monitoring and the employment of calibrated infusion pumps. Determination of the proper dose and its infusion rate is not only tedious and time-consuming, but often confusing as well, with possible grave consequences for the patient. The administration rate is often expressed in micrograms per kilogram body weight per minute, while the infusion pump is calibrated in milliliters per hour. Furthermore, the amount of drug and amount of diluent solution is important, for the infusion rate is not only related to the dose, but also to the concentration of the solution.

A second, but equally important difficulty occurs with the use of certain drugs, particularly the antiarrythmics. These drugs require a loading dose, an amount of drug necessary to establish a clinically effective concentration. It usually exceeds multiples of the maintenance dose which is the amount that maintains the drug level in the circulation in the optimum range. Making the problem even more difficult is the fact that for some drugs there are several acceptable ways to obtain an appropriate loading dose.

Finally, to round out the problem, the intensive care situation is often a stressful one, with personnel who are often tired and under pressure to quickly calculate doses and infusion rates. The possiblities for error, even in a calm relaxed atmosphere, are legion; in a typical intensive care setting, it is sometimes a wonder that the right dose gets calculated at all. The propensity for error was pointed out quite clearly by Lamb et al. (1) in a study in which ten surgical house officers and 23 experienced critical care nurses were asked to manually compute a drip rate of dopamine for a patient of a particular weight, given the ordered dose. Three of ten house officers and none of the nurses were able to calculate the right answer within five minutes. When additional time was allowed, only 50% of the staff was able to make the appropriate calculation.

Lamb (1), Neu (2) and others (3,4,5) have all published programs for programmable calculators in order to alleviate these problems. However, the memory and computing power available to these machines are quite limited. Even the program by Goyette (6) which employs a "pocket computer" is only able to solve one type of problem at a time and forces the user to key in data multiple times. In the authors' opinion single-keystroke data entry is far preferable, since fewer errors are likely to result. Finally, there has been no program to date that is able to output results in an attractive, easily readable format, suitable for placement in a patient's chart. Such a format presents not only the result (the infusion rate) but also all data which were keyed in or keystroke-selected to allow a manual check, if desired. This last

has medico-legal ramifications as well; it is a good idea to record the
amount of drug and its concentration in order to demonstrate that proper
procedures had been carried out.

For all these reasons a computer program was designed to meet the
designed objectives and considerations enumerated above. Named DOSECALC
it offers versatility, simultaneous application of loading and
maintenance doses of multiple drugs, simplicity, safety, and convenient
final interpretation and execution. To obviate common user-generated
errors, the DOSECALC is "menu" or option driven. Since this program is
designed for use by nurses and physicians alike, a list of indications,
contraindications, and cautions, as specified by various authorities
(7,8,9), is included. As an added feature, the usual supply form and
amount is displayed. Only regularly used dilutions, easily recognized
by hospital personnel, are allowed. If a drug has multiple loading dose
schedules, the user has the opportunity to examine them and select one.
Finally, printer capability is obligatory to satisfy the need for
hard-copy for use elsewhere.

The Apple II+ Version

The Apple II+ is a microcomputer originally manufactured in 1977
(as the Apple II) as a home and hobbyist computer. In the past six
years, more than any other "personal computer" it has probably been
responsible for the virtual explosion of computer consciousness and
"computer literacy" in North America. This is due to the intrinsic ease
of use afforded by the Read-Only-Memory (ROM)-based BASIC programming
language, and, beginning in 1979, the DOS 3.3 disk operating system. By

efficient and clever use DOS and commercially available "utilities" (machine-language programming aids), the Apple can be induced to function at an extremely sophisticated level, to the point that some applications that are not practical for a mini-or mainframe computer (without a great deal of programming time and effort) can easily be executed on the microcomputer.

The original design impetus for DOSECALC came from an early dissatisfaction with the manner in which various application programs were loaded into Random-Access-Memory (RAM) by DOS. It so happens that when a particular program is called from disk, a previously called program is eliminated. What was originally desired was a "controller program" which would call up various other programs as needed. However, the controller would be destroyed and, at the end of a given program, would have to be recalled. Apple DOS does have a certain so-called "chaining" ability. That is, the variables of a given program may be inserted into a portion of RAM and preserved while a second program appears, after which they may then be used.

Either of the above options, while useful in themselves, are inadequate for an application such as DOSECALC. What is desired is not a multiplicity of programs, which is wasteful in terms of time, programming effort and disk space (the 5¼" floppy disk has only 140K of useful storage). Chaining is not a viable alternative, either. What is needed is a master program which would be able to access a "procedure file" for each drug. Each file would contain all the program information about a drug needed by the user. BASIC in and of itself, unlike some other languages (such as Pascal), does not lend itself easily to such applications. However, by manipulating DOS, this problem could be solved.

In order to understand the solution, a short explanation of DOS in general and the "EXEC" command in particular is necessary (10): the Apple II Disk Operating System allows BASIC programmers to make use of disk files. DOS files can be programs, such as Integer or Applesoft Basic programs, or binary information, such as machine language programs or pure data, or Textfiles of ASCII text. The first three of these filetypes are used to store programs; their contents may not be accessed for manipulation by running a BASIC program. On the other hand, textfiles contain text or pure information. Programs may create such files, and open, close, read and write them.

Apple DOS has the capability of reading commands to itself from textfiles as well as from the keyboard. The obvious application is to create a semi-automatic turnkey system activated by one keystroke. Furthermore, Apple DOS is so constructed that whole programs can be converted (captured) into textfiles. Since a BASIC program executes line by line, it is, as far as the computer is concerned, no different than a line, of plain text, since both are read sequentially. The EXEC commands allows this process to occur. When DOS reads a line that starts with a line number from an EXEC textfile, it "knows" that the line must contain a BASIC statement, so it passes the line to the BASIC interpreter. Therefore, if a captured program is EXECed, the program is ultimately fed back into memory, statement by statement.

As mentioned before, the LOAD or RUN commands cause a single file containing a BASIC program to be read into memory. A second such command will cause any program already in memory to be destroyed. It

would seem impossible to store a program in more than one given file.
With textfiles, this can be accomplished. If the first program contains
EXEC commands, and the line numbers of the program contained within the
textfile are different from that of the first program, then
the textfile portion can be neatly appended , with no destruction of
program information. By having the very last line of each textfile (one
for each drug) read PRINT "RUN 2000" it is not only possible to append
the file to the controller program but to activate it at that point as
well.

A last point: since what is being done constitutes multiple
appending, it is for obvious reasons critical to ensure that each and
every textfile is of exactly the same length. Smaller files have REM
statements (REMarks which were ignored by the program) for "place
takers".

One of the problems with DOSECALC is the fact that a great deal of
text needs to be displayed on the screen. In order that an attractive,
professional-quality product be portrayed, it has become necessary to
consider a method of screen display other than the PRINT statement.
Fortunately, several commercial products are available (of which
"Utility City" is one*) which have been developed to satisfy similar
needs. The "Screenwriter" utility enables one to format screens
essentially at will, and stores them in binary format on disk. In order
to display a given screen, all that is required is to employ the BLOAD
(binary load) command. This expedient is able to save hundreds of lines
of program code, and greatly enhances the loading speed of both the
controller program and the textfiles. For hard-copy, a four-line
screen-dump subroutine is used.

*Beagle Bros. 4315 Sierra Vista, San Diego, CA 92103 USA

The final product is a relatively short (27 sector) controller program which is able to load completely from disk into memory in seven seconds. The user first sees the title screen followed by a menu which displays categories of drugs. When a key is pressed, a second menu with the specific drugs comes into view. When the key is now pressed, the screen will blank out and the textfile is called up. Two to three screens of text showing indications and contraindications are now at the user's disposal. The last screen will generally indicate how the drug is supplied and the permissible dilutions. Finally, the acceptable dosage range is displayed. When the RETURN key is pressed the screen blanks and the user is prompted for the patient's weight, desired dose and, if indicated, the desired loading dose and/or loading dose format. When the user has entered the last datum, a "results screen" will appear, containing not only the desired answers, but also all the previously keyed or keystroke-selected information. The user has now the options to 1) recalculate infusion rate of the same drug, 2) activate the printer for hard-copy, 3) return to the main menu for selection of another drug, or 4) quit the program (Figure 1).

THE PCS (IBM 3031) VERSION:

Adapting the DOSECALC program to a mainframe computer operating in a hospital environment demanded radical changes in program strategy. University Hospital at the Health Sciences Center of the State University of New York at Stony Brook utilizes an IBM 3031 mainframe computer which services over a hundred terminals and printers. Patient Care System (PCS) is an IBM-designed computer system designed to aid all

departments in a hospital by linking the functional areas of the
hospital and by providing these areas with a means of entering and
reviewing data about a patient. PCS is comprised of programs, screen,
files, and "procedures" called Data Collection Lists (DCLs) (11,12).

Routines for the creation of screens an quite straightforward and
easy to accomplish. Using the Panvalet Editor (PANE) ** routines,
screens were made up for each drug. An added feature is that commands
for influencing screen flow could be appended to a particular screen
"out of sight". Furthermore, drug information could also be placed in
subsequent screens and operations. It soon became clear that such an
approach would rapidly become unwieldy and inefficient. Another way was
sought and found, using the flexibility and power of the DCL.

A DCL is a series of instructions to gather data and process them
in a predefined sequence. In many respects, it acts as a controller
program rather than a subroutine; since DCLs are used to process a
procedure in stages, the whole DCL is not executed at one time.
However, unlike a controller program in BASIC, a DCL cannot stand alone;
it must receive a command from a control screen, giving a specific name
and "Target Status" (T-Status). The T-Status is a numeric value that is
compared against each line of the DCL to determine if the line should be
processed.

While the name of the DCL remains constant as it is called to
execute the various stages of processing, the T-Status numeric value
changes. It increases as successive stages are processed. As data are
collected and/or processed at each stage of the DCL execution, they are

**Pansophic Systems, Inc. 709 Enterprise Drive, Oak Brook, IL 60521 USA stored in a temporary (i.e., for the duration of the complete execution of the DCL) data base. These data are retrieved from the data base each time a succeeding stage of the DCL is executed. When all the processing is completed, the data are automatically destroyed.

For the purpose of DOSECALC, automatic deletion/destruction of data would not do. To get around this limitation, small files were created and entered directly into computer permanent memory. When such a file is accessed, its contents can be duplicated on the temporary data base. When processing is complete, data base information will be deleted, allowing the data base to accept new data following the appropriate screen command. In this way, the "program overwriting" function of Apple II+ DOSECALC was emulated.

The PCS version of DOSECALC operates in the following manner: after logging on to the computer, the operator, using a light pen, probes the master screen to call up the "help screen", upon which is the initiating command for DOSECALC. The first program screen to appear is a menu which lists all options. At this point one screen is available, but the menu may have as many "pages" as needed. Upon probing the desired drug, a second screen displaying indications, contraindications and cautions is displayed and the DCL is activated. By probing the screen again, a function screen is displayed, showing how the drug is supplied, as well as all the dilution options. The user probes one such option and presses the ENTER key. The next screen called prompts the user to key in the patient weight and the desired dose (the probe selected dilution data are automatically displayed). The screen is reviewed, and the ENTER key is pressed again. The final screen is the "results screen", re-displaying all the data (weight, dose, drug weight

and dilution volume) as well as the calculated answer in ML/MIN,
MICRODROPS/MIN on ML/HOUR. Options at the bottom of the screen allow
the user to RETURN to the Master Screen, RECALCULATE a dose for the same
drug, or go to the MAIN MENU to select another drug. The terminal
keyboards are supplied with an automatic DUP key which allows one to
print data which is displayed on the screen.

ERRORPROOFING

Among other considerations, errorproofing a program is perhaps the
hardest and most important task a programmer must accomplish. The more
experienced a programmer is, the less likely will he make common
mistakes. It then becomes a task to imagine what mistakes or errors a
typical user might make. The Apple program uses, as much as possible,
keystroke driven commands, which are placed in the INPUT mode. That is,
only a single letter or number is usually needed and the user has to
press the RETURN key to have the program actually execute the command.
This gives the user an opportunity to review the selection and change it
if necessary. At various points in the program it is possible to go
directly back to the main menu and start again. In order to keep the
format tidy, data entry may be any symbol, but limits are imposed by
data type and by range. If a keyed datum falls outside these limits, it
automatically erases and the cursor returns to its original position.
The limits imposed in the program are quite generous and serve primarily
to eliminate obviously inappropriate data. The PCS version, by dint of
the light-pen probe capability, allows the user directly to point at
what is desired. Except for selecting dilution options (v.i.), however,
all probes are "immediate detectable" which means that command execution

begins right away. In order to give the user an opportunity to get out of a wrongly-selected routine, every screen has a provision to RETURN to the main menu. In contrast, delayed-detectable fields on a screen imply that until either the ENTER key is pessed or an immediate detectable field is probed, no program/DCL execution will occur. The user can change the selection of dilution options at will, secure in the knowledge that no uncontrolled program execution will happen. Like the Apple version, keyed-in data can be alphanumeric, but limits are set.

FUTURE DEVELOPMENTS

The original DOSECALC program is written in BASIC. Because of its very nature, it is rather slow in execution. Furthermore, since it does depend on disk access, a very real limitation exists in the amount of drugs which can be included. The typical Apple Disk II with 140K of storage capacity allows 15 drugs. A second disk, with about another 10 drugs is currently in preparation, and can be run completely independently of the present program. Eventually, however, the programs will be combined and revised. The main revision will be a change in programming language, from BASIC to Pascal. Since Pascal is a compiled language, rather than an interpreter (like BASIC), it will execute much faster. Also, Pascal offers far more flexibility and power; instead of creating text files to be EXECed, these files can be directly written as "procedures" which can be accessed via a "linker" subroutine. The final advantage is portability. Since the actual working program (unlike the source code) is in compiled (machine language) form, it can be used on any machine provided it can be accessed (i.e., the DOS must be compatible). For those mini or mainframe computers with resident Pascal compilers, the program source code can be sent by modem as a text-file, compiled on the spot and run.

Since the IBM 3031 only accepts compiled languages, it runs at maximum speed. No radical change in programming language is necessary. PCS, however, has particular developmental possibilities of its own.

At present, a program with only 12 drugs is available. A second menu page can be added with essentially no change in the DCL. Drugs with unusual requirements (loading doses, for example)need only to activate an alternate DCL to run. In order to enhance flexibility, a printing DCL subroutine can be added for automatic printout of results on command at the terminal's "home printer" or at any printer destination selected by the user.

Finally, the program structure can be used for interactive applications other than drug dose management. Fluid balance calculations, acid-base interpretation and/or management can all be set up in a similar manner. The user thus has many opportunites to utilize the computer as a helper rather than a demanding master, and so interact with the system in a positive fashion.

SODIUM NITROPRUSSIDE RESULTS

PATIENT WEIGHT   =   73   KG

DESIRED DOSE   =   5   MCG/KG/MIN

DRUG WEIGHT   =   50   MG

SOLUTION VOLUME   =   250   ML

DRIP RATE   = 1.825   ML/MIN

                         = 109.5   MICRODROPS/MIN

                         = 109.5   ML/HR

PRINT RESULTS   RECALCULATE

MAIN MENU   QUIT

FIGURE 1

REFERENCES

1)   Lamb J, Rose EA, King TC, et al: A simple programmable calculator technique for dosage determination and administration of drugs by continuous infusion. Heart & Lung 10 (1): 72-74, 1981

2)   Neu T, Mahoney C, Wilson AD, et al: Calculator assisted determination of dilutions for continuous infusion medications. Crit Care Med 10:610-612, 1982

3)   Ruiz BC, Tucker WK, Kirby RR: A program for calculation of intra-pulmonary shunts, blood-gas and acid base values with a programmable calculator. Anesthesiology 42:88-95, 1975

4)   Finlayson DC, Yin A: Calculator assisted cardiorespiratory monitoring. Crit Care Med 9:604-606, 1981

5)   Shabot MS, Shoemaker WC, State D: Rapid bedside computation of cardiorespiratory variables with a programmable calculator. Crit Care Med 5:105-111, 1977

6)   Goyette RE: A simple means of assuring proper drug dosage. Anesthesiology 58:202-203, 1983

7)   Gilman AG, Goodman LS, Gilman A, eds: The Pharmacological Basis of Therapeutics, 6th Ed., New York, MacMillan, 1980

8)   Physician's Desk Reference, 37th Ed., Oradell, NJ, Litton Industries, 1983

9)   American Hospital Formulary Service, American Society of Hospital Pharmacists, 1980

10)   The DOS Manual--Disk Operating System, Cupertino, CA, Apple Computer Inc., 1981 pp 73-81

11)   Patient Care System Application Coding--Student Text, Atlanta, IBM Corporation (Marketing Support Publications) 1981

12)   Patient Care System Application Development System--Design and Coding Guide, Atlanta, IBM Corporation (Marketing Support Publicatins) 1981

COMPUTER ASSISTED LEARNING IN ANAESTHESIOLOGY

Dr. J.W.R. McIntyre
Department of Anaesthesia
University Hospital, Edmonton, Alberta, Canada

Definitions are important and in this presentation the word education means the mastery of skills and an understanding of their underlying principles. The word computer refers to a tool - or instructional device - that can be used by teacher and learner during the educational process. My task now is to discuss the role of the computer in instructional development, the process of improving instruction, in anaesthesiology. To help do this I will describe an instructional model (fig. 1), which will be used to indicate the possible role of the computer in educating trainee anaesthetists. This model is a combination of those described by De Cecco[1] and Blondin[2]. First it introduces the entering behaviour of the trainee and then follows a sequence dealing with identification of educational problems, instructional objectives, instructional procedures of which computer assisted learning is the one concentrated on, and lastly performance assessment.

Physicians learning about anaesthesia vary in their attitudes and previous professional experience. The knowledge base of recent medical graduates is predictable and the course content can be easily planned. The content for continuing education of anaesthetists already in practise is unpredictable and must be planned on the basis of new knowledge selected by instructors and needs indicated by morbidity and mortality reports[3] as well as formal audit[4].

A statement that an educational problem exists is only justified if

the assessment of the trainees final competence is valid. Written and
oral national examinations in most English speaking countries are believed
to be valid assessments. Even if they are not they represent educational
objectives that are clearly defined. Each year some trainees fail to pass
these examinations at the end of the statutory training period. This constitutes an educational problem. Related problems may be insufficient
good teachers in the Faculty or insufficient funds to pay instructors.
Additionally some teaching requirements are repetitive as successive groups
of trainees pass through the instructional process or should be repetitive
for certain trainees to learn satisfactorily. These last processes are
likely to be perceived by teachers as intellectually unrewarding and in
some instances a denial of more rewarding time spent in academic endeav-
ours with gifted trainees. These problems apparently do not have a serious impact on society as a whole though it might have a dilatorious effect
on the overall quality of a nation's anaesthesia services. However, they
certainly have financial and lifestyle implications for some trainees and
for some faculty. I believe we can conclude that there are educational
problems in anaesthesiology. Except perhaps in developing countries they
may not be acute but they merit further consideration.

An instructional objective describes the intended outcome is not a
description of course content.[5] It is stated in behavioural or performance
terms that describe what the trainee can do when demonstrating his or her
achievement of the objectives. This has been documented for anaesthesia
and later attention will be drawn to certain examples.

The computer assisted learning tool is usually a place where each
student has access to two visual displays for graphics and other material,
an audio output and a keyboard via which the user can interact with the
program and indirectly with the persons that prepared the course content

and mode of delivery. This is in the form of statements, questions, and explanations that can be presented in many different ways. The learner is forced to interact much more frequently than is possible during a lecture, seminar, or tutorial. Similarly calculations associated with clinical management can be requested and presented to the learner much more quickly than the conventional blackboard slide or transparency permits. Thus the drill and practice aspect of learning can be accomplished more efficiently.

Anaesthesia training presented as educational objectives is a vast undertaking. Now I shall choose a very few objectives, relate them to certain educational problems, and suggest where computer assisted learning may play a useful role for certain students or certain training centres.

Instructional objectives:

"The trainee can usefully relate knowledge of the basic sciences to the management of anaesthetised patients."

This can be broken down to two new objectives:

(i) "The trainee can use specified physiological measurements to derive other physiological data."

(ii) "The trainee can use specified data about a patient to predict drug dosage necessary to produce a specified change in the patient's condition."

Educational problem:

Some trainees taught in our environment with conventional instructional methods do not reach these objectives.

Educational solution:

The problem might be solved by increasing tutorial time for these students. Alternatively computer assisted learning programs explain how calculations and predictions are made, provides factual knowledge, and engages in dialogue with the trainee regarding predictions of pharmacological or physiological change. Drill and practice protocols can be set up to meet a specified educational objective.

The complex pharmacological interactions that occur clinically can be simulated rapidly and, in the same fashion that Mapleson[6] has described sophisticated anaesthetic vapour delivery systems so computer programs can provide planned discussion with the learner about drug uptake distribution and excretion illustrated graphically and numerically. The next stage of learning - or perhaps a parallel instructional procedure - is clinical experience in the operating room.

Another example of an instructional objective is:
"The trainee can inject 4 ml of fluid into the immediate vicinity of a stellate ganglion."

This can be further broken down:

(i) "The trainee can identify the surface markings necessary for performing a stellate ganglion block."

(ii) "The trainee can predict accurately the whereabouts of anatomical structures in the vicinity of the route to the ganglion and the ganglion itself."

Educational problem:

Our trainees do not seem to know all the structures that they should be looking for when they examine skeletons and dissections or when they are getting practical experience doing blocks. Indeed not all the relevant structures are present in laboratory exhibits.

Solution:

Appropriate computer based programs can ensure that the trainee has acquired prerequisite anatomical knowledge before they begin other instructional procedures with faculty examining dissections, discussing video tapes, and clinical experience.

In contrast however there are other important educational objectives and problems for which computer assisted learning does not seem to have a role. For example: teaching a trainee to be consciously aware of every unexpected event during anaesthesia: teaching a trainee to communicate effectively in a verbal fashion regarding patient management with physicians, nurses and aides.

The most obvious objective for a trainee in anaesthesia is that "The trainee can assemble appropriate information about a specified clinical situation; analyse it; and plan management." The educational problem is that some trainees are slow to learn this. The danger of using computer assisted learning rather than skilled tutorials to cope with this problem is that the trainee will merely learn certain patterns to deal with specified situations and not be able to cope with the variety of clinical situations that confront a specialist anaesthetist and which require the application of concepts. The trainee may become a programmed anaesthetist rather than an educated one and less able to participate in verbal case discussions that should be an integral part of his or her professional life. In addition computer based patient management problems in anaesthesia must be elaborately complex if they are to accommodate a variety of management patterns and be representative of professional opinions throughout a large geographic area.[7] A fundamental question regarding relying for instructional purposes on computer based patient management problems is comparison between the importance of restrictions imposed by them compared with the results of conventional instructional procedures performed perfunctorily or for insufficient time.

Medical educators have been interested in computer assisted learning for many years. A recent background report[8] emphasises what are perceived

as positive aspects of applying computer technology to medical education
and assessment but does not discuss the experimental findings presented
or address controversial issues. Under the heading 'Implications' thir-
teen potential changes are listed. These include the development of individual testing for physicians, improved continuing medical education, a
changing role of faculty members, and improved understanding of health
and disease. Another recent review concludes that thoughtful and observ-
ant testing has not tempered the early and uncritical optimism for computer assisted learning in medical education.[9] Publications about its
use in anaesthesia education are few though exhibits at meetings indicate a burgeoning interest in it. A critical question is "Is it better
in practice than existing methods?" Such a question must be preceded by
a careful definition of educational objectives and any associated educational problems. At the present time assessment of the performance of
computer assisted learning in anaesthesia education based on published
material is impossible because these reports[10-14] rarely consider all the
facts relevant to the testing of an instructional device. The situation
apparently has not changed since Campeau[15] stated ".... media research
in post school education has not provided decision makers with practical
valid, dependable guidelines for making instructional technology choices
on the basis of instructional effectiveness", and Staettler[16] remarked
that "The present state of the art does not solve the persistent problem
of instructional design media selection." However, we must be cautious
about assessment regarding anaesthetists based on experience with other
categories of learner. Education in anaesthesia has widely varying fac-
ets and choices of learning method vary from individual to individual.[17]
Similarly we must be cautious about the use of computer programs to test
certain aspects of clinical competence. Computer based education is most

frequently applied to test knowledge and skills in areas in which correct responses do not involve an effective component such as attitudes or preferences.[8] This presumably refers to 'professional opinion'. In an-aesthesia this varies[18] and content and program design for anaesthesia problems for widespread use must have informed input from a wide variety of anaesthesia centers.

In conclusion published data is insufficient to evaluate computer assisted learning in anaesthesiology. However on theoretical grounds there is a useful place for computer assisted learning in anaesthesia ed-ucation. Certain tasks can be delegated to the instrument. The weaker trainee will be helped and for the superior trainee learning will be more time effective. Existing faculty will have more time to devote to other academic interests - in association with trainees if this is appropriate. However, before adopting computer assisted learning as an instructional system the wise educator will carefully analyse his or her educational problems and the available ways of solving them. One of the benefits of the existence of computer assisted learning is that it encourages in-structors to think analytically about their teaching committments.

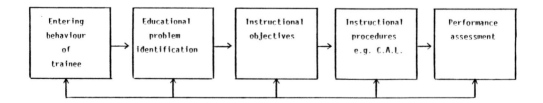

References

1. DeCecco, John P. Psychology and Instructional Technology In Training Research and Education. Robert Glaser, Ed. Univ. of Pittsburgh Press 1962.

2. In: Gustafson, Kent L. Survey of Instructional Development Models. ERIC Clearing House on Information Resources. Syracuse University 1981.

3. Evolution of a Provincial Committee on Anaesthetic and Operative Deaths. Alberta 1952-72. McIntyre, J.W.R., Can. Anaes. Soc. J. 20.578.1973.

4. A formal audit as continuing medical education: anaesthesia for neurosurgery. McIntyre, J.W.R. and Purdell-Lewis, J.G., Can. Anaes. Soc. J. 29.174.1982.

5. Preparing Instructional Objectives. Robert F. Mager, Fearon Publishing Inc., Palo Alto, California, 1962.

6. From Clover to Computer. Mapleson, W.W., Anaesthesia 34.163.1979.

7. Some aspects of computer assisted instruction and evaluation in the practice of anaesthesia. McIntyre, J.W.R., Skakun, E.N. Proc. 3rd Canadian Symposium on Instructional Technology, 1980.

8. Computer Technology in Medical Education and Assessment. Congress of United States, Office of Technology Assessment, Washington, D.C. Library of Congress 79-600146. September 1979.

9. Computer Assisted Learning. Editorial, Lancet 1.293.1980.

10. Computer assisted learning in the teaching of anaesthesia. Kenney, Gavin N.C., Schmulian, Carol. Anaesthesia 34.159.1979.

11. Computer aided instruction as a part of an undergraduate programme in anaesthesia. McIntyre, J.W.R., Can. Anaes. Soc. J. 27.68.1980.

12. The micro computer in self assessment for examinations in anaesthes-
    ia. Parbrook, Geoffrey D., Davis, Paul D., Parbrook, Evelyn O.
    Anaesthesia 36.1136.1981.

13. Evaluation of a computer simulation program for teaching halothane
    uptake and distribution. Heffernan, P.B., Gibbs, J.M., McKinnon,
    A.E. Anaesthesia 37.43.1982.

14. The micro computer in self assessment for examinations. Kenyon, N.G.,
    Newby, D.M., Edbrooke, D.L. Anaesthesia 37.606.1982.

15. Campeau, P.L. Selective Review of the Results of Research on the
    Use of Audio Visual Media to Teach Adults. A.V. Communication
    Review 22, 1 Spring 1974, pp. 5-40.

16. Saettler, Paul. An Assessment of the Current Status of Educational
    Technology. ERIC Clearing House on Information Resources, Syra-
    cuse University 1979.

17. Purkis, I.E. Continuing Medical Education: Learning Preferences of
    Anaesthetists. Can. Anaes. Soc. J. 29.421.1982.

18. Measuring agreement between anaesthetists. Wilson, M.E., Skene,
    A.M. Br. J. Anaesth. 51.61.1979.

TEACHING WITH "ATTENDING": TUTORIAL USE OF AN EXPERT SYSTEM

PERRY L. MILLER M.D., Ph.D., DENISE ANGERS, M.D., J. ROBERT KEEFER, M.D.,
NALIN SUDAN, M.D., GUY TANNER, M.D.

DEPARTMENT OF ANESTHESIOLOGY, YALE UNIVERSITY SCHOOL OF MEDICINE

ABSTRACT

The ATTENDING computer system is being developed to critique a physician's
plan for anesthetic management. Although still under development, the system
is being used experimentally for teaching with hypothetical patients, using
the teaching format of an interactive "mini case conference". In addition to
its educational value, this tutorial use of ATTENDING has the further
advantage of allowing the system's anesthetic knowledge to be tested and
"debugged" while in its formative stages.

1. INTRODUCTION

The ATTENDING computer system (1, 2) is being developed using Artificial
Intelligence techniques to critique a physician's plan of anesthetic
management. This approach to the design of a medical computer-advisor differs
from that taken in other medical systems.

The traditional approach to computer-assisted medical decision-making
involves developing a computer system which simulates a physician's
decision-making process. Such a system gathers information as a physician
would, and then tries to arrive at similar conclusions. From a clinical
standpoint, such a system has the effect of trying to tell a physician what to
do.

The ATTENDING system, in contrast, takes a different approach. This
approach might best be described as "Medical Plan-Analysis" by computer.
Here, instead of trying to tell a physician how to practice medicine, the
system first asks the physician how he proposes to manage his patient. It
then critiques the proposed plan, discussing the risks and benefits of that
plan as compared to reasonable alternatives.

As a result, whereas the traditional computer-advisor tells the physician,
in effect: "This is how I think you should manage your patient.", ATTENDING

says, "This is what I think of your management plan."

There are a number of potential clinical advantages of Medical Plan-Analysis as a modality for medical computer advice. 1) It accommodates the inherent variation of medical practice. 2) It leaves the primary responsibility for formulating patient management with the physician, and allows the computer to play a secondary role, providing feedback to help evaluate and optimize his approach. 3) It casts the computer in the role of an ally, rather than as a potential competitor.

The ATTENDING system is a developmental prototype, still undergoing expansion and refinement. This paper describes how the system is being used experimentally for teaching while still in its formative stages.

2. ARTIFICIAL INTELLIGENCE AND EXPERT SYSTEMS

The ATTENDING system is designed using Artificial Intelligence (AI) techniques. Artificial Intelligence (3) is the science of what might be loosely called "making machines think." In practice this involves trying to make machines behave, respond, or perform tasks in ways which appear to exhibit intelligence. AI techniques have been applied to many problems, including: 1) playing games such as chess, 2) "understanding" written or spoken language, 3) recognizing objects in a visual scene, and 4) performing medical diagnosis.

One recent direction in AI research has been the development of "expert systems" (4). An expert system is a problem-solving system which contains knowledge ("expertise") about a practical, real-world domain. Examples of domains are medicine, computer system design, and geologic analysis. The system's knowledge is usually gathered from one or more human experts, whose problem-solving behavior the system attempts to simulate. Thus an expert system might perform medical diagnosis, design computer systems, or perform geologic analyses, depending upon the domain of its "expertise." Two surveys of medical expert systems are referenced. (5, 6)

3. ATTENDING'S KNOWLEDGE BASE

ATTENDING is an expert system whose domain is anesthetic management. To allow it to critique anesthetic management, ATTENDING has an anesthetic "knowledge base" which guides its analyses. ATTENDING's knowledge base has two components.

1. Knowledge of alternative anesthetic agents and techniques. ATTENDING is designed to critique a central but circumscribed component of anesthetic management: the choice of agents and techniques to be used for premedication, induction, intubation, and maintenance of general or regional anesthesia. ATTENDING's knowledge base currently contains approximately 50 agents and techniques. These include many of the commonly used management alternatives.

2. Knowledge of the anesthetic implications of a patient's medical problems. Each underlying medical problem implies certains risks for a patient's anesthetic management. A given technique may be harmful in the presence of a certain problem, or may be beneficial. In complicated patients with several underlying problems, risk tradeoffs often exist; techniques which are good for one problem may be bad for another, and vice-versa. Thus, to critique anesthetic management, ATTENDING must know the anesthetic implications of each underlying medical problem. In particular, ATTENDING must know the risks or benefits of each agent and technique in the presence of that problem. ATTENDING currently contains this information for 25 problems. This constitutes the system's major present knowledge limitation.

4. CONSULTATION VS. TEACHING

The ATTENDING system can be used in two ways: for consultation and for teaching.

Consultation: Here an anesthetist describes an arbitrary patient, together with a proposed management plan, for the system to critique. To be able to do this, ATTENDING must be familiar with all the patient's medical problems. As a result, this consultative use of ATTENDING is restricted by the modest number of medical problems presently known to the system.

Teaching: Despite ATTENDING's current knowledge limitations, the system can still be used for teaching with a variety of challenging patients. The 25 problems known to ATTENDING include a good number of the most important, common, interesting problems, and by combining these in different ways, many interesting risk tradeoffs can be explored. Thus, the system can be used productively as a teaching tool while its knowledge base is still under development.

5. THREE TEACHING MODES

ATTENDING can be used for teaching in three modes. Each mode has certain advantages and allows certain types of management issues to be explored. In all three modes, a short paragraph describing a patient is first presented by ATTENDING, as illustrated in the Appendix.

"BEST PLAN" mode: Here an anesthesia resident is asked to propose a reasonable plan for ATTENDING to critique. This mode can help explore interesting management issues in both common and uncommon diseases. If, however, a standard anesthetic approach is satisfactory (such as thiopental, succinylcholine, ethrane, nitrous), certain interesting management issues may frequently not be confronted in this mode.

"CRITIQUE" mode: Here ATTENDING presents the resident with a proposed plan containing management errors. The resident is asked to critique that plan himself, and then compare his critique with ATTENDING's. This mode can help explore the anesthetic implictions of less commonly used techniques, as well as specific management features of particular diseases.

"WORST PLAN" mode: Here the resident is asked to propose a deliberately poor plan. He then lists the errors he perceives and compares this list to ATTENDING's analysis. This mode is useful from two standpoints: 1) It serves to test and "debug" the system's knowledge. 2) It allows the resident free rein in exercising his knowledge of the risks and benefits of different approaches to the patient's management.

Using these three modes, interesting anesthetic management issues can be explored in an interactive fashion. A resident can gain experience in formulating his anesthetic approach to complicated patients, and at the same time receive feedback to help him evaluate his approach.

6. INTERACTIVE "MINI CASE CONFERENCES"

In experimenting with ATTENDING as a teaching tool, we have found it useful to provide an organized structure for the teaching sessions. One way to do this is to create teaching modules, each structured around a theme.

For instance, the Appendix shows part of a teaching session structured around the theme of "emergency inductions." Here the computer first introduces the topic by discussing certain important issues. Then three interesting patients are described in turn, and the resident is asked to propose a plan for each (in either BEST PLAN or WORST PLAN mode) or to critique a plan outlined by the computer (CRITIQUE mode). Finally, the computer types out a few questions for the resident to think about.

In this fashion, an interactive tutorial session with ATTENDING is organized around a clinical theme, using the format of a "mini case conference" in which the management implications of several interesting patients are explored.

7. SUMMARY

The ATTENDING project is a major undertaking as, indeed, is the development of most expert systems. An ultimate goal is a system which could be used for consultation with a fairly broad range of patients. There are, however, productive milestones which can be achieved short of this eventual goal. One of these is tutorial use of the system while its knowledge base is still modest in size.

Tutorial use of ATTENDING serves several functions. First, it can be of educational value. Also, it can help to exercise, test, and "debug" the system's knowledge base in its formative stages.

In addition, it is anticipated that Medical Plan-Analysis, ATTENDING's approach to computer-assisted medical decision-making, can be productively extended to many other areas of medical management. Experimental use of the system for teaching can provide practical experience with the approach, and thereby give insight as to domains where the approach might most profitably be applied, and as to the type of advice such a system might most usefully provide.

REFERENCES
1. Miller PL. 1983, in press. Critiquing anesthetic management: The "ATTENDING" computer system. Anesthesiology.
2. Miller PL. 1983, in press. ATTENDING: Critiquing a physician's management plan. IEEE Trans. PAMI.
3. Winston PH. 1977. Artificial Intelligence. Reading: Addison-Wesley.
4. Davis R. 1982. Expert Systems: Where are we? And where do we go from here? The AI Magazine 3:3-22.
5. Kulikowski C. 1980. Artificial intelligence methods and systems for medical consultation. IEEE Trans. PAMI, PAMI-2:464-476.

6. Shortliffe EH: Buchanan BG, Feigenbaum EA. 1979. Knowledge engineering for medical decision making. A review of computer-based clinical decision aids. Proc. IEEE 67:1207-1224.

APPENDIX

TEACHING WITH ATTENDING: A SAMPLE "MINI CASE CONFERENCE"

This Appendix shows part of a sample teaching session, and illustrates the "mini case conference" format that can be used. In this example, responses typed by the resident are underlined. Comments inserted to explain features of the session are enclosed in brackets.

Welcome to the ATTENDING system.

Please answer by typing numbers on a single line:
    COMMAS or SPACES may separate the numbers.

PLEASE SELECT A TEACHING MODULE:
1.   EMERGENCY INDUCTIONS
2.   INCREASED ICP
3.   AIRWAY PROBLEMS
TYPE 0 TO QUIT

*** TYPE ONE ***1

[First, ATTENDING introduces itself and asks which of three teaching modules the resident would like to use. In this case, the module entitled "emergency inductions" has been chosen. Next the system types out a brief discussion of emergency induction of anesthesia, and then describes the first of three hypothetical patients.]

EMERGENCY INDUCTIONS

Induction of anesthesia for emergency surgery can be fraught with many risks depending on the acute situation and on the patient's underlying medical problems. In planning an induction for an emergency case, two considerations are particularly important:

1. the possibility of a full stomach,

2. the patient's volume status.

The interaction of these two central considerations with a patient's other problems can lead to a host of potential risks and risk trade-offs. At times the optimal anesthetic approach to one problem may also be beneficial for another, but often it is not.

case 1: Here a particular agent can be beneficial for two problems.

- PATIENT HISTORY -

A thirty four year old male with a history of asthma requiring several past hospitalizations comes to surgery after an auto accident for repair of a likely fractured spleen. His blood pressure is 90/50. He ate dinner earlier in the evening.

[Next the resident proposes a plan for this patient's management. This is the "BEST PLAN" mode.]

- PLEASE OUTLINE A PLAN -

PREMED: 1-NONE   2-ATROPINE   3- GLYCOPYRROLATE   4-MORPHINE
5-DEMEROL   6-FENTANYL   7-VALIUM   8-PENTOBARBITAL   9-SECONAL
10-VISTARIL   11-DROPERIDOL   12-PHENERGAN

```
*** TYPE ONE OR MORE ***7

*** TYPE 1 IF GENERAL ... 2 IF REGIONAL *** 1

    INDUCTION:  1-THIOPENTAL  2-KETAMINE  3-HALOTHANE  4-ENFLURANE
*** TYPE ONE *** 2

    INTUBATION:  1-NONE  2-CONVENTIONAL  3-RAPIDSEQ  4-AWAKE_ORAL
    5-AWAKE_NASAL  6-MASKCRICOID  7-SUCCINYLCHOLINE  8-CURARE
    9-PANCURONIUM  10-FLAXEDIL  11-METOCURINE
*** TYPE ONE OR MORE *** 3,7

    MAINTENANCE:  1-HALOTHANE  2-ENFLURANE  3-N2O  4-O2  5-MORPHINE
    6-DEMEROL  7-FENTANYL  8-CURARE  9-PANCURONIUM
    10-FLAXEDIL  11-METOCURINE
*** TYPE ONE OR MORE *** 1,3,4,9

- YOU HAVE SELECTED -
    1 GENERAL
    2 PREMED - (VALIUM)
    3 INDUCTION - (KETAMINE)
    4 INTUBATION - (RAPIDSEQ SUCCINYLCHOLINE)
    5 MAINTENANCE - (HALOTHANE N2O O2 PANCURONIUM)
*** TYPE  0 IF OK ... ELSE NUMBER FOR CHANGE ***0
```

[ATTENDING critiques this plan as shown below.]

There are a number of basic principles involved in this patient's management. First, a patient with asthma must be protected from bronchospasm. Second, in the presence of hypovolemia, one must attempt to prevent hypotension. Third, in a patient with a full stomach, one must consider the problem of aspiration.

Intubation of this patient is certainly necessary because of a full stomach. Rapid sequence intubation is a reasonable approach. This, however, could have the conceivable risk of bronchospasm. An alternative approach to rapid sequence intubation would be intubation after mask induction with cricoid pressure.

In regard to maintenance, inhalational technique has the advantage of preventing bronchospasm by keeping the anesthetic level deep. On the other hand, it involves the risk of hypotension in the presence of hypovolemia. An alternative approach to inhalational technique would be balanced anesthesia. This might have the risk of possible bronchospasm due to light anesthesia. It does, however, have the advantage of maintaining blood pressure.

Looking at other aspects of the proposed plan, for a patient with asthma, induction with ketamine has the advantage of suppressing bronchospasm since ketamine is a bronchodilator. Also, in the presence of hypovolemia, induction with ketamine has the advantage of helping avoid hypotension since ketamine is supportive of blood pressure.

[This concludes ATTENDING's critique of the first teaching case. Next two more cases are explored using one or another of the system's teaching modes. Finally a short series of questions are typed out for the resident to think about, involving the mechanisms and clinical use of ketamine and of thiopental. Once this is done, the "emergency induction" teaching module is finished, and the resident is given the option of choosing a different module if he wishes.]

INTRODUCTORY COURSES IN COMPUTING FOR ANAESTHETISTS

J.H. KERR, B.J. HARRISON and W.L. DAVIES,
Nuffield Department of Anaesthetics,
John Radcliffe Hospital, Oxford, England.

The remarkable reduction in the real cost of computing power seen in the last 5 years or so has upset earlier cost/benefit evaluations and made it necessary to re-examine the role of the computer within the hospital. Tasks which would previously have been prohibitively expensive are now worth considering because of the availability of cheap, flexible and ever more powerful micro-processors. These expanding possibilities have lead to a widespread demand for computing expertise particularly among established clinicians.

In 1978, the Nuffield Department of Anaesthetics appointed an electronic engineer who was experienced in the design of equipment using microprocessors. At that time there was one desktop calculator in use in the department and no direct link to the University mainframe computer. Since then, there has been a rapid increase in the number of microprocessors and microcomputers and early in 1983 there were 3 mainframe terminals and 34 active microprocessor systems. These range from a dedicated wordprocessor primarily for secretarial use to embedded microprocessors monitoring and controlling blood gas electrodes and infusions of analgesics and anaesthetics. Since the late 1960's, the research interests of the department had been such that a statistician had been employed part-time who mainly used the large University computers. In 1979, a full time computing and statistics assistant was appointed who was interested in the use of small computers.

In 1981, because of the availability of this expertise in both hardware and software and of practical experience gained in the application of computers within anaesthesia, the authors (a clinician with computing interests, the programmer and the electronic engineer) decided to organise an introductory course in computing. It was hoped to attract fairly senior anaesthetists (Consultants and Senior Registrars) principally from smaller district hospitals who might be considering whether to acquire a computer for departmental use.

This paper describes the structure of the first two courses held in 1981 & 2 together with the immediate reactions of the students and the longer term effects on their computing activities.

AIMS

The aims of the course were to provide an introduction to (a) a range of microcomputer applications within an anaesthetic department, (b) running a microcomputer system and (c) programming [in BASIC]. At the end of the course it was hoped that the students would be able to estimate the approximate time and costs involved in a particular application.

It was felt necessary to have a minimum of a one-week residential course to allow sufficient time to achieve these aims. The course would consist of a mixture of lectures, demonstrations and practical sessions. The approach was to be essentially non-technical, but the necessary technical aspects of computing would be approached from the clinical and research viewpoints. The number of participants was limited to 24 because the planning group felt it was vital to allow all those attending to have a reasonable amount of hands-on experience.

INSTRUCTORS & STUDENTS

Lecturers on the courses included academic and commercial computer professionals and electronic engineers and clinicians from Oxford and elsewhere. Demonstrators at the practical sessions were drawn from departmental scientific staff.

Students were anaesthetic consultants and senior registrars from teaching and district hospitals throughout the United Kingdom. On each of the courses most of the students were district hospital consultants (29/47), a few came from teaching hospitals (7/47) and the remainder were senior registrars (11/47). Each year there was a 'waiting list' of applicants for whom there was no space on the course.

COURSE STRUCTURE

Before arriving in Oxford, course members were sent and asked to read a simple introductory text called "The Computer - How it works" (David Carey, Ladybird Books). An introduction to the course over an informal supper on Sunday evening enabled a prompt start to be made on Monday.

Introduction.

The first morning was devoted to a general overview of computing, illustrated with demonstrations of text, graphics and sound using a personal microcomputer. This gentle introduction was followed by a lecture on methods of communicating with the machine leading to the concept of a computer language. After coffee, the manager of the Medical School Data Centre described mainframe computers and minicomputers. He referred to the services provided at the Data Centre and took the course on a visit to it.

The afternoon was occupied with an introduction to the practical sessions and will be discussed in more detail later.

On Tuesday morning, the first lectures and demonstrations on various Applications of computers to clinical and research problems were given. These were structured so that the application was considered first and then a discussion of the relevant computer technique followed (Table 1).The concept of a software "package" was introduced and it was stressed that most computer users were likely to spend much of their time using such programs. On-line information processing was demonstrated as was the ability of a computer to control equipment. The sessions included a good deal of valuable commercial participation, both from clinical equipment manufacturers who utilise computers in their instruments (e.g. Oxford Computer Systems) and from microcomputer manufacturers and distributors who have been extremely helpful in supporting the course by loaning computers and providing literature (e.g. Research Machines Ltd.).

Practical, Technical and Clinical Sessions.

For three sessions, the course was divided into three groups of 8 persons. In each period one group obtained hands-on experience, the second group were shown and discussed various computer applications on-site in the Intensive Therapy Unit (ITU), and the third group went a little further into some aspects of computer hardware. On each of the first three evenings (Monday to Wednesday), one group were allowed a further hands-on session. The duration of this session was greatly increased from one hour in the first course to an extended 3 hour session (until 21.00) on the second course, in response to the apparently insatiable appetite for "hands-on" experience. Each year approximately one third of the participants admitted to some previous computing experience (ranging from programmable calculators to mainframe computers) and they were allocated to the group which had their first hands-on session on the Monday evening.

TABLE I. Lecture and demonstration topics

Year	Subject	Computing Aspect	Type
1981	Pain relief studies Pharmacodynamic calculations	Data crunching, statistical packages	Lecture
	Mass spectrometry	On-line processing.	Demonstration
	Unibed-patient monitoring system. (Oxford Medical Systems)	"Embedded" Microprocessor software controlled monitoring.	Demonstration
	The 'Mac' physiological simulations.	Modelling.	Lecture.
	Predicting anaesthetic problems.	Specialised use of data-base.	Lecture & demo.
	Controlling anaesthesia.	Systems engineering.	Lecture & demo.
	Controlling intracranial pressure.	" " "	Lecture.
	Looking ahead.	Possible hardware developments.	Lecture & demo.
1982	"Problems in the data jungle", pharmacological studies.	Statistical packages. Number crunching Modelling	Lecture.
	Multifunction electrodes.	On-line processing and control.	Lecture & demo.
	Mass spectrometry	On-line processing.	" "
	Gas mixing valves	Embedded microprocessor.	" "
	"Looking ahead"	Computer system and interface developments	Lecture & demo.
	Teaching programs for anaesthetic self-assessment.	Software package.	Lecture.
	ITU data collection and information. Teaching programs for nurses.	Software packaging – importance of user friendliness. Data collection and use.	Lecture & demo.

Practical Experience

The aims of these sessions were 1) to overcome the fear of interacting with the computer, 2) to demonstrate the principal ideas of problem solving via programming, 3) to relate these ideas to a particular programming language (BASIC), and 4) to help students write simple programs

The Monday afternoon session called "Getting to Grips with the computer" was aimed at dealing with the first two aims. The format was essentially the same in both courses, when the first part of the afternoon was spent demonstrating the operation of the microcomputer. This was followed by a quick run through of some computer commands, mainly to illustrate the sort of responses that the computer makes, and what happens when mistakes are made. It was noticeable that many students still felt that typing errors somehow 'broke' the computer!

The second half of the session was devoted to problem solving. Simple problems, for example converting Fahrenheit to Centigrade, were analysed in guided class discussion, and broken down into logical steps. Most beginners found difficulty in understanding the amount of analysis needed for even the most simple and straightforward of programs. Towards the end of the afternoon the discussion returned to the expression of the problem in a computer language. The problems analysed previously were translated from their component steps into BASIC and typed into the computer. The need for precision was demonstrated and the program was run after the necessary syntax corrections had been made.

At the end of this session, each student was given information leaflets about how to operate the microcomputer and the simpler BASIC commands and syntax rules, plus a book ('Computing Using BASIC: an interactive approach' by Tonia Cope, published by Ellis Horwood, Chichester. 1981) to help them in the practical sessions later in the week. They were also given a sheet of problems in an increasing order of complexity with hints which either pointed to a new command in BASIC, or explained a programming technique that the user might find helpful.

The "Hands-On" sessions on Tuesdays and Wednesdays were informal. In 1981 there were 4 computers so each group was divided into 4 pairs, but the immediate feed-back from this course indicated that this arrangement was unsatisfactory. In 1982, 8 computers were available in a Local Area Network so that each course member was able to work separately.

The problem sheets were intended only as guidelines and several students brought specific problems to tackle. Some of these were enormous projects and the participant's ambition had to be restrained, but usually it was possible to select aspects of these ideas which were simple enough for a beginner to tackle, but sufficient to give them an idea of the work involved. At each session there were 3 or 4 demonstrators present who were experienced BASIC programmers to assist students on a one-to-one basis. This arrangement allowed everyone to work at their own speed and while some students were able to work happily on their own, others found the concepts harder to grasp and needed more help.

In 1982 the timetable was rearranged to allow a second 3 hour session for each group during an(other) evening. The full BASIC manuals were made available, and several people experimented with the uses of some more obscure commands, especially those for colour graphics while others tried their hands at word processing.

ITU Sessions. Since computers have been used widely and for a relatively long time in Intensive Care, several students had come on the course hoping to apply computer techniques within their units. During the session in the ITU four microprocessor applications were demonstrated. Most of these were based on a microcomputer located in a small room off the unit which was linked to an intelligent terminal placed between two of the beds. Students were divided between the computer room and the ITU proper and each sub-group of 4 was accompanied by a clinician who demonstrated and discussed the applications displayed in each location.

The sub-group in the ward were first shown the enhanced capabilities of equipment within which microprocessors were embedded (Patient monitors and balloon pump). Most of the time, however, was spent "playing with" an on-line system for the collection, manipulation, storage and display of fluid balance data. The system had been designed to allow nursing staff to enter information about the patient's fluid intake and output via a modified (splash-proofed and simplified) keyboard situated close to the bed. Students were encouraged to experiment with the entry procedure and then to examine and comment upon the updated information displays. Features intended to improve the "friendliness" of the system (e.g. the use of machine-code routines to generate displays quickly) and factors which had adversely affected the system's acceptability (e.g. the hospital engineers' habit of testing the mains emergency back-up without warning!) were pointed out and discussed.

While in the computer room, students were shown the unit's statistical

data-base and its development was described from edge-punched cards, through
forms which were batch processed on a remote main-frame computer, to the
current system which involved entry, updating and storage of information upon
the Unit's microcomputer. After often lively discussion, the suite of programs
developed to aid clinical activities within the Unit were demonstrated. These
included programs for deriving the usual physiological indices (Riley analysis,
renal function tests), for calculating drug dilutions in infusions, and for
exploring pathophysiological behaviour (e.g. the effect of changing haemoglobin
concentration on arterial oxygenation). Print-outs of these programs proved
extremely popular.

Technical Aspects

In these sessions an attempt was made to improve the students'
understanding of the internal workings of a computer. While it was accepted
that most anaesthetists will not require a detailed knowledge of electronics,
it was hoped that some insight into the general structure and organisation of
computers would prove useful in certain applications.

Most clinicians are familiar with analogue electrical signals, so this
was used as the starting point. It was explained that it is necessary to
convert physiological and other data to a digital form to allow the information
to be handled by the common (digital) computer, which only works with binary
numbers. This was followed by an description of the organisation of the memory
"pigeon-holes" and the internal architecture of the computer. The operation of
storing and moving information between registers and memory showed the use of a
logical rule and a similar rule for the addition of binary numbers was
demonstrated. Each logical rule was presented to the computer by a code word,
or machine code instruction and sequences of these instructions were combined
to represent more complex actions and so developed into higher level languages.
In this way, the concepts involved in compilers and interpreters were
approached.

In the first course, the students' reactions indicated that too much
technical detail was presented despite the use of laymans' terms. The emphasis
in the second year was moved further towards clinical aspects. The interfacing
of a microcomputer with a digital syringe pump to control and record the
infusion of an analgesic) was discussed and demonstrated in the presence of a
computer-naive clinician who had used the equipment on the ward. She explained
the clinical aspects of the project and provided valuable comment on the

problems she had encountered, stressing the need to present a "friendly" interface to clinical users. This application was also used to introduce the need for comprehensive and effective safety devices. Students were given graphic warnings about the hazards of knob-twiddling or key-pressingbystanders and of environmental conditions (e.g. transients in the power supply, plaster dust in the disc drives!). At the end of the session, students were encouraged to examine and handle loose microprocessor chips and floppy disks removed from their protective covering and rules for the correct treatment of computing equipment re-inforced.

More applications - clinical and non-clinical.

On the Thursday morning in 1981 a further series of lecture /demonstrations with outside speakers was organised with the aim of presenting a wider range of applications (see Table I) and of computing techniques such as modelling and data collection and handling. In the second course the morning was utilised to consider languages in more depth and to allow a fairly lengthy hands-on session (shared keyboards) working with a word processing package. Coffee was followed by a demonstration and discussion about likely computing developments, particularly in the field of interfacing equipment.

On Thursday afternoon, participants were given a break from computing and taken on a very popular conducted tour of some of the older Oxford Colleges. At 5.30 a Guest Lecture was arranged which was opened to any other interested members of the Department. In 1981 Mr David Price lectured on "Closing the loop", describing his experiences in neurosurgical intensive care and in devising a system to control intracranial pressure. In 1982 Dr Gavin Kenny described the development and use of a set of teaching programs for self assessment and discussed data collection within the ICU. After the guest lecture there was a formal dinner in one of the College Halls which was attended by everyone who had been connected with the course. Discussion was notably technical and went on long into the night!

Course Review and Discussion.

On Friday (after a slightly later start!), a further Guest Lecture was followed by a panel discussion. The panel was made up of guest lecturers and other clinical users, academic and commercial computer professionals, and the course organisers and it considered questions put by the students. The organisers hoped that the discussions generated would help students understand unresolved problems and give them an opportunity to raise matters which were of particular importance to them. Most of the questions related to the choice of hardware and software, and a number of people wanted a simple answer to the question: "What computer should I buy?". However, by the end of the morning, it was hoped that most people would recognise that the variety of factors relevant to such a decision made it impossible to give one common answer.

Over coffee and after lunch a small microcomputer show was mounted at which as many different types of microcomputer as possible were set up and demonstrated (table II). Course participants were encouraged to try as many types as possible. At least one user familiar with each microcomputer was present throughout to guide course members (and load the games!).

TABLE II. Microcomputer types demonstrated at Computer Shows.

1981	1982 (as 1981 plus the following)
Research Machines 380Z	Altos 3 user with 5 Mbyte disk
Nascom 2 and 3	Merlin
Sinclair ZX80	Dragon
Compukit 101	Osbourne 1
PET	Sinclair Spectrum
Sharp Pocket Computer	Sinclair ZX81
	BBC 'B' microcomputer
	Superbrain
	Sharp MZ80B
	Apple II
	Research Machines 480Z
	Commodore VIC
	Hewlett Packard 97
	Wang (circa 1948)
	Brunsveiga (circa 1937)

ASSESSMENT

Immediate. On the final day, course members were asked to complete a short questionnaire to help the organisers improve any subsequent course. Twenty of the twenty three students returned the form in 1981 and all twenty four in 1982. After some organisational questions, they were asked to indicate whether they felt that the time allotted to different types of session (lectures, demonstrations and hands-on) was too little, too much or about right. Results, with the actual number of hours, are indicated in Table III.

TABLE III. Immediate reactions to course structure.

R E S P O N S E
(> = too much time. < = too little time.)

	1981 (19 replies)				1982 (24 replies)			
	Hours	OK	>	<	Hours	OK	>	<
Lectures	11	13	6	1	10	21	1	2
Demonstrations	12	11	5	4	12	17	4	4
Hands-On	4.5*	4	-	15	9**	19	-	5

* 1 keyboard/2 students.   ** 1 keyboard/student

In 1981, 15/20 gave a negative answer to the question "Do you think you were adequately prepared before being let loose on the computers?", indicating that it was necessary to spend more time developing the pre-course literature, and to slow down the pace of the introductory sessions. In 1982 the number of negative replies had fallen to 9/24 suggesting that these problems had been partly solved although there was still room for improvement. The answers to other questions, and our responses to them, have been referred to earlier in the paper.

Table IV. Current and projected computing activities of former course members.(36 replies)

APPLICATION	ACTIVE	PROJECTED
Record keeping *	13	6
Word processing	11	2
Computer assisted teaching	10	1
Calculations and statistics	9	1
Intensive Care	3	1
Research	3	
Teaching own children	3	
Control of equipment	2	
Patient management	2	
Departmental rotas		4
Theatre anaesthetic records		2

* includes reference catalogues, junior staff experience register, equipment inventory, pain clinic records.

Longer term follow-up.

Further questionnaires were sent out to all students about a year after the first course, and six months after the second. It was hoped to gain information about whether their computing activities had been influenced by the course and about their current areas of interest and progress. The response was good, with 17 replies coming from the 1981 course and 19 from 1982. From these it was seen that about half of 1981 respondents, and more than 3/4 of those from 1982 now have access to a computer at work or at home and that most had been involved in the purchasing process. Quite a number of those without computers pointed out that it was lack of funding rather then lack of interest that was holding them back. Others stated that the rapid rate of development in hardware had persuaded them that things would only get better and cheaper if they waited. A wide range of activities, both current and proposed, were reported (Table IV). A major cause for concern was the time taken to develop software, especially as the students were having to learn more advanced programming techniques as they went along.

DISCUSSION

With the widespread availability of small computers and the plethora of introductory computing books, it may be argued that it is unnecessary to offer introductory courses to anaesthetists. Responses from the two courses have been emphatically positive (18/23 in 1981 and 23/24 in 1982) when asked if we should run further courses of this type, and there have been requests from within and without the Department that we should provide something similar for clinicians working in Oxford. When students were challenged to explain why they could not have achieved the same result in terms of computing expertise by themselves, several asserted that the most important factor was being isolated from their normal responsibilities and thus being able to concentrate on the subject for prolonged periods without distractions. Others had clearly gained confidence both from the closely supervised formal teaching and from the sight of other beginners experiencing the same problems as themselves. It has been striking how hesitant beginners to computing have been to start operating the micro and how slowly the inexperienced have taken to programming. Regular users (even if using a 'black box' approach themselves!) must be restrained from the temptation to rush the initial introductory stages.

Students now seem to have greater awareness of the time required to develop software and of the non-interchangeability of programs between machines. It is obviously sensible to promote schemes through which clinically relevant programs may be advertised and encouraging to see recent developments to this end (e.g. The Intensive Care Society's Computer Group and the program register in Anaesthesia).

THE USE OF COMPUTER-GENERATED NUMBERS IN INTERPRETING THE EEG

N. TY SMITH
IRA J. RAMPIL

INTRODUCTION

The EEG holds great promise as a monitor in the operating room, particularly for estimating the depth of anesthesia and detecting the presence of cerebral ischemia. This promise has not yet been realized, however. The main obstacle to the realization of these goals has been the raw EEG itself. The tracing is difficult to interpret without considerable training. Only a few seconds of raw EEG are available for inspection at any one time, making it difficult to follow trends. The standard written EEG record during a case is voluminous, being generated at the rate of up to 300-600 pages per hour. For these and other reasons, additional personnel are usually required if one wishes to record the conventional EEG in the operating room.

Several attempts have been made to overcome these obstacles to the routine use of the EEG in the operating room. In general, these attempts have used computerized techniques to transform and compress one pattern, the raw EEG, from its original squiggles to another, more readable, compact pattern. (In this compression some - ideally mostly redundant - information is lost.) Most of the analysis techniques popular in anesthesia today explore the amplitude and frequency aspects of the EEG waveform, ignoring other characteristics such as waveshapes, and correlations between signals from different anatomical sites. The major types of compressed displays have been the amplitude analysis (Cerebral Function Monitor, CFM), compressed spectral array (CSA), the density modulated spectral array (DSA), aperiodic analysis (the Neurometrics EEG Monitor), and zero-crossing analysis (the Klein Analyzer).

Although even ostensibly complex patterns, such as those presented by the aperiodic display or by some spectral displays, can be easily learned by the anesthetist, a quantitative description of patient condition, given the present level of development in the use of computers, is best dealt with by using discrete numbers, analogous to blood pressure or heart rate. Fortunately, these numbers can be extracted through the same computational techniques that produce the patterns. As a matter of fact, the history of EEG analysis is replete with examples of attempts to extract single numbers or sets of numbers from the EEG. Many of the resulting techniques have been developed by engineers for neuroscientists. A surprising number, however, have been developed primarily for monitoring the anesthetized patient.

It is the purpose of this paper to outline some of the numbers which have been extracted from the EEG; to describe

how they have been derived; to relate them to other, more
familiar, physiologic numbers; to discuss how they have been
applied to monitoring or to a better understanding of anesthetic
agents; to bring this information into perspective; and to
anticipate what the future holds - or what we feel it should
hold.

SOME NUMBERS OF INTEREST
    Cerebral Function Monitor. One of the early attempts to
compress the EEG for monitoring purposes occurred in 1969,
when Maynard[1] described a device which evolved into
the commercially available Cerebral Function Monitor (CFM). The
original device displayed a single EEG parameter derived from a
single channel of raw EEG, via a rather complex sequence of
filtering, logarithmic range compression and rectification. The
predominant filter had a rising slope over the pass band, thus
emphasizing the higher frequency activity to a certain extent.
Another way of explaining this filtering process is to say that
the device produces an output which is the product of the predominant amplitude and power over the pass band (2 - 12 Hz).
There have been anecdotal reports on the use of the original
device over a wide range of applications in anesthesia, neurology,
and intensive care.[2] Unfortunately, the mapping from
EEG to CFM output in the original device was not unique, and
the device could not easily distinguish between mid frequency
low-amplitude signals and low-frequency high-amplitude signals.
Moreover, the device was relatively insensitive to frequencies
from 16 - 32 Hz and above, which are of considerable interest
for monitoring. Recently, a variant of the CFM device has been
introduced. This new CFM separates out the amplitude and mean
frequency (a zero crossing frequency, see below) and displays
each value on both an instantaneous and a trended basis. The
device appears to be somewhat less sensitive to ischemic changes
than either CSA or DSA. As noted below, Grundy et al[3,4]
using paired CFM's (one for each hemisphere) found that
the devices missed three episodes of cerebral ischemia in a
series of 34 carotid endarterectomies. This agrees with our
experience. In a preliminary series of 10 carotid endarterectomies simultaneously monitored with CFM, CSA, and DSA, each
using comparable electrodes, the CFM failed to demonstrate an
appreciable change in its readings during the two ischemic EEG
changes noted in the series, each clearly demonstrated by both
spectral displays (Rampil IJ: unpublished data). A large controlled study of the clinical utility of this new device has
not yet been reported.
    Analog filters. Another early attempt to extract numbers
from the frequency content of the EEG for monitoring during
anesthesia occurred in 1970, in the laboratories of Lopes da
Silva,[5] We used a bank of 20 analog band-pass filters,
with band widths of 1 or 2 Hz. The output of these filters
was averaged for 1 minute on a computer of average
transients. The resulting histogram was, in a way, a pattern,
which changed with changes in halothane concentration. To
simplify and quantify the output for comparison with anesthetic
concentration, we used the outputs of individual filters, for

example the 20 Hz filter output voltage, or the outputs of different combinations of filters, for example, the sum of the outputs of the 2 and 3 Hz filters. There was a linear relation between the end-expired concentration and the 20 Hz or 2+3 Hz outputs. Changes in concentration of as little as 0.5% were easily detected with these numbers. If the inspired halothane concentration was changed in a sinusoidal fashion, the changes in these numbers resembled a sinusoidal pattern. Thus the numbers seemed to reflect halothane concentration in the brain. The major problem with the technique, however, was that each new set of numbers was available only every minute. It was apparent that the numbers changed much faster than that.

The Klein Analysis. Another technique, which displays numbers alone, was developed by Klein,[6,7] who uses a zero-crossing technique. The zero-crossing technique counts the number of times the EEG crosses the isoelectric (zero-voltage) line in a given time period, giving an estimate of the mean frequency of the EEG, called the zero-cross frequency (ZXF). The Klein analysis displays the ZXF along with a measure of the average EEG amplitude, the mean rectified voltage (MRV). The third number of the basic, three-number display is the spontaneous EMG activity (see below), derived as the rectified output of a bandpass filter centered at 100 Hz. Klein has also differentiated the raw EEG signal twice and derived a ZXF and MRV each from the first and second derivatives to generate four additional numbers for a more elaborate display. With this many numbers (seven), it is difficult to say whether one has a set of numbers or a pattern. Each of these numbers can be easily displayed, observed and used individually, however, or used in any size combination.

Levy et al[8] have pointed out theoretical disadvantages to the zero-crossing technique: it is mathematically appropriate only in the case of narrow bandwidth signals, which the EEG generally is not. Furthermore, in practical terms it is excessively sensitive to minor changes in the EEG, and the ZXF that is generated by an EEG is not uniquely related to that EEG, that is, widely different EEG waveforms produce the same ZXF. Yet it seems to work. Harmel et al[9] have reported on its extensive use in many situations with many different anesthetic agents. It has given them information useful for the care of patients. We have examined its use with pure morphine, fentanyl, or sufentanil in O_2[10] and with alfentanil or thiopental as induction agents.[11] In each situation, one can see changes in the numbers which seem to reflect changes in brain concentrations of the agents. Recently, Klein and Davis studied depth of anesthesia with the predictive accuracy of the ZXF ranging from 60 - 97% for halothane and 53 - 97% for enflurane.[7]

Median power frequency (MPF). The median power frequency (MPF) is defined as the frequency which divides the spectral histogram into two equal areas. In other words, the MPF is the frequency above which one half the EEG power resides, and below which the other half resides. It is computed using a power spectrum obtained from a fast Fourier transform of the raw EEG data.

We have explored the MPF over the past several years. As with so many numbers, it has demonstrated itself particularly useful with halothane. Step, pulse, and sinusoidal changes in inspired halothane concentration produce very rapid, appropriate changes in MPF. The rapid changes are detectable because we re-compute the MPF every 4 seconds. The higher the frequency of the sine wave, however, the less capable is the EEG, as reflected by the MPF, of following changes in anesthetic concentration.(Fig.1) Thus a frequency-response curve shows decreasing MPF response amplitude with increasing frequency. This low pass filter effect may be due as much to the inability of the ventilating equipment to produce very rapid changes in anesthetic concentration, as to an intrinsic inability of the brain and the circulation to response to the rapid changes which are delivered. The MPF is very sensitive to changes in the high-amplitude, low-frequency range particularly when there are several simultaneous bands of EEG activity. Therefore, to allow the MPF to focus on the relevant frequency band with halothane, we usually filter out the information below 4 Hz.

We have also compared the EEG effects of thiopental and Althesin, using the DSA and the MPF.[1,2] These techniques indicate that Althesin is slower in both onset and decay. The latter was determined by calculating the mean rate of decay of the MPF.

Peak power frequency. The peak power frequency (PPF) is the frequency which contains the most energy during a given epoch. In a statistical sense, it is a modal distribution. As with so many other numbers, with halothane there is a good linear relation between end-expired concentration and the PPF. We have examined this relation and developed the regression equation:

$$PPF = -2.8[H]_A + 13.4 \quad (r=0.9)$$

This equation implies that given the value of the PPF, one should be able to predict the alveolar concentration of halothane. This is true, within an error of about ± 0.2 vol%. In addition, we have developed equations showing that changes in CO_2 or the passage of time can change PPF independently of halothane concentration. The first equation states that PPF increases by 0.1 Hz for every torr increase in $P_A CO_2$. It is not clear whether these changes represent true changes in anesthetic depth, although CO_2 can influence MAC. The second equation states that PPF increases by 0.2 Hz for every MAC-hour. This is consistent with the fact that in man, anesthetic depth, as reflected by the cardiovascular system, lightens with time.[13]

The PPF for enflurane or isoflurane is not as useful as that for halothane, since the slope of PPF vs. end-expired concentration is so steep. There are interesting relationships between the PPF's of four anesthetic ethers, however. The concentration vs. PPF curve moves progressively further to the right for diethyl ether, fluroxene, enflurane, and isoflurane. This sequence is the same as that of increasing sensitivity to seizures and of decreasing basicity of the ether oxygen. The latter phenomenon is caused by the presence of fluorine, which withdraws electrons from the oxygen, thus making the oxygen less basic and making the compound behave less like an ether. Thus, the closer the fluorine atoms are to the oxygen, the less basic it is.[14]

Spehr and Gotze recently reported a statistically significant decrease in PPF following open heart surgery in those patients with neurological complications.[15]

Spectral edge frequency. The spectral edge frequency (SEF) is conceptually based on a simple model of the frequency spectrum of the EEG. The model is not meant to emulate any true physiologic process, but only to provide a framework with which to simplify the characterization of the complex EEG signal observed. This model hypothesizes a truly random (infinite bandwidth) internal EEG generator, the output of which is modified by various filtering processes between the point of origin and the point of measurement. The properties of the filters, in turn, are affected by the state of the brain. The spectral edge frequency then, may be defined in terms of this model as the high frequency cutoff of these intrinsic filters. In other words, the spectral edge frequency is the highest frequency present in a significant quantity in the spontaneous EEG on an epoch by epoch basis.

Currently reported implementations of the spectral edge frequency are all based on examination of power spectra.[16,17,18,19] The examination may be accomplished by manual inspection, in which case the spectral edge frequency is defined as the highest frequency visually apparent in a spectral array type display.[17] Alternatively, automated evaluation of spectral edge frequency has been reported, using a variety of algorithms ranging from the 97th percentile power frequency[18] the frequency obtaining the best match against a predefined spectral pattern template. A commercially available version of the SEF has been implemented in the Neurotrac EEG Spectral Analyzer using a combination of the 97th percentile and then a pattern match to reduce susceptibility to extraneous noise. The Neurotrac plots the SEF superimposed on the corresponding CSA display. While this may appear somewhat redundant, in practice, some changes in the spectral pattern are accentuated and easily visible at a glance from across the room, while preserving the underlying data.

The spectral edge frequency has been examined both as an indicator of the depth of anesthesia and as an indicator of cerebral ischemia. The results to date are described below.

The initial studies of the relationship between depth of anesthesia and spectral edge frequency examined the effects of halothane or enflurane in a canine model.[16] A change in the end-tidal concentration of anesthetic agentin either of these agents alone in O_2 produced a rapid, repeatable change in SEF. An increase in end-tidal anesthetic concentration produced slowing and hence a decrease in SEF. There was variability between dogs in the sensitivity of the spectral edge frequency to concentration, although the measure was repeatable in individual dogs. In the clinical range of anesthetic depth, typical sensitivities were 8 Hz/MAC for halothane and 20 Hz/MAC for enflurane. The magnitude of these changes is considerably more than the changes seen with MPF. The addition of N_2O did not interfere with the

SEF response, and the SEF also proved insensitive to large variations in mean arterial pressure produced by alpha-adrenergic agonists.

Recently, Stanski and coworkers[20] have correlated the spectral edge frequency with serum concentrations of thiopental in normal human volunteers. The definition of SEF used in this study was the 95 percentile power frequency. A nonlinear regression was used to fit the SEF versus concentration data to a sigmoid curve. They observed an average baseline SEF of 24.5 $\pm$ 4Hz and an average SEF of 12.7 $\pm$5.4 Hz at the time of maximum thiopental effect. The average serum concentration (IC50) of thiopental which produced a shift in SEF from baseline to midway between the baseline and the SEF at maximal effect was 15.9 $\pm$5.1. The IC50 measurement was used to assess individual sensitivity to thiopental and was repeatable in individuals with an inter-subject variability of 30%. This group has suggested[19] that, on the basis of a lack of significant change in the IC50 with repeated doses, acute tolerance does not occur over the duration of their monitoring interval of one hour. Changes in spectral edge frequency apparently related to ischemia have been used to predict the occurrence of new neurologic deficits[17] following surgery. In a recent study by Rampil[17] of patients undergoing carotid endarterectomy, an ischemic EEG event was defined as a sudden (less than 30 seconds) drop in SEF, unrelated to anesthetic manipulations, to below 50% of the average SEF during the preceding minute. The patient population was divided, based on preoperative neurological status, into two groups: neurologically intact (78 patients) vs. preoperative cerebral infarction (33 patients). The study revealed that in neurologically intact patients, only those with an ischemic EEG event persisting 10 min or longer had a new neurological deficit postoperatively. The spectral edge frequency did not appear reliably predictive of new neurological deficits in the 33 patients with prior cerebral infarction. It should be emphasized that these neurological changes were quite gross, and that more subtle changes - psychological or neurological - may be associated with shorter ischemic events.

Numbers from aperiodic analysis. Of all the pattern displays, the aperiodic (Neurometrics) display retains the most information. It was also designed to "read" the frequency and amplitude content of the EEG in a manner analogous to the way an electroencephalographer does it. In aperiodic analysis, the amplitude and period of each wave encountered in the EEG are used to generate a continuously scrolling color display of vertical lines plotted against frequency and time. In addition to being displayed on a screen, the information is stored on a floppy disk and is available for retrieval and manipulation. Michael Quinn, of our group, has developed a program which allows us to select an epoch of any duration and print out 153 numbers which characterize that epoch (Fig. 2). For each of 30 1-Hz bins (0.5-1.5, 1.5-2.5, etc.) the following numbers are printed out: number of waves, total power (TP) of these waves in mcV squared, the mean power of each wave, the per cent power in each bin, and the cumulative per cent power (CP) in each bin. Also printed out are the total number of waves and the total power for all 30 bins, as well as the mean power for all bins.

There is an enormous amount of information available for quantitative analysis from this method. This superabundance can be both an advantage and a disadvantage. On the one hand, it may allow us to characterize the effects of anesthetics in a more detailed manner than has been previously possible. It has become clear that each agent has its own detailed pattern, or signature. This pattern may change with changing depth. It is also possible that each combination of agents has its own pattern, and that this pattern changes as the relative portion and absolute amount of each agent changes! If this is true, the more detailed the method, the greater the likelihood of classifying these relationships. On the other hand, plowing through say 50 sheets with up to 153 numbers each and trying to detect relationships, or selecting the right number or combination of numbers optimal for that set of situations can be an formidable task. Remember that the number of combinations and permutations of these 153 numbers is enormous.

Nevertheless, we have applied this technique in a preliminary examination of several anesthetic agents. Using the ever reliable halothane, we note that two distinct bands appear during halothane anesthesia, and that the higher frequency band decreases in frequency (shifts down) and narrows with increasing concentration. Thus the numbers reflecting cumulative per cent power, the bins with the greatest total per cent power, and/or the frequencies below which 90% (F90) or 50% power resides, may be the best to examine with halothane.

A much more difficult problem for the EEG has been assessment of depth of anesthesia with narcotic agents, such as morphine, fentanyl, sufentanil, or alfentanil. The Neurometrics seems to offer hope for the analysis of these difficult agents. Many of the individual variables which we selected from the Neurometrics matrix showed marked changes with induction of and emergence from the narcotics. In addition, these variables seemed to give different information at different depths of anesthesia. For example, at one extreme, CP3 is apparently very sensitive to small concentrations or light levels of anesthesia, as indicated by the fact that nearly maximum changes were seen very early in the anesthetic, before insertion of the oral airway. We speculated that CP3, TP4, and F90 should be useful for low-to moderate-dose fentanyl or sufentanil, while TP1 should be more useful for moderate-to high-dose fentanyl or sufentanil anesthesia. In general, the same considerations apply to alfentanil, that is, the emphasis is on the low-frequency information.

We have also examined thiopental and have observed that the higher frequency bins can also give useful information. These include the sum of the average power of bins 14-16 and 17-19, as well as the sum of the total power of bins 17-19.

Comparisons of numbers. Grundy et al,[3,4] have compared several EEG numbers under clinical conditions. As mentioned above, to detect cerebral ischemia they have used paired CFM's, one for each hemisphere. From each of these devices, they derive maximum, minimum, and average amplitudes, in microvolts, and zero-crossing frequency, in Hz. Although the digital readouts from the paired CFM's (new version) were the easiest to read clinically, they did miss three changes detected by an independent, standard spectral analysis (MED 80) in the small series of 34 patients undergoing carotid endarterectomy surgery under general or regional anesthesia. They also examined the relative power and frequency in 4 frequency bands, as determined by a MED 80, a special-purpose computer which performs a fast-Fourier transform and displays the CSA, as well as a small set of numbers from the aforementioned power bands. In this group of 34 patients the printout from the MED 80 had the greatest success in detecting episodes of cerebral ischemia. These investigators have also computed the ratio of alpha power on the operated side to alpha power on the unoperated side, and detected asymmetry during episodes of cerebral ischemia.

Asymmetry ratios. Asymmetry ratios have also been used by van Huffelen and coworkers[21] to assess patients who have clinical signs of cerebral ischemia but whose standard EEGs are read as normal. They examined the difference between hemispheres (left to right) of the alpha band PPF (normal inter-hemispheric difference is quoted as less than 0.4 Hz), and the difference in power between the two sides in the delta2 sub band (2-3.4 Hz). Analysis by their criteria revealed abnormality in 14/20 symptomatic patients with "normal" EEG, and 1/20 abnormalities in a group of controls.[21]

The electromyogram. A final, interesting number which can be derived from scalp electrodes is the spontaneous muscle activity or EMG. The EMG is usually considered an artifact by electroencephalographers but in fact, the EMG can be quantified to provide information on resting muscle tone which relates both to the depth of anesthesia and to the degree of neuromuscular blockade. This relationship was studied first by Fink,[22] and later by Harmel.[9] Generally speaking, the EMG may be distinguished from the EEG by the observation that the EMG tends to have a wider bandwidth, containing energy of substantially higher frequency than the EEG. Hence the approach of Harmel, Klein and Davis was to take the amplified signal from the scalp and pass it through a bandpass filter with frequency limits of 95-105 Hz. The filtered signal contains mostly EMG activity which is then rectified and averaged. This group reported typical EMG values of 4.0 mcV in awake patients and 0.7 mcV in patients with good surgical relaxation. Another approach being investigated (Rampil IJ: Unpublished data, 1983) is to connect an otherwise unused channel of an EEG spectral analyzer to electrodes placed on the right neck and shoulder. The electrodes in this configuration pick up mostly EMG from the underlying muscle groups, some ECG, and an infinitesimal amount of EEG. Processing this signal as though it were an EEG produces a corresponding spectral array, optimally including frequencies to 30 Hz and higher. The EMG analyzed in this manner may be quantified by measuring the total power in the alpha + beta frequency ranges.

CONCLUSIONS

A great many schemes have been proposed to quantify and thereby simplify the analysis of the intraoperative EEG. Thus far the clinical experience with any of the techniques described above is very limited. The display of information derived from EEG analysis is a continuum from raw EEG tracings, to aperiodic or spectral array displays, to single numbers which vary with time. It is difficult at this time to assess where along the continuum the optimal point for EEG interpretation lays. Currently we seek the best tradeoff between legibility and loss of relevant data. Certainly, the type of display must match the sophistication of the operator, and must suit the clinical situation at hand. Perhaps combinations of trend patterns and trended numeric parameters displayed together as in the CSA with a highlighted SEF may prove optimal.

Clearly, we are just beginning to scratch the surface of what should be a fertile field. For example, we know how to tell computers to watch numbers as they flash by, but not so well how to scan patterns. Extracted numbers therefore will be used in the first generation of alarms based on EEG. Whether this represents a compromise remains to be determined.

Artifact. The clinical usefulness of any of the of the EEG numbers described above will remain extremely limited until reliable automatic detection of artifacts can be implemented. Two classes of artifact plague EEG monitoring in the operating room and intensive care unit. The first class includes those stereotypic, patently obvious sources of extrinsic interference which a computerized monitoring system should be able to manage relatively easily: Faulty electrode contacts, excessive power line pickup, electrosurgical pickup, electrode motion, or improper settings of the amplifiers. The second class contains the intrinsic, biologic sources of error and includes superimposed ECG, EMG, and electro oculograms. In addition, if spectral analysis of underlying rhythms is of primary concern, then spike waves may be considered an artifactual addition to the background EEG. (Aperiodic analysis, by its very nature, includes spikes in its recognition algorithm.) These artifacts are more difficult for a computer to recognize and probably will require heuristic algorithms in the time domain, as well as filtering in the frequency domain to detect and minimize their presence in the analysis.

The recognition of artifact is important, since artifact will be with us for a long time, given the low level of the EEG signal, and those who monitor will have to appreciate the fact of its existence, as neurologists do today. Any EEG analyzer intended for general clinical use should not only indicate when artifacts are present, but should also assist the operator in diagnosing and correcting the sources of artifact. Since the aperiodic display retains so much information, one can detect and classify most artifacts on it and know when to disbelieve the display, as well as how to procede with the elimination of the artifact, eg, 60 Hz.

In summary, computer-derived numbers have helped quantify the EEG, and, on occasion, have helped monitor the depth of anesthesia or the presence of cerebral ischemia. However, pattern displays will not be replaced by numbers for a long time - until the computer can replace the eye as a competent pattern recognizer. Perhaps the combined use of patterns will enhance the information presented to the physician.

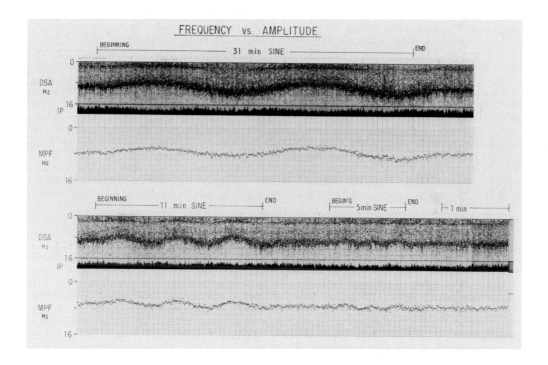

FIGURE 1.

The response of the DSA and MPF to sine wave variations in inspired concentrations of halothane. Note that as frequency increases (the period decreases), the peak-to-peak variation in MPF also decreases.

PATIENT: AGE: 21

PROCEDURE: AST/BEN/PLA-SUBJ.7
                                        DATE: Tuesday   1 /25/1983

RECORDING STARTED AT : 11:28   FILE LENGTH =   36 MINUTES AND 3 SECONDS

POWER SUMMED FROM 21:00 TO   24:30 FOR A TOTAL OF   210 SECONDS.

POWER UNITS = MICROVOLTS SQUARED   GAIN = 2

FREQUENCY BIN	WAVES IN BIN	SUM OF POWERS OF THOSE WAVES	AVERAGE POWER OF THOSE WAVES	PER CENT POWER OF THOSE WAVES	CUMULATIVE PER CENT POWER
1	7*	79102#	11300$^{\perp}$	1.85$^{\perp\perp}$	1.85+
2	49	238548	4868	5.59	7.44
3	95	439480	4626	10.30	17.75
4	101	442184	4378	10.36	28.12
5	91	354064	3890	8.30	36.42
6	31	102308	3300	2.39	38.82
7	11	34984	3180	.81	39.64
8	42	192212	4576	4.50	44.14
9	117	611952	5230	14.34	58.49
10	150	809840	5398	18.98	77.48
11	84	417424	4969	9.78	87.27
12	28	128968	4606	3.02	90.29
13	16	70550	4409	1.65	91.95
14	44	76100	1729	1.78	93.73
15	45	84762	1883	1.98	95.72
16	34	45561	1340	1.06	96.79
17	24	39631	1651	.92	97.71
18	28	35315	1261	.82	98.54
19	11	11038	1003	.25	98.80
20	9	10740	1193	.06	99.06
21	8	5081	635	.11	99.18
22	8	8864	1108	.02	99.38
23	9	7591	843	.17	99.56
24	6	5753	958	.13	99.70
25	6	3747	624	.08	99.78
26	1	324	324		99.79
27	2	1586	793	.03	99.83
28	4	1538	384	.03	99.86
29	1	324	324		99.87
30	14	5356	382	.12	100
TOTAL	1076††	4264960▲	3963 x		

0 NOISY SECONDS (0   % OF INTERVAL)

0 SECONDS WITHOUT ANY WAVES (0   % OF INTERVAL)

      * Number of Waves   + Cumulative % Power (CP)
      # Total Power (TP)   ++ Total Number of Waves
      $\perp$ Mean Power   ▲ Total Power of 30 Bins
      $\perp\perp$ % Power   x Mean Power of 30 Bins

FIGURE 2. A printout of the Neurometrics matrix in a healthy, male patient.
Note the alpha predominance at 9 and 10 Hz. Examples of the
variables discussed in the text are marked and keyed. (above)

REFERENCES

1. Maynard D, Prior P, Scott DF: Device for continuous monitoring of cerebral activity in resuscitated patients. Brit Med J 4:545

2. Prior P: Monitoring Cerebral Function. Amsterdam, Elsevier/North Holland, 1979.

3. Grundy BL, Sanderson AC, Webster MW: Hemiparesis following carotid endarterectomy: Comparison of monitoring methods. Anesthesiology 55:462-466, 1981.

4. Grundy BL, Webster MW, Nelson P: Brain monitoring during carotid endarterectomy. Anesthesiology 55:A129 (abstr.), 1981.

5. Lopes da Silva FH, Smith N Ty, Zwart A, et al: Spectral analysis of the EEG during halothane anesthesia. Input-output relations. Electroenceph Clin Neurophysiol 33: 311-319, 1972.

6. Klein FF: A waveform analyzer applied to the human EEG. IEEE Trans Biomed Eng BME-23:246-252, 1976.

7. Klein FF, Davis DA: The use of the time domain analyzed EEG in conjunction with cardiovascular parameters for monitoring anesthetic levels. IEEE T-BME 28:36-40, 1981.

8. Levy W, Shapiro HM, Maruschak G, et al: Automated EEG processing for intraoperative monitoring. Anesthesiology 53:223-236, 1980.

9. Harmel MH, Klein FF, Davis DA: The EEMG - a practical index of cortical activity and muscular relaxation. Acta Anaesth Scand 70(Suppl):97-102, 1978.

10. Smith N Ty, Silver H, Sanford TJ, et al:The EEG during high- dose fentanyl, sufentanil, or morphine-oxygen anesthesia. Anesth and Analg, 1983, submitted.

11. Smith N Ty, Westover CJ, Jr, Silver H, et al: Induction with thiopental or alfentanil: EEG effects. Anesthesiology, 1983, submitted.

12. Smith N Ty, Baker AB: The human EEG during thiopental or althesin induction. Anesthesiology 51:S6, 1979.

13. Eger EI, II, Smith, N Ty, Cullen DJ, et al: A comparison of the cardiovascular effects of halothane, fluroxene, ether, and cyclopropane in man: A resume. Anesthesiology 34:25-41, 1971.

14. Stockard JJ, & Bickford RG: The neurophysiology of anaesthesia. In Gordon (Ed): A basis and practice of neuroanaesthesia. Elsevier/North Holland, 1981, p43.

15. Spehr W, Gotze P: Computerized EEG and prediction of psychopathology after open heart surgery. In: Lechner H, Aranibar A (Eds) EEG and clinical neurophysiology. Amsterdam, Excerpta Medica, 1980, pp603-610.

16. Rampil IJ, Sasse FJ, Smith NT, Hoff BH, Flemming DC: Spectral Edge Frequency - A new correlate of anesthetic depth. Anesthesiology 53(suppl):s12, (abstr.), 1980.

17. Rampil IJ, Holzer JA, Quest DO, Rosenbaum SH, Correll JW: Prognostic value of computerized EEG analysis during carotid endarterectomy. Anesth Analg (Cleve) 62:186-92, 1983.

18. Epp RL, Negin M, Lee KJ: Performance specification of a microcomputer-based compressed spectral array system. IEEE Frontiers of Computers in Medicine, 1982, pp32-39.
19. Hudson RJ, Stanski DR, Meathe E, Saidman LJ: Does acute tolerance to thiopental exist? Anesthesiology 57(3):A501 (abstr.), 1982.
20. Stanski DR, Hudson RJ, Meathe E, Saidman LJ: Estimation of brain sensitivity to thiopental with the EEG. Anesthesiology 57(3):A502 (abstr.), 1982.
21. van Huffelen AC, Poortvliet DCJ, van der Wulp CJM, Magnus O: Quantitative EEG in cerebral ischemia - A) Parameters for the detection of abnormalities in "normal" EEGs in patients with acute unilateral c cerebral ischemia. In: Lechner H, Aranibar A (Eds) EEG and clinical neurophysiology. Amsterdam, Excerpta Medica, 1980, pp 125-130.
22. Fink BR: Electromyography in general anesthesia. Br J Anaesth 33:555, 1961.

AUTOMATIC EEG MONITORING DURING ANESTHESIA.

A.J.R. SIMONS
HEAD OF THE DEPT. OF CLINICAL
              NEUROPHYSIOLOGY
ST. ANTONIUS HOSPITAL
J. VAN SCORELSTRAAT 2
UTRECHT, THE NETHERLANDS

R.A.F. PRONK
A.Z.V.U.
DE BOELELAAN 1117
AMSTERDAM, THE NETHERLANDS
(FORMERLY M.F.I.-T.N.O., DA COS-
TAKADE 45, UTRECHT, THE NETHER-
LANDS).

INTRODUCTION.

EEG monitoring means that the spontaneous electroencephalogram is used as a parameter to evaluate brain function during critical conditions of the patient in order to prevent irreversible damage of the brain. The method has been used already for a long period (Gibbs et al., 1937; Bickford, 1950; Meyer and Gastaut, 1961; Shapiro, 1978; Prior, 1979; Pronk and Simons, 1982; Simons and Pronk, 1982). There are a number of circumstances in which this type of monitoring may be very succesful. A good review may be found in Prior (1979). Concerning anesthesia one may distinguish between EEG monitoring of the anesthesia itself (Bimar et al., 1977; Eger, 1978) in which one tries to determine the depth of anesthesia and especially the moment at which the patient looses consciousness and EEG monitoring during anesthesia under conditions which may lead to serious risks to the brain. To determine the depth of anesthesia a number of sophisticated methods based on the spontaneous on-going EEG have been developed (McEwen et al., 1975; McEwen, 1976; Berezowski et al., 1976). In a routine setting these methods have not been succesful up to now (Saunders, 1981) (Fig. 1). A combination with other EEG techniques such as evoked responses may be promising in future (Grundy et al., 1982). By means of the EEG one may easily follow global alterations of brain function during anesthesia (Faulconer et al., 1960; Sadove et al., 1967; Uhl, 1977; Prior, 1979). This may be of help to stabilize the anesthesia. It still needs intermediate action of the anesthesiologist. Servo-anesthesia with the help of the EEG has been investigated (Bickford, 1950; Verzeano, 1951; Belville et al., 1954), but routine methods have not been realised up to now.

The second reason for EEG monitoring during anesthesia has obtained clinical significance. As the brain is very sensitive to alterations in metabolism, it is possibly the organ most sensitive to hypoxia. A circulatory arrest of more than three minutes may lead to irreversible damage of the neurons (c.f. Tulleken, 1978). Of importance is that the brain generates continuously electrical signals which are in direct relation to that metabolism (Ingvar, 1976). Thus the measuring of the EEG is a potent method to control the level of metabolism of the brain during cardio-vascular surgery and to determine whether the condition becomes marginal. A number of patient parameters such as bloodpressure are of importance to stabilize brain function (Juneja et al., 1972[1]) so are temperature, PO_2 and to a lesser extent PCO_2 and electrolytes (Juneja et al., 1972[2]). Deterioration of one of these parameters does not necessarily have clinical importance as brain function concerns, unless the EEG is also deteriorating: the EEG reflects whether or not the combined effect of all those factors is still sufficient to a good brain function and whether one may tolerate the worsening of a certain parameter for some time.

THE EEG.

The EEG is the result of the combined effect of synchronised, mostly rhythmic potentials of very many apical dendrites of cortical neurons (Brazier, 1977; Niedermeyer and Lopes da Silva, 1982). The frequency of the variation of the potentials is between 0.5 and 25 c/sec. The amplitude of the potentials on the scalp is between 10 and 200 µV. The synchronisation is likely to be a result of the entrainment (Dewan, 1969), by which oscillating systems of nearly the same frequency having a mutual relation gradually show the development of a common rhythm. The amplitude at the scalp is a function of the amount of synchronisation.

The most important task of the brain is information processing during which synchronised activity of the neurons diminishes. This means that during active functioning of the brain measurable rhythmic potentials nearly disappear. With lowering of information processing the synchronisation returns. One may see this for example in the occurence of occipital alpha rhythm, in closing of

the eyes and disappearing of this rhythm with open eyes.
Diminished information processing occurs:
- in a resting state with eyes closed.
- during certain phases of sleep.
and also during a number of non-physiological conditions as:
- diminishing of consciousness.
- under the influence of sedatives.
- under the influence of anesthesia.
- during hypoxia.
Not only is the amplitude of the signals augmented, but also one
sees a lowering of the frequency: the mean frequency of the
potentials is proportional to the cortical metabolism (Ingvar,
1976). This may be due to diminished circulation or a lowered
oxygen availability. Also lowering of the temperature of the brain
leads to a strong diminishing of metabolism and thus to a slowing
of the EEG (Boba, 1960; Parks, 1961; Stokhof, 1976; Pronk, 1982;
Simons and Pronk, 1982). It is also a well established fact that
deepening of anesthesia leads to a slowing of the EEG (Fig. 2).
The alterations of the EEG follow within seconds those which occur
as a result of alterations of cerebral metabolism and this makes
the EEG very useful as parameter in judging brain function. The
EEG however gives no direct information concerning the function of
deep brain systems (brain stem, thalamus), but only indirect information because of the very strong influence of these systems on
cortical functions (Niedermeyer and Lopes da Silva, 1982). These
systems maintain a regulating influence on cortical functions
during unconsciousness and anesthesia, which is probably the reason
that during these situations a close symmetry between both
hemispheres is observed. Asymmetry proved to be an important
parameter in the judgement of a possible alteration in one of the
hemispheres. Amplitude is of relative importance. In general a
lowering of the amplitude in a situation where mostly very low
frequences occur, is an indication of an important deterioration
of cortical neurons (Simons and Pronk, 1982). Regional differences
of the potential fields are very pronounced during waking and
sleeping conditions and diminish during disturbances of conscious-

ness, hypoxia, anesthesia and cooling (Simons and Pronk, 1982) (Fig. 2). This means that relatively simple electrodemontages may be used in monitoring brain function during this situation.

EEG MONITORING.

Because EEG monitoring is essential non-invasive it does not mean any extra burden to the patient. There are however a number of handicaps to the use of EEG monitoring, i.e. the rather complex instrumentation, the interference-sensitive EEG registration and the expert knowledge which is needed to interpret the EEG information. All those difficulties are prohibitive in the routine use of EEG monitoring during small surgery

With major interventions it is different. They may be threatening to the patients brain. In cardiovascular and carotid surgery there are a number of important reasons to monitor the EEG during anesthesia. The possibility of a worsening of brain function due to a diminished cerebral blood and oxygen supply is great. Irreversible cerebral alterations resulting in neurological and psychopathological postoperative disturbances still occur (Speidel et al., 1980; Sotaniemi, 1982, 1983). The usual anesthetic parameters (bloodpressure, PO_2, PCO_2, pH, etc.) do not give indications as to the adequacy of the blood supply to the brain. Moreover, most of the functions which are measured and which may be of importance to a good brain function are artificial:

1. Heartaction has stopped.
2. Circulation, oxygenation and bloodpressure are determined by extracorporeal circulation.
3. The temperature is externally regulated.
4. Biochemical factors are artificial.
5. There is no good autonomous regulation.

The only source of real and continuous information on brain function is the EEG (Simons and Pronk, 1982; Pronk, 1982). This observation already led to EEG monitoring during the very early period of cardiac surgery (Arfel et al., 1961).

The most useful aspects of EEG monitoring during surgery with respect to the prevention of brain damage are:

1. The detection of EEG abnormalities at the time of their
   occurrence.

2. The prediction of postoperative neurologic outcome.

The immediate recognition of unexpected and unacceptable changes makes possible the prevention or limitation of postoperative morbidity, that is, neurologic or psychopathological complications, by applying early intraoperative therapeutic measures. When abnormal EEG activity occurs during surgery and persists to the end of the operation, there is a risk that postoperative cerebral complications may occur (Pronk, 1982).

In the last decades, several investigators have reported on EEG monitoring during open heart surgery (Arfel et al., 1961; Storm van Leeuwen et al., 1961; Fischer-Williams and Cooper, 1964; Prior et al., 1971; Wright et al., 1972; Simons, 1973; Weiss et al., 1975; Prior, 1979; Salerno et al., 1978). Nearly all of these authors report on the electroencephalographic changes during the extracorporeal circulation.

Since the task of EEG monitoring during anesthesia and surgery requires visual interpretation when carried out in the conventional way of EEG strip chart recording of very long duration, computer-assisted EEG monitoring methods were developed. The main characteristic of these methods is the data reduction of the EEG to features which permit a faster and easier detection of abnormalities and trends in the brain activity.

Bickford et al. (1971) developed a spectral analysis system which transforms the on-going EEG into a series of autospectra called a "Compressed Spectral Array" (CSA). This method was adapted and implemented into a microprocessor system by Smith and Fleming (1974) to produce so-called "Density Spectral Array" (DSA). Uhl and Meathe (1976) also used Bickford's method for the development of a system for EEG monitoring during anesthesia. Similarly, Butler (1975) developed a spectral analysis system.

The Berg Fourier Analyzer was one of the first commercially available EEG spectral analysis systems to be used for monitoring purposes. Experiences with the system were published by Bricolo et al. (1978) and Weber et al. (1979). Computerized EEG processing based on period/amplitude analysis was developed by Tonnies (1959),

Klein and Davis (1975, 1981), Pronk et al. (1975), Cohen et al. (1976) and Demetrescu (1976).

Some techniques process the EEG into simple measures of an averaged frequency and/or amplitude. Hjorth (1970) introduced the normalized slope descriptors. Prior and Maynard (1971) developed an EEG filtering device, the Cerebral Function Monitor (CFM). Levy et al. (1980) compared several EEG monitoring methods (spectral analysis (CSA and DSA), Cerebral Function Monitor, period/amplitude analysis) and found the spectral analysis with DSA presentation to be the most promising for monitoring during anesthesia.

All methods of EEG monitoring during anesthesia up to now present the EEG parameter without reference to the parameters of anesthesia, bloodpressure, temperature, perfusion etc.

However, they influence brain metabolism and the EEG pattern in such a way that it resembles the alteration which occurs as a result of hypoxia. To be able to determine the condition of the brain the other parameters have to be taken into account with the EEG interpretation (Simons and Pronk, 1982). EEG analysis also proves to be very difficult to relate EEG alterations to the other parameters. A great experience in EEG is necessary. The lack of this experience in most centres of cardiovascular surgery may be an important reason why up to know EEG monitoring has scarcely been applied.

THE CHOICE OF AN EEG ANALYSIS TECHNIQUE.

Automatic monitoring of brain function by means of the EEG during anesthesia is much more than automatic EEG analysis alone. On EEG analysis and quantification much research has been done already (c.f. Pronk, 1982). This author did a comperative study to the value of different EEG analysis methods. The results indicated that the period-/amplitude analysis gave almost equivalent results as the method of Hjorth (1970) and as spectral analysis. The way in which an expert judges the EEG is comparable in a certain way with the method of period-/amplitude analysis. In the development of an automatic EEG monitoring system we therefore choose for the period-/amplitude analysis.

THE CHOICE OF EEG CRITERIA.

In practice it proves that only a very restricted number of all the alterations of the EEG which may occur during cardiovascular surgery is important to determine a deterioration of brain function (Simons and Pronk, 1982, 1983). These alterations are:

1. Diminishing of the number of fast waves.
2. An increasing number of slow waves.
3. A lowering of the amplitude during a slow EEG period and eventually the occurrance of a silent EEG.
4. A constant asymmetry.

There are a number of special EEG features which occur during these situations such as suppression burst activity during very deep cooling (Storm van Leeuwen et al., 1961; Simons and Pronk, 1982), which are not pathological. They only indicate a strongly reduced brain function (Fig. 3).

The relatively small number of important EEG criteria gave the possibility to automate the decisions which have to be made on the interpretation of the brain function.

AN AUTOMATED EEG/ANESTHESIA MONITORING SYSTEM.

Because the number of waves in the EEG per unit of time has a strong relation with brain function (information processing and metabolism) the period-/amplitude analysis gives a good indication about this function. However, this number (N) changes continuously because the EEG during anesthesia or comparable situations shows no regular rhythm, but only very irregular waves with frequencies between 0.5 and 25 c/sec. (Fig. 2).

From our research it proved that in general an integrating period of 15 seconds is long enough to average strong fluctuations of N (Pronk, 1982; Simons and Pronk, 1982).

Clinical neurophysiological experience shows moreover that EEG alterations under these circumstances only have importance if they occur during a period of at least 10 to 15 seconds.

The determination of the number of waves from right and left
hemisphere gives the possibility to compute in a rather simple way
the amount of asymmetry of both hemispheres. The value of one integration period of 15 seconds is slightly weighted in relation to
some preceding periods of 15 seconds (Pronk, 1982).
Because we found a changing asymmetry of about 5% (SD 1.8) during
non-pathological conditions the decision of a possible pathological state is only taken if a constant asymmetry to one side of
7% and more at least two minutes occurs. Of course an amplitude
asymmetry has also to be taken into account. As already mentioned
hypoxia is a very threatening situation and leads to a slowing of
the EEG. The measurement of the amount of slowing and the
signaling of the point where on empirical grounds one may expect
that a marginal situation is reached, is a very important requirement of an automatic EEG monitoring system.

THE MARGINS OF SAFETY.
The margins which we determined in case of slowing, low amplitude
and asymmetry are the following:
1. A mean of 30 waves or less per 15 seconds.
2. A mean amplitude of 15 µV or less (up to a silent EEG), also
   over a period of 15 seconds. However, only if at the same time
   the conditions sub 1 have been fulfilled.
3. A constant asymmetry of more than 10% during at least two
   minutes (Simons and Pronk, 1982, 1983; Pronk and Simons, 1982;
   Pronk, 1982).

If the above mentioned critical values are surpassed, a number of
important parameters of the patient and of the anesthesia have to
be checked to be sure that a real risk to the brain may exist. If
the EEG is slow with or without low amplitude these are:
1. The amount and kind of anesthesia and the moment it has been
   applied. Anesthesia diminishes cerebral information processing
   and thus metabolism. As a result there occurs an important
   slowing of the EEG, which is related to the kind and dosis of
   the anesthetic. A slowing of the EEG during anesthesia is not
   abnormal, but to take a decision on this feature the above

mentioned data have to be accounted for.

2. The perfusion and body temperature. Cooling diminishes and
   slows down the biochemical processes. The oxygen need is very
   much lowered and therefore cooling is used to protect the brain
   against the effect of an insufficient circulation. During
   cooling the EEG slows in accordance with the perfusion temperature. However, because of the protecting properties of cooling
   there is only a very small chance for the brain to suffer and
   the slowing has then no pathological significance. During
   rewarming the brain needs at once much more oxygen, especially
   if the rewarming is very fast (Simons and Pronk, 1982, 1983).
   Because this need cannot always be fulfilled, a hypoxia
   develops, still worse as a result of low bloodpressure and the
   possible appearance of micro-bubbles in the blood caused by
   temperature rise (Bethune, 1980; Longmore, 1980). This
   situation leads in our experience to a very slow EEG
   (2 c/sec.) during fast rewarming at a level of approximately
   34° C. It is assumed that this may have harmful effects on
   brain function.

3. Cerebral autoregulation may be lacking if bloodpressure drops
   beneath 50 mm Hg (Juneja, 1972[2]; Bethune, 1980; Longmore, 1980).
   It is possible that this occurs even at a higher bloodpressure
   during anesthesia and it is practically certain that this is
   the case in patients with hypertension (Gelmers, 1982). During
   a rather deep anesthesia with a slow EEG and with a perfusion
   temperature not below 27° C a low bloodpressure may have
   consequences for the brain function because circulation may be
   lacking. Because the EEG is already slow this may not be at
   once clear. Under these circumstances bloodpressure has also
   to be taken into account in the judgement of a possible risk
   to the brain.

PROBLEM SOLUTION.

It is possible to monitor brain function by means of a simple
stripchart recording of the EEG together with a periodic collection of information on anesthesia. It may be clear that with an
increasing number of complex (cardiovascular) operations an

insufficient number of EEG experts will be available to supervise ↓
this type of simple monitoring. The very low margins of safety,
the need for fast decisions, the huge amount of information in the
EEG and other patient parameters and the necessity of continuous
observation call for a fully automatic monitoring and warning
system. The automatic EEG monitoring system which we developed
(Pronk, 1982; Simons and Pronk, 1982, 1983) fulfills or provides
the following conditions:

1. Automatic acquisition and recording of the EEG of both
   hemispheres and the bloodpressure and temperature of the
   patient.
2. Suppression of EEG signal interference.
3. EEG datareduction and extraction of clinically relevant
   features.
4. Interactive use for manual input of anesthetic information
   and for review of patient data.
5. Automatic warning and alarm at the occurrence of abnormal EEG
   activity.
6. Synoptic presentation of trends in the patient data in
   graphical form.
7. Numerical display of instantaneously measured patient data.
8. Documentation of patient data and anesthetic information.

An outstanding feature of the monitoring system is the
possibility of automatic generation of warnings and/or alarms
if the EEG activity falls below the acceptable limits for the
patient. Since the system is intended for usage in the operating
theatre, it was necessary to develop a small computerized system
with interactive facilities (Fig. 4, 5). This development was
based on experience with a pilot study for EEG monitoring (Pronk
et al., 1975). The development of the system was achieved in a
joint project of the department of Clinical Neurophysiology of
the St. Antonius Hospital and the Institute of Medical Physics
of TNO in Utrecht. During 1976 to 1978 the development was
supported by a grant of the Dutch Heart Foundation.

A block diagram of the EEG monitoring system is presented in fig. 6. The monitored patient signals are four EEG derivations, the arterial bloodpressure (systolic and diastolic values), the nasopharyngeal temperature and, during cardiopulmonary bypass, the pump generated pressure and the temperature of the perfusion blood of the heart-lung machine. The signals are amplified and low pass filtered before automatic processing.

A detailed description of the whole system may be found in Pronk (1982) and Simons and Pronk (1982).

Warning and alerting signals which are generated in plain language on the display screen, tell the anesthesiologist about the kind and severity of the EEG disturbance in the same way as an expert would do. Because asymmetry is a very important parameter, priority warnings are given if the amount - for a period of two minutes - is > 10-15% (SLIGHT ASYMM.) or > 15% (SEVERE ASYMM.).

The decision about a diffusely deteriorating brain is more complex. Diminishing of the number of positive and negative going $\emptyset$-crossings to less than 120 in 15 seconds is a significant criterium, based on experience. After detecting this or lower values the computer program looks for:

- Temperature of the perfusion and body; the rising and falling of these and the difference between these two temperatures.
- Anesthesia: kind and decay-time.
            quantity.
            moment of administration and point of time there-
            after.
            duration of continuous administration.
- Special neurotropic agents: i.e. Lidocaïne.

Only if these factors cannot explain the excessive slowing of the EEG, the warning SLOW EEG appears. If at the same moment the bloodpressure is below 50 mm Hg and the perfusion temperature > 27° C an extra warning occurs: LOW PRESS.

At a very low amplitude (< 15 µV) with a slow EEG and normal temperature indicating a deteriorating brain, LOW EEG is signaled.

The warning SILENT EEG occurs when the mean amplitude of a
15-second period stays below 8 µV.

The information on anesthesia introduced by the anesthesiologist
via a special keyboard is important to the function of the system
(Fig. 4). Without this information every above mentioned change
of the EEG generates a warning signal.
Of course quite a lot of measures have been taken to prevent the
system reacting on every EEG instability or abrupt fluctuation in
the trend. Electrocautery is signaled so it is possible to
evaluate these artefacts from real EEG changes.
On a video display the anesthesiologist may observe the information on the results of the EEG analysis, the bloodpressure, the
temperature, special events and anesthesia in numerical and
graphical form including also the trend (Fig. 7, 8).
After a warning signal the anesthesiologist may block the
releasing of more penetrating alarms by pressing a so-called
attention key. The specific warning stays displayed on the screen
as long as the abnormality exists.
All the preceding information may be recalled on the display
(Fig. 9) and at the end of the surgical procedure within minutes,
there is a complete hard-copy available to be put into the patients
documents. Also the information is permanently stored on mass
memory (Fig. 7).

EXPERIENCE AND RESULTS.
It proved that the aim to computerize the detection and decision
procedure used by the clinical neurophysiologist for all practical
purposes has been realised. Apart from the information on the
existence and the kind of a marginal situation to the brain of the
patient on which the anesthesiologist may then react with
appropriate measures, the used method of EEG monitoring also has
given more precise insight into the trend of the alterations of
brain function under the influence of different kinds of
anesthetics and also of temperature and bloodpressure (Fig. 8).
Concerning the definition of the exact moment at which consciousness diminishes to such an extent that surgery may be applied, it

is of importance that we found that many patients shortly before
the induction of anesthesia and with eyes closed showed a very
pronounced peak in the curves at a frequency of 8-9 c/sec., which
is about the frequency of the normal waking alpha rhythm. This
peak directly disappears after the introduction of anesthesia. This
is probably the moment that consciousness is very much diminished
(Fig. 10). During surgery there may again appear a peak at the
frequency of 8-9 c/sec. In such a case it seems appropriate to us
to add more anesthetics. If the patient really awakes however,
there is a big chance that because of high activation the above
mentioned peak again disappears. As a rule we may see then a
relative or absolute augmentation of the amount of fast activity
and there will be very few slow activity.

In our opinion a great amount of slow activity is a sign of poor
information processing and thus in general an indication of
sufficient anesthesia.

Different kinds of anesthetics show a certain specificity in the
EEG analysis profile (Fig. 8). During cooling and rewarming the
EEG analysis profiles are also very specific and it appears that
the brain reacts as sensitive to cooling and rewarming as it does
to anesthetics and hypoxia: Many action of the anesthesiologist
reflect well in the trend of the EEG analysis profiles (Fig. 8).
The use of automatic EEG monitoring during anesthesia is therefore
of much broader importance than only to prevent possible cerebral
calamities. By frequent application the anesthesiologist may learn
to be much more efficient which without doubt will promote quality.
Moreover, the monitoring and documentation system is very useful in
a didactic respect.

The system functions now several years and has been used during
more than 2000 operations in 4 rooms. A special version with the
accent on fast and sensitive asymmetry detection was developed to
monitor patients during carotid surgery. Parallel to the monitoring
system a stripchart recording is made with very low paperspeed to
control the quality of the EEG signal, which is done by an
EEG technician. The cost is not prohibitive, if one takes into
account that most of the time no trained EEG specialist has to be

present. Research is now underway to evaluate the impact on the anesthetical procedure and the outcome of cerebral function after surgery.

CONCLUSIONS.

The most important advantages are:

1. Independent of the presence of an expert clinical neurophysiologist continuous EEG monitoring is possible during any surgery in which there may develop a critical situation to the patients brain.

2. The decisions which are taken automatically evolve from objective measurements and follow criteria based on a very large experience in EEG monitoring.

3. Different from visual interpretation the exactness is independent of the duration of the procedure. Sampling of parameters is regular and frequent. With visual monitoring this can never be done in an equal way.

4. The anesthesiologist may be sure that no cerebral calamities occur, if no warning signals are generated and therefore he has not to pay attention to the brain function continuously. Because there is a steady display of the (EEG) parameters and the trends, he may get a good insight into the result of his actions.

5. Within minutes one knows which important alterations have occurred and thus one is able to react at once to prevent permanent cerebral dysfunction, which otherwise is only detected long after the end of the procedure.

6. If postoperative neurological or psychopathological complications exist, there may be determined at which moment something happened to the brain during surgery and how severe it was.

7. A good documentation of the whole procedure is available a few minutes after surgery and may be an aid in later decisions. To a large degree it may do away with the usual anesthesia documentation.

8. The information of every 15-second period is permanently stored on data-file and is available for research purposes.

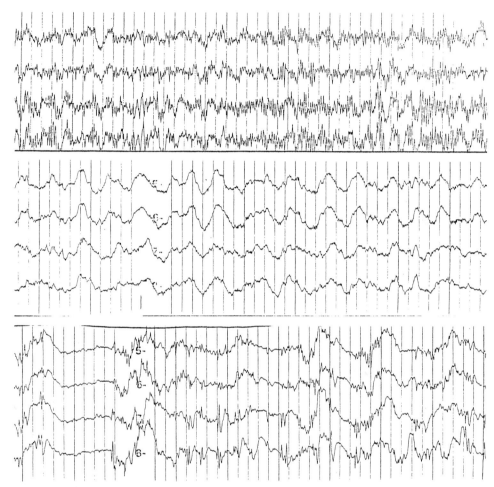

Fig. 1. This picture shows one of the reasons why determination of the level of anesthesia by means of the EEG is so difficult: 3 EEG patterns from about the same level of anesthesia but with different anesthetics: N_2O, Fentanyl, Etomidate.

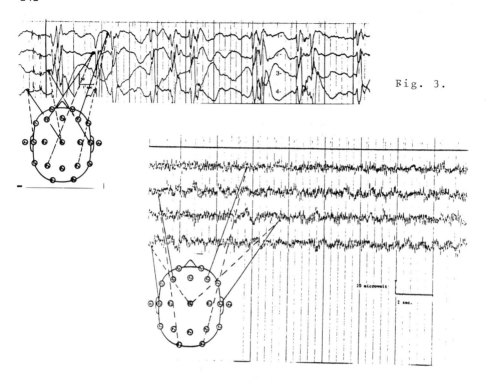

Fig. 3.

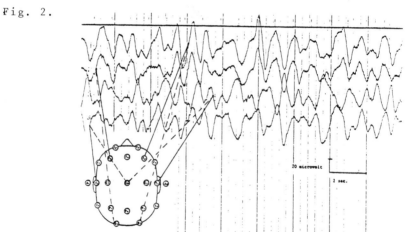

Fig. 2.

Fig. 2. EEG pictures at a low and a deep level of anesthesia.
The symmetry is presented, but regional differences
disappear.

Fig. 3. Suppression burst activity during deep cooling
(T < 20° C). Still deeper cooling leads to longer
intervals of the bursts and eventually electrical
silence.

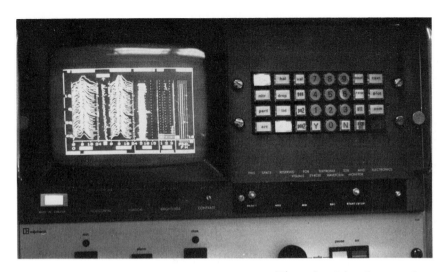

Fig. 4. Display and
keyboard built into
anesthesiologists
front end.

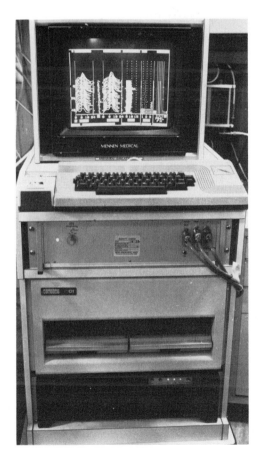

Fig. 5. Microcomputer
system in
technicians room.

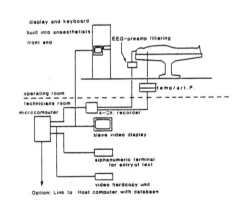

Fig. 6. Block diagram of
the monitoring
configuration.

244

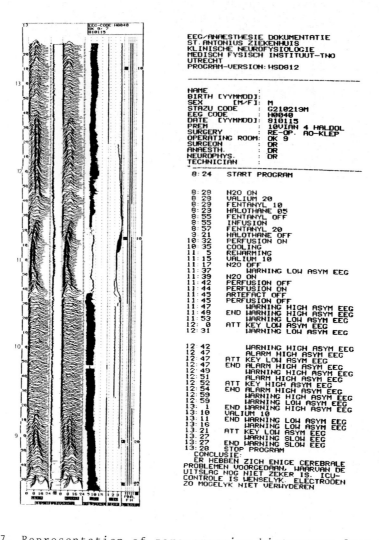

Fig. 7. Representation of zero-crossing histograms from both
hemispheres of a patient during open heart surgery.
The histograms were computed every minute; the time
scale (from 8:24 hours to 13:28 hours) is vertically.
On the right of the EEG histograms, the arterial
blood pressure, temperature values and anesthetic
data (P, F, N, H and L) were plotted. The text at the
right side refers to the graphical data at the left.
Notice that at 11:47 a warning was given about an
asymmetry in the EEG which occurred a few minutes
after stopping the artificial perfusion and persisted
to the end of the operation.

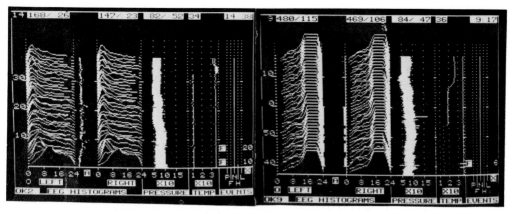

A. Anesthesia with N_2O (N) and Fentanyl (F).

B. Identical anesthesia in a child.

Fig. 8 A - D. Example of a number of displays which may appear on the video screen.

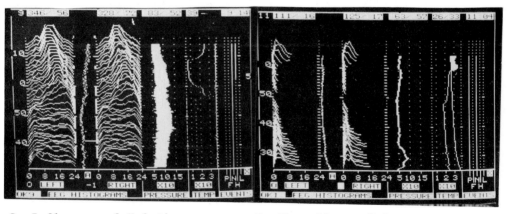

C. Influence of Halothane given at about 9.00.

D. The effect of deep cooling/rewarming with a short period of a silent EEG at 10.50.

246

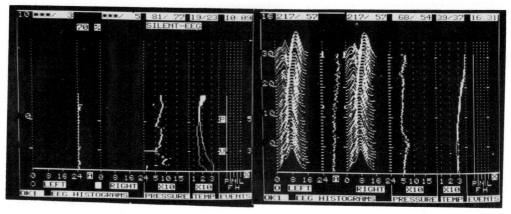

E. Indication of SILENT EEG as
   a result of very deep
   cooling (13° C). V = Valium,
   P = Pentothal.

F. Typical picture during
   slow rewarming.

Fig. 8 E - H.

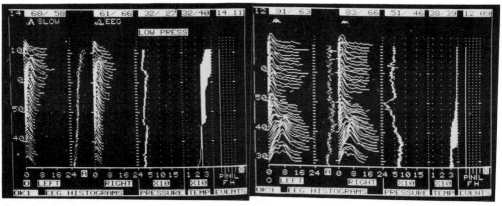

G. Typical picture during
   fast rewarming.

H. The effects of low
   blood pressure during
   rewarming.

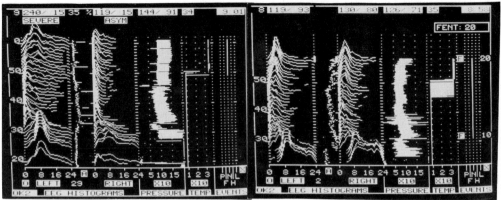

I. SEVERE ASYMMETRY in a patient
with right sided cerebro-
vascular abnormalities.

J. FENT: 20 appears during
3 minutes after
introducing this
information.

Fig. 8 I - K.

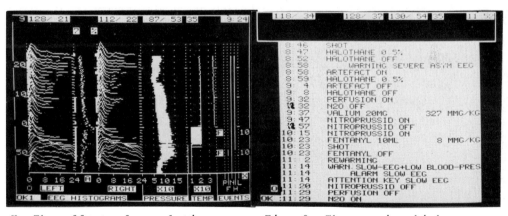

K. The effect of cumulative
dosis of Fentanyl (F).

Fig. 9. The way in which
the events are
documented and may
be recalled during
the procedure.

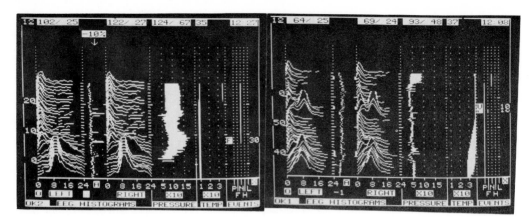

Fig. 10. The disappearance of the "alfa-peak" after the
         induction of anesthesia, indicating the moment
         consciousness is greatly diminished.

         At the end of the rewarming period and without
         anesthesia the "alfa-peak" reappears. This may
         indicate the returning of consciousness.
         After the appropriate reaction (Fentanyl, Valium)
         the peak disappeared again.

REFERENCES.

Arfel, G.; Weiss, J.; DuBoucet, N.
EEG findings during open heart surgery with extra-corporeal circulation.
In: Meyer, J.S.; Gastaut, H. (Eds.). Cerebral anoxia and the Electroencephalogram.
Thomas, Springfield, Ill., 1961: 231-249.

Bellville, J.W.; Artusio, J.F.; Bulmer, M.W.
Continuous servo-motor integrator of the electrical activity of the brain and its application to the control of cyclopropane anesthesia.
Electroenceph. Clin. Neurophysiol. 1954, 6: 317.

Berezowski, J.L.; McEwen, J.A.; Anderson, G.R.; Jenkins, L.C.
A study of anesthesia depth by power spectral analysis of the electroencephalogram (EEG).
Canad. Anesth. Soc. J. 1976, 23: 1-8.

Bethune, D.W.
The life span of gaseous emboli and organ damage.
Speidel, H.; Rodewald, G. (Eds.).
Psychic and neurological dysfunction after open heart surgery.
Proc. Int. Symposium, Hamburg, 1978.
Georg Thieme Verlag, Stuttgart, New York, 1980.

Bickford, R.G.
Electronic control of anesthesia.
Electronics, 1950, 23: 107-109.

250

Bickford, R.G.; Fleming, N.; Billinger, Th.
Compression of EEG data.
In: S.A. Trufant (Ed.), Transaction of the American Neurological
Association, Vol. 96.
Springer, New York, 1971, 118-122.

Bimar, J.; Bellville, J.W.
Arousal reactions during anesthesia in man.
Anesthesiology, Vol. 47, No. 5: 449-454, 1977.

Boba, A.
Hypothermia for the neurosurgical patient.
Charles C. Thomas, Springfield, Ill., 1960.

Brazier, M.A.B.
Electrical activity of the nervous system.
The Williams and Wilkens Company, Baltimore, 1977.

Cohen, B.A.
Period analysis of the electroencephalogram.
Comput. Progr. Biomed., 1976, 6: 269-276.

Demetrescu, M.
The aperiodic character of the electroencephalogram (EEG): a new
approach to data analysis and condensation.
Physiologist, 1975, 18: 189.

Eger, E.I.
Monitoring the depth of anesthesia.
In: Monitoring in anesthesia. Saidman, L.J.; Smith, N.T. (Eds.).
John Wiley and Sons, 1-14, 1978.

Faulconer, A.; Bickford, R.G.
Electroencephalography in anesthesiology.
Charles C. Thomas, Springfield, Ill., 1960.

Fischer-Williams, M. and Cooper, R.A.
Some aspects of electroencephalographic changes during open heart surgery.
Neurology (Minneap.), 1964, 14: 472-482.

Fleming, R.A.; Smith, N.T.
An inexpensive EEG processor for operating room and intensive care use.
In: Proc. San Diego Biomed. Symp., 1974: 13.

Gelmers, A.J.
The neurology of hypertension: a neurologists view.
Clin. Neurol. Neurosurg. 1982. Vol. 84 - 2.

Gibbs, F.; Gibbs, E.; Lennox, W.
Effect on the electroencephalogram of certain drugs which influence nervous activity.
Arch. Int. Med., 1937, 60: 154-166.

Grundy, B.L.; Procopio, P.T.; Boston, J.R., Doyle, E.
Sensory Evoked Potentials for intraoperative monitoring.
IEEE Trans. Biomed. Engng., Vol. BME-29, No. 8, 1982.

Hjorth, B.
EEG analysis based on time domain properties.
Electroenceph. Clin. Neurophysiol., Vol. 29: 306-310, 1970.

Hjorth, B.
Time domain descriptors and their relation to a particular model for generation of EEG activity.
In: Computerized EEG analysis (Eds.: Dolce, G.; Kuenkel, H.): 3-8. 1974.

Ingvar, D.H.; Sjölund, B.; Ardö, A.
Correlation between dominant EEG frequency, cerebral oxygen uptake and bloodflow.
Electroenceph. Clin. Neurophysiol., 1976, 41: 268-276.

252

Juneja, I.; Flynn, R.; Berger, R.
The arterial, venous pressures and the EEG during open heart
surgery.
Acta Neurol. Scandinav. 48, 163-168, 1972.

Juneja, I.; Flynn, R.; Berger, R.
The arterial pH, pCO_2 and the electroencephalogram during open
heart surgery.
Acta Neurol. Scandinav. 48, 169-175, 1972.

Kinichi, S.; Vijaya, K.; Keshav, K.; Vajubhai, S.; Vibhavary, S.
Detection of neurological abnormalities during open heart surgery.
In: Anesth. Congress, San Francisco, Calif., 1978.

Klein, F.F.
A waveform analyzer applied to human EEG.
IEEE Trans. Biomed. Engng, 1976, BME-23: 246-252.

Klein, F.F.; Davis, D.A.
A further statement on automated EEG processing for intraoperative
monitoring.
Anesthesiology, 1981, 54: 433-434.

Levy, W.J.; Shapiro, H.M.; Maruchak, G.; Meathe, E.
Automated EEG processing for intraoperative monitoring.
Anesthesiology, 1980, 58: 223-236.

Longmore, D.
Causes of cerebral complication after open heart surgery.
Speidel, H.; Rodewald, G. (eds.)
Psychic and neurological dysfunction after open heart surgery.
Proc. Int. Symposium, Hamburg, 1978.
Georg Thieme Verlag, Stuttgart, New York, 1980.

McEwen, J.A.; Anderson, G.B.; Low, M.D.; Jenkins, L.C.
Monitoring the level of anesthesia by automatic analysis of
spontaneous EEG activity.
IEEE Trans. Biomed. Engng, Vol. BME-22, No. 4, July 1975.

McEwen, J.A.
Estimation of the level of anesthesia during surgery by
automatic pattern recognition.
Ph.D. Thesis, Vancouver, 1976.

Niedermeyer, E.; Lopes da Silva, F.H.
Electroencephalography: Basic principles, clinical applications
and related fields.
Urban and Schwarzenberg, Baltimore-Munich, 1982.

Parker, A.S. (ed.)
Hypothermia and the effects of cold.
British Medical Bulletin, 1961, Vol. 17, No. 1.

Prior, P.F.
Monitoring Cerebral Function.
Elsevier/North-Holland Biomedical Press, Amsterdam, 1979.

Prior, P.F.; Maynard, D.E.; Sheaff, P.C.; Simpson, B.R.;
Strunin, L.; Weaver, E.J.M.; Scott, D.F.
Monitoring cerebral function: clinical experience with new
device for continuous recording of electrical activity of the
brain.
Brit. Med. J., 1971, 2: 736-738.

Pronk, R.A.F.; Simons, A.J.R.; De Boer, S.J.
The use of the EEG for patient monitoring during open heart
surgery.
In: IEEE Proc. Computers in Cardiology, Rotterdam, 1975, 77-82.

254

Pronk, R.A.F.
EEG processing in cardiac surgery.
Thesis, 1982.
Vrije Universiteit, Amsterdam.

Pronk, R.A.F.; Simons, A.J.R.
Automatic recognition of abnormal EEG activity during open heart
and carotid surgery.
In: The Kyoto Symp., Electroenceph. Clin. Neurophysiol., Suppl. 36.
Elsevier Biomedical Press, Amsterdam, 1982.

Sadove, M.S.; Becka, D.; Gibb's, F.A.
Electroencephalography for anesthesiologists and surgeons.
J.B. Lippincott Company, Philadelphia, 1967.

Salerno, T.A.; Lince, D.P.; White, D.N.; Beverly, L.R.;
Charette, E.J.P.
Monitoring of electroencephalogram during open heart surgery.
A prospective analysis of 118 cases.
J. Thorac. Cardiovasc. Surg., 1978, 76: 97-100.

Saunders, D.
Anesthesia, awareness and automation.
Br. J. Anesth., 53, 5: 1-3, 1981.

Shapiro, H.M.
Monitoring in neurosurgical anesthesia.
In: Monitoring in anesthesia. Saidman, L.J; Smith, N.T. (Eds.)
John Wiley and Sons, New York, 171-204, 1978.

Simons, A.J.R.
Aspects of EEG control during open heart surgery.
Electroenceph. Clin. Neurophysiol., 1973, 35: 105-106.

Simons, A.J.R.; Pronk, R.A.F.
Les données électroencéphalographiques pendant la chirurgie à
coeur ouvert. Leur analyse automatique en relation avec les

paramètres anesthésiques et son utilisation pour la surveillance
peropératoire de la fonction cérébrale.
Rev. E.E.G. Neurophysiól., 1982, 12: 243-252.

Simons, A.J.R.; Pronk, R.A.F.
EEG analysis in monitoring anesthesia.
In: Objective Medical Decision-making; Systems Approach in Acute
Disease.
Proc. Workshop: SWG/COMAC-BME. Commission of the European
Communities, 1983 (in press).

Sotaniemi, K.A.
Prediction of cerebral outcome after extracorporeal circulation.
Acta Neurol. Scandinav. 66, 697-704, 1982.

Sotaniemi, K.A.
Cerebral outcome after extracorporeal circulation. Comparison
between prospective and retrospective evaluations.
Arch. Neurol. Vol. 40, 75-77, 1983.

Speidel, H.; Rodewald, G. (Eds.)
Psychic and neurological dysfunction after open heart surgery.
Proc. Int. Symposium. Hamburg. 1978.

Georg Thieme, Stuttgart, 1980.

Stokhof, A.A.
Left ventricular bypass-assisted hypothermic circulatory arrest in
the dog.
Thesis, 1976.
University of Utrecht.

Stockard, J.J.; Bickford, R.G.; Schauble, J.F.
Pressure-dependent cerebral ischemia during cardiopulmonary bypass.
Neurology (Minneap.), 1973, 23: 521-529.

Storm van Leeuwen, W.; Mechelse, K.; Kok, L; Zierfuss, E.
EEG during heart operations with artificial circulation.
In: Meyer, J.S.; Gastaut, H. (Eds.), Cerebral anoxia and the
electroencephalogram.
Thomas, Springfield, Ill., 1961: 268-278.

Tönnies, J.F.
Automatische EEG-Intervall-Spektrumanalyse (EISA) zur
Langzeitdarstellung der Schlafperiodik und Narkose.
Arch. Psychiat. Nervenkr., 1969, 212: 423-445.

Tulleken, C.A.F.
Circulation of the brain.
In: Oxygen supply of heart and brain, 34-46.
Dutch Heart Foundation, The Hague, 1979.

Uhl, R.R.; Meathe, E.A.; Maruchak, G.F.; Saidman, L.J.; Ozaki, G.T.
Correlative monitoring of brain activity and perfusion during
anesthesia.
In: Proc. San Diego Biomed. Symp., 1977: 425-428.

Verzeano, M.
Servo-motor integration of the electrical activity of the brain
and its application to the automatic control of narcosis.
Electroenceph. Clin. Neurophysiol., 1951, 3, 25.

Weber, B.; Echter, E.; Couegnas, J.
Monitorage des spectres de fréquence, complément de la
surveillance électroencéphalographique en réanimation.
Agressologie, 1979, 20: 183-192.

Weiss, M.; Weiss, J.; Cotton, J.; Nicolas, F.; Binet, J.P.
A study of the electroencephalogram during surgery with deep
hypothermia and circulation arrest in infants.
J. Thorac. Cardiovasc. Surg., 1975, 70: 316-329.

Witoszka, M.M.; Tamura, H.; Indeglia, R.; Hopkins, R.W.;
Simeone, F.A.
Electroencephalographic changes and cerebral complications in
open heart surgery.
J. Thorac. Cardiovasc. surg. 1973, 66: 855-864.

Wright, J.S.; Lethlean, A.K.; Hicks, R.G.; Torda, T.A.; Stacey, R.
Electroencephalographic studies during open heart surgery.
J. Thorac. Cardiovasc. Surg., 1972, 63: 631-638.

COMPUTERIZED EMG AND EEG CORRELATES OF CONSCIOUSNESS

H.L. EDMONDS, JR., Y.K. YOON, S.I. SJOGREN, H.T. MAGUIRE, C.P. McGRAW

1. INTRODUCTION

Changes in the levels of consciousness and cerebral function are major concerns in anesthesia and critical care. Although diminution of conscious reactivity is sought during anesthesia, pronounced decreases signifying prolonged cerebral hypoperfusion or hypoxia must be avoided. Thus, reliable, convenient monitors are needed to assess the level of consciousness and integrity of cerebral processes. Recently, Levy compared the existing techniques for computerized EEG analysis (6). He concluded that a combination of zero-cross frequency (ZXF) and mean integrated amplitude (MIA) offered a simple, useful approach to intra-operative monitoring. However, at that time no such commercial device was available. In the past year the Anesthesia and Brain Activity Monitor (ABM^R) has been developed. Currently, only one brief evaluation of the monitor has been made (8). This device provides fundamental information on the adequacy of cerebral function in the complex, electrically hostile environs of the operating room (OR) and intensive care unit (ICU). The purpose of this report is to present a more extensive evaluation of the ABM.

2. PROCEDURE

2.1. Instrumentation

The ABM (DATEX/Puritan-Bennett) measures frontalis muscle EMG amplitude, mean EEG frequency and amplitude. The broadband biopotential obtained from skin electrodes attached to the temporal and mid-forehead regions is both high- and low-pass filtered to obtain EMG (60-300 Hz) and EEG (1-25 Hz), respectively. Using discrete analog devices, filtered signals are full-wave rectified and integrated to obtain mean rectified voltage/sec (MRV presented as digital values). Ten sec averages are then displayed as histograms in a series of vertical bars with the aid of a Z-80 microprocessor. Mean frequency of the EEG is determined by use of the ZXF. As noted by Levy (6) and others, ZXF is excessively sensitive to minor changes in EEG pattern. Small decreases in EEG amplitude may lead to marked increases in ZXF without actual changes in the underlying rhythm. Futhermore, several distinct EEG patterns may have the same ZXF. Therefore, evaluation was limited to analysis of EEG/EMG amplitudes.

2.2. Subjects

EMG and EEG recordings were obtained from 41 surgical patients ranging in age from 6 months to 76 years. These patients were scheduled for a wide range of surgical procedures lasting from a few minutes to many hours. Premedication and anesthetic technique were not standardized. Thus, some younger patients received no premedication. Anesthesia was induced and maintained by mask. In contrast, older patients generally received analgesics, tranquilizers, anti-sialagogues and neuromuscular blockers prior to induction and intubation with thiopental and succinylcholine. Maintenance anestheisia utilized halothane, isoflurane, or enflurane. Additionally, seven comatose patients and 4 student sleep-study volunteers were studied.

2.3. Experimental Design

2.3.1. Surgical patients. A period of EMG/EEG amplitude was quantified in awake patients in the OR immediately prior to induction of anesthesia. Continuous recording was then made during induction and maintenance of anesthesia. During each procedure, vital signs, drug administration and the nature of surgical status were coded on permanent record by an integral event marker.

2.3.2. Coma patients. The ABM was used to monitor 7 comatose patients for periods of up to 24 hr. ICU nursing staff recorded time of drug administration and interactions with the patient. In 5 of these patients, intracranial pressure (ICP) was also monitored.

2.3.3. Sleep study volunteers. EMG/EEG records were obtained during normal drug-free sleep in 4 student volunteers.

2.4 Analysis

EMG/EEG amplitudes were recorded in each state of consciousness. Baseline amplitude was defined as the average minimum obtained in 5 successive 90 sec epochs. Amplitude variability was determined by the average difference between maximum and minimum values. Average values for minimum amplitude and variability in the awake, conscious state were compared to those in the anesthetized or sleeping subject by paired Student's t-test. In the former group, anesthetized values were obtained beginning 15 min after induction. This 4.5 min period was the least likely to be contaminated by the effects of the short-acting induction agents or by marked surgical stimuli. The initial appearance of slow wave sleep (SWS or non-dream sleep), characterized by sustained low voltage EMG, was chosen as the 4.5 min period of

unconsciousness for sleep subjects. Since the conscious
state was absent in comatose patients, two 4.5 min periods
separated by a 60 min interval were compared.

3. RESULTS

3.1. Surgical Patients

Typical effects of isoflurane on EMG and EEG are
depicted in Fig. 1. The variable high amplitude awake EMG
markedly diminished during induction and maintenance of
anesthesia, even in the absence of neuromuscular blockers.

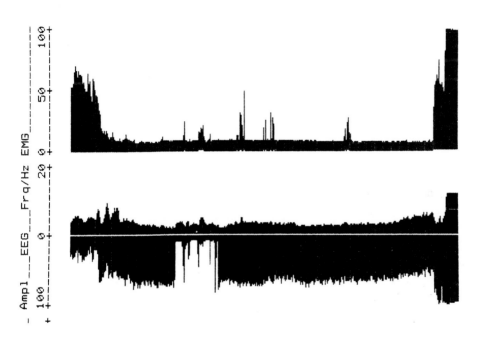

Figure 1

MRV of the EEG initially increased in amplitude and decreased
in variability during anesthesia. However, the magnitude of
the amplitude change following induction was dependent, in

262

part, on the conscious values. Large increases were seen in patients with low amplitude awake values, while little or no change was noted in individuals with high amplitude awake baselines. In this trace, the precipitous decline in EEG MRV amplitude accompanied a period of marked hypotension. Prompt restitution of adequate cerebral perfusion resulted in an immediate increase in MRV.

EMG respones to the volatile anesthetics are summarized in Fig. 2. All three agents produced significant decreases in EMG amplitude and variability. In contrast, the MRV of the EEG, (Fig. 3), was not appreciably altered by the anesthetics. These agents all significantly decreased MRV variability, however.

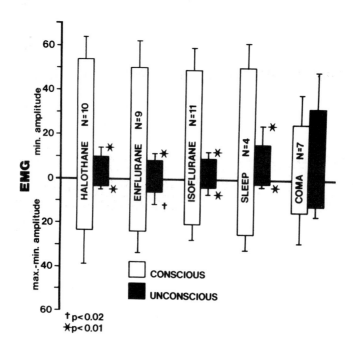

Figure 2

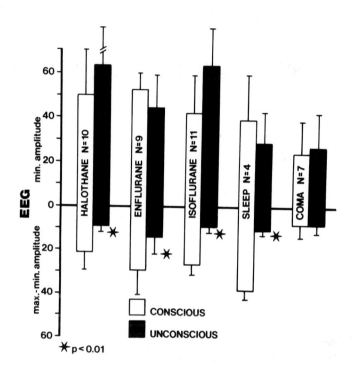

Figure 3

3.2. Coma Patients

Fig. 4 illustrates the appearence of the EMG and EEG in
an unresponsive comatose patient. Paroxysmal bursts of
variable high amplitude EMG activity are superimposed on a
low voltage baseline. These bursts were associated with
marked elevations in the ICP. In the absence of increased
ICP, EMG amplitude remained low for many hours (Fig. 2). EEG
MRV was usually of low amplitude (Fig. 3). However, the lack
of amplitude variability was the more consistant finding.
This unique stability of EEG amplitude proved to be a
hallmark of the comatose state.

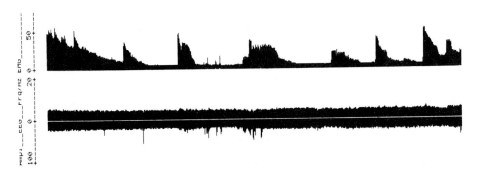

Figure 4

3.3 Sleep Patients

Since the frontalis muscle EMG records activity associated
with rapid eye movement (REM), it is useful in distinguishing
dream (REM) and non-dream (SWS) sleep.

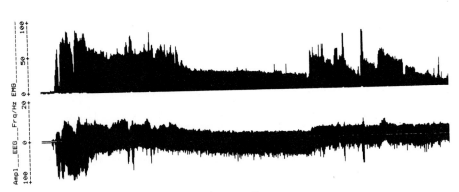

Figure 5

Fig. 5 clearly depicts EMG and EEG changes associated with
transition from awake, through initial REM to SWS. High and
variable EMG amplitude of the awake state was moderately
decreased. Continued variability appeared to be coupled with
periods of activity of extraocular muscles. EEG amplitude
decreased markedly. During SWS, EMG was further diminished
and variability virtually abolished. Increases in EEG MRV
and decreases in variability were consistent with the well-

known synchronous high voltage slow activty of SWS. These EMG/EEG changes from awake to SWS are summarized in Fig. 2 and 3.

4. DISCUSSION

Sulg (7) appears to have been the first to suggest that a combination of ZXF and MRV could be useful in anesthetic monitoring. This technique, later termed period-amplitude analysis (PAA) by Klein and Davis (5), seemed to offer advantages over existing methods. PAA was more powerful than the cerebral function monitor (CFM) (2) since the former displayed frequency and amplitude separately. Futhermore, changes in PAA during anesthesia were more easily interpreted by the anesthesiologist than those produced by power spectral analysis (PSA). However, until now the lack of a commericially available PAA device has hampered clinical evaluation of the technique.

Fortunately, earlier studies on the use of MRV in quantifying EEG changes offer valuable insight into its effective application (4). Extensive filtering employed in the CFM and PSA eliminate much of the variability inherent in the EEG. In contrast, MRV clearly represents this variability and uses it to advantage. That is, Goldstein (3) noted that the time-course of the variability of the distribution of amplitudes was at least as important as changes in the MRV value itself. We therefore chose to compare amplitude and variability changes in drug and non-drug state to "minimize the otherwise bewildering inter-subject variations" (3).

By adhering to Goldstein's precepts, we have found EEG amplitude analysis to reliably differentiate consciousness from unconsciousness. Even though MRV did not differ significantly in the awake vs. anesthetized or awake vs. sleeping states, MRV variability in anesthetized or sleeping subjects was less than half the corresponding awake values. The use of successive 90 sec. epochs for quantification of MRV variability in this study was necessary for statistical analysis. Yet, the histogram display of the ABM provides an adequate visual estimation of this variablity for intra-operative monitoring.

It is obviously impossible to obtain awake values from comatose subjects. Even though comatose MRV values tend to be lower than those seen in awake or anesthetized subjects, inter-subject differences make such distinctions unreliable. Again, however, variability of the MRV over time is the key. Without exception, MRV variability in comatose patients was remarkably low. During continuous recordings of up to 24 hr, MRV varied little in unresponsive patients. Clinical improvement, as indicated by increasing Glasgow Coma Scores paralleled increases in EEG amplitude variability.

Although amplitude analysis can differentiate consciousness from unconsciousness, it is unclear whether the actual depth of anesthesia can be reliably ascertained. It's major utility, therefore, is its ability to monitor the adequacy of cerebral oxygenation or perfusion. It is well-established that the EEG change most often seen in hypoperfusion is an attenuated amplitude. Marked frequency changes may or may not occur (1). Furthermore, the pattern of amplitude changes is of paramount importance in differentiating hypoxia from deep anesthesia. Transition between adequate and inadequate oxygen supply is abrupt and so are amplitude changes. Since deep inhalational anesthesia requires time to develop, markedly diminished MRV will be similarly paced. Unanticipated cerebral hypoxia can thus be detected immediately.

In the absence of high doses of neuromuscular blockers, the frontalis muscle EMG offers additional information on the level of consciousness. Volatile anesthetics produce a marked and consistent decrease in EMG amplitude and variability. Abrupt increases in these values indicate that the patient is either responding to surgical stimuli or is emerging from anesthesia.

In the non-drugged sleeping subject, the EMG correlates with eye movement and serves as an indicator of REM or SWS sleep. Unresponsive comatose patients generally have low amplitude EMG activity with little or no variability. Such a pattern is reminiscent of surgical anesthesia. However, in 5 patients with ICP monitors, we noted paroxysmal increases in the EMG associated with a rising ICP. The precise physiological basis for this observation is unclear, but enhanced restlessness is a well-known clinical sign of increased ICP.

In summary, the EEG and EMG displays of the ABM provide valuable information for operating room and ICU personnel. Compared to the awake state, the diminished variability of EEG amplitude reliably reflects the synchronizing effects of volatile anesthetics on the EEG. Similar comparisons of EEG amplitude provide a measure of the adequacy of cerebral oxygenation/perfusion. Changes in EMG activity in comatose patients may offer a non-invasive index of ICP.

REFERENCES

1. Chiappa, K.H., Burke, S.R., Young, R.R.: Results of EEG monitoring during 367 carotid endarterectomies -- use of a dedicated mini-computer. Stroke 10:381, 1979.

2. Dubois, M., Savege, T.M., O'Carroll, T.M., et al: General anaesthesia and changes on the cerebral function monitor. Anaesthesia 33:157, 1978.

3. Goldstein, L.: Psychotropic drug-induced EEG changes as revealed by the amplitude integration method. In: Psychotropic Drugs and the Human EEG (Ed. T.M. Itil) Karger, Basel p. 131 1974.

4. Goldstein, L. and Beck, R.A.: Amplitude analysis of the electroencephalogram. Internat Rev Neurobiol 8:265, 1965.

5. Klein, F.F., Davis, D.A.: The use of the time domain analyzed EEG in conjunction with cardiovascular parameters for monitoring anesthetic levels. IEEE Trans Biomed Engineer BME 28:36, 1981.

6. Levy, W.J., Shapiro, H.M., Maruchak, G., et al: Automated EEG processing for intraoperative monitoring: A comparison of techniques. Anesthesiology 53:223, 1980.

7. Sulg, I., Hollmen, A., Breivik, H., et al: A novel computerized device for monitoring of brain, muscle tension and pCO_2 in anesthesia, recovery and in intensive care. Proc. 6th Europ Cong Anesthesiol 1982.

8. Sulg, I.A.: Manual EEG analysis. Acta Neurol Scand. 26:31, 1969.

COMPUTER CONTROL OF ANESTHESIA DELIVERY

DWAYNE R. WESTENSKOW, Ph.D., WILLIAM S. JORDAN, M.D.,
JOHN K. HAYES, M.S. M.S., THOMAS D. EAST, Ph.D.

The basic design of the anesthesia machine has changed very little in the past 10 years.[1,2,3] The means of providing gas flows to the breathing circuit remains essentially unchanged. Because of the variable effect which fresh gas flows rates have on the breathing circuit gas concentrations, training and experience are necessary before one can deliver a smooth and controlled anesthesia, with existing equipment, particularly when using closed circuit anesthesia. The anesthesia machine can be made easier to use by adding computer control. The anesthetist may then adjust the inspired oxygen concentration, the end-tidal anesthetic concentration, the circuit volume, and the end-tidal carbon dioxide concentration; the computer will set the fresh gas flows. By letting the user set these primary parameters, the machine becomes function oriented and anesthesia safety may improve.

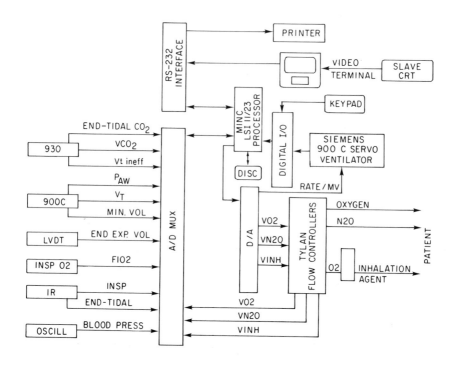

EQUIPMENT DESCRIPTION

The computer system shown in Figure 1 has been added to an anesthesia machine to control the fresh gas flows and to adjust mechanical ventilation. It includes a MINC microcomputer, Tylan mass flow controllers, and a Siemens 900C ServoVentilator.

The MINC 11 microcomputer (Digital Equipment Corp, Mynard, Ma) uses the PDP 11/23 microprocessor with the hardware floating point math package, 64K MOS 16 bit memory, 2 1/2 megabyte disc drives, 4 programmable clocks and a graphics terminal. The D/A outputs (12 bit) control the flow of oxygen (0-1 l/min) and nitrous oxide (0-1 l/min) through mass flow controllers (Tylan Corporation Carson, Ca). The flow of inhalational agent is controlled by a third Tylan controller which adjusts the oxygen flow through a copper kettle vaporizer. D/A channels also control the respiratory rate and minute volume of the 900C servo ventilator (Siemens-Elema, Solna, Sweden) through the ventilators computer interface.

Analog inputs enter through the 16 channel 12 bit A/D convertor. Inputs include end-tidal CO_2, CO_2 production, and ineffective tidal volume (Siemens 930 CO_2 analyzer module); airway pressure, tidal volume, and minute volume (Siemens Servo Ventilator); volume of the anesthesia circuit (Transducer Systems Incorporated, North Bradford, Conn.); inspired oxygen concentration (Critikon, Tampa, Florida); inspired and end-tidal inhalation agent concentration (IR analyzer Siemens Elema, Solna, Sweden); and mean arterial blood pressure (Critikon, Tampa, Florida). A video terminal with slave video display and a dot-matrix printer are interfaced through RS232 ports. A dedicated keypad is interfaced through a 16 bit digital I/O port. The servo ventilator start of inspiration signal enter through an interrupt channel.

The software consists of a main frame program to run the graphics display, coordinate data collection, and handle I/O. This main frame program supports a number of different feedback control modules in order to allow a wide variety of anesthesia protocols. The main frame consists of three main parts. The first part requests information about the patient as well as the desired values for the inspired oxygen concentration, end-tidal inhalation agent concentration, end tidal CO_2 concentration and tidal volume. The second section includes user input-output routines. It updates the trends on the video display, stores 10 breath averages on disc, and services the keypad. Keypad input includes changes in the desired setpoints, the selection of trending variables, entry of blood gas values or program termination. The third portion handles data collection and feedback control. This interrupt driven routine collects 16 parameters each breath, stores these parameters in the appropriate work space, applies feedback control algorithims and sends control signals to the D/A output channels. Feedback control is based on either proportional-integral-derivitive (PID) or self-tuning adaptive techniques, depending on the desired response time and application. Five feedback control loops adjust the fresh gas flows and ventilation.

The software also includes routines to handle offline data collection and calculations. The text editor is used to enter and edit the following data: venous and arterial blood gases, pulmonary artery pressure, pulmonary arterial wedge pressure, central venous pressure, body temperature, and cardiac output. Calculations include venous admixture, alveolar-arterial oxygen content difference; arterial, mixed venous, and alveolar oxygen content; arterial, mixed venous, and alveolar oxygen saturation; and alveolar as well as mixed venous temperature corrected oxygen and CO_2 partial pressures.

TESTING THE CONTROL CONCEPT

Inspired Oxygen

One of the main objectives in implementing computer control was to provide better control of the inspired oxygen concentration. The feedback controller for the oxygen control loop was adjusted with sufficient integral gain to keep the inspired oxygen concentration within 0.1 % of the desired value. The actual oxygen concentration, however, remained at the desired level only if the oxygen sensor and the reference voltage remain in calibration. The sensor was found to drift less than 0.5 %/hr and the reference voltage less than 0.3%/hr.[5,6] With worst case conditions, the oxygen concentration was 4% from the desired value after 4 hrs. Using a prototype system, we found that it required approximately 1.7 min to make a 10% change in the inspired oxygen concentration. The system returned to a true steady state in 6.2 min.[6,7]

When a constant inspired oxygen concentration was maintained in a closed leak tight circuit, the fresh gas oxygen flow provided a continuous measure of the patient's oxygen consumption (VO_2).[8,9] The accuracy of the VO_2 measurement was found to be within 5% of reading. There were several sources for error in this measurement of VO_2. The temperature of the rebreathing circuit had to be constant, if it changes by 1° C/hr, VO_2 was in error by 0.4 ml/min. A leak in the closed circuit caused an error in the VO_2 reading which was directly proportional to the leak and the oxygen concentration. Drift in the oxygen sensor caused a worst case error of 4 ml/min (sensor drift of .8%/hr at 60% oxygen). Finally, changes in functional residual capacity (FRC) caused an error in VO_2 which was proportional to the volume of oxygen moved into or out of the FRC.

Circuit Volume

When using a closed circuit to deliver anesthesia, the fresh gas flows must be properly adjusted to maintain a constant circuit volume. This function was performed automatically by the computer system. A linear variable displacement transducer (LVDT) attached to the top of a standing bellows ventilator was used to adjust the N_2O flow to keep the end expiratory circuit volume constant. The nearly infinite resolution of the LVDT sensor allowed very precise control of the volume. However, the surgeon's elbow on the chest, shifting of the patient's position, movement of the extremities, etc, each caused the FRC and circuit volume to change. In our clinical experience with an analog controller, we found that the nitrous oxide flow varied considerably to keep the volume constant. Changes in the circuit volume of 100 ml were no uncommon and, as a result, the nitrous oxide flow was not constant but had a standard deviation of approximately 30 ml/min. These fluctuations had to be averaged to give a mean value for nitrous oxide uptake.

End-Tidal Inhalation Agent

Feedback control automatically adjusted the inspired vapor concentration of an inhalation agent to maintain the desired end-tidal concentration. This technique, which provides an automated "over-pressure" induction, was studied in dogs (20 kg) during 4 hours of closed circuit anesthesia.[9] Using enflurane with oxygen and nitrous oxide, the end-tidal concentration was held within .037 $\pm$ .067 vol% (mean $\pm$ SD) of the desired concentration. The end-tidal concentration overshoot the desired value by .28 $\pm$ .067 vol% three minutes after induction. After 8 min the concentration remained within 0.1 vol% of the desired value.

Ventilation

The ventilation control algorithm adjusted the 900 C ServoVentilator's inspired minute volume to keep the end-tidal PCO_2 at the desired level. Using a traditional PID prototype controller in an animal study, $PaCO_2$ was kept within 1.25 mm Hg of the desired value, even with an average increase in CO_2 production of 44%.[10] Using a similar controller end-tidal PCO_2 was maintained within 0.1 $\pm$ .17 torr (mean $\pm$ SEM) of the desired value in 12 dogs following a hydrochloric acid injury.[11]

Rapid Induction

During induction of anesthesia, the inhalational agent inspired concentration was automatically adjusted under computer control to produce the desired end-tidal concentration. Initially, the inspired concentration was well above the desired final concentration, thus speeding the induction process. The initial inspired concentration depended on the gain of the feedback controller. Our system gain was adjusted so that the initial inspired concentration was approximately twice the desired end-tidal concentration. This approach was an attempt to match the traditional "over-pressure technique".[12]

A prototype end-tidal controller was used in two studies to validate the concept. Seven dogs were studied during a four hour period of enflurane-nitrous oxide anesthesia.[9] Following a sodium thiopental induction, the animals were intubated and the necessary monitors placed. After 10 minutes of oxygen breathing, the controller was initiated and the end-tidal concentration brought to 2.0 vol%. The inspired concentration began with a maximum of 3.7 vol% 3 min after induction. It gradually decreased until it reached 2.1 vol% after 4 hours. In a second control group of 7 animals, the inspired concentration was held constant at 2.0 vol%. There were no statistically significant differences between the two groups of animals with regard to enflurane uptake, heart rate, blood pressure, or cardiac output. The uptake of enflurane was greater in the end-tidal group only during the first 6 min. The end-tidal induction technique appeared to have no adverse cardiovascular effects beyond those found during induction with a constant inspired concentration.

In a second study, 23 patients were monitored during general anesthesia.[13] Following endotracheal intubation, these patients were connected to the closed rebreathing circuit with the end-tidal concentration held at 2.0 vol%. The mean inspired enflurane concentration reached a maximum of 3.5 $\pm$ .35 vol% (mean $\pm$ SD) 6 min after induction. The inspired concentration decreased to 2.4 $\pm$ .25 vol % after 60 min. Though there was considerable variability in enflurane uptake between patients, the controller properly adjusted the inspired concentration to compensate for these changes resulting in variability in the end-tidal concentration of less than 0.1 vol%.

Although a rapid "over-pressure" induction can be given according to a model of anesthesia uptake, the model must be tailored to the individual patient and careful clinical judgement is needed.[14-18] With the computer controlled system described here, it is not necessary to rely on a model or recipe, rather the gas concentrations are measured and controlled automatically.

MONITORING TRENDS IN GAS UPTAKE

The computer controlled anesthesia system was designed for use with either closed circuit or nonrebreathing anesthesia circuits. The control function remained the same with either circuit. Pulmonary mechanics and CO_2 production were monitored in each case. Oxygen uptake, N_2O uptake, and inhalational agent uptake were monitored only during closed circuit anesthesia.

Though it is difficult to evaluate the importance of gas uptake monitoring during anesthesia, certain correlations have been found. Significant changes in VO_2 have been identified with the following conditions.

1) Endotoxic shock was found to cause a 71% decrease in VO_2 when monitored during an endotoxin infusion in Rhesus monkeys.[19] The fall in VO_2 may have been due to reduced cardiac output or to reduced tissue metabolism.

2) Bolus infusions of fentanyl and thiopental given in patients undergoing general anesthesia caused an average decrease in oxygen consumption of 8.7 and 8.8 % respectively.[20] These changes were not seen in patients already at a level of deep anesthesia.

3) Blood pressure and heart rate were elevated using dopamine, atropine, an electrical pacing and phenalephrine and the accompaning changes in VO_2 studied in dogs.[21] VO_2 increased by 14% with dopamine, 17% with atropine, 16% with pacing, 14% with phenalephrine. All changes were significantly different from the control values.

4) Painful stimuli increased VO_2 during light anesthesia but not during deeper levels of anesthesia.[22] This relationship was studied during changing levels of nitrous oxide-fentanyl, and nitrous oxide-thiopental anesthesia in 24 dogs. Dose dependent relationships between VO_2, blood pressure, and cardiac output were found.

5) VO_2 and VCO_2 have been used to calculate the patient's metabolic rate by indirect calorimetry.[23,24] When interpreted in light of the patient's substrate utilization, the RQ may indicate hyperventilation or CO_2 retention.

Nitrous oxide uptake and inhalation agent uptake both follow muti-exponential curves with components for vessel-rich tissue, vessel-poor tissue, and blood and lung.[16,25] It would seem that there is useful information in an individual's uptake curve. With the alveolar ventilation controlled, the rapid uptake phase becomes a function of the patient's cardiopulmonary status. When the rapid uptake phase is complete, one has greater confidence that the patient has reached equilibrium with the selected gas concentration and may respond more predictably to surgical stimulus.

SUMMARY

An anesthesia machine has been developed with computer control of the fresh gas flows. Oxygen, nitrous oxide, and vaporizer flows are automatically adjusted by a microcomputer using mass flow control devices. Flow rates are optimized by the computer using feedback techniques. Flow rates are adjusted to achieve a "user selected" inspired oxygen concentration, end-tidal volatile agent concentration, and circuit volume. Ventilation is adjusted to a user-selected end-tidal CO_2 concentration and tidal volume.

With a computer controlling the fresh gas flows several advantages resulted. The overpressure induction was automated, the inspired oxygen concentration was controlled, the circuit volume was held constant during closed circuit anesthesia, computerized records allowed instant recall of trends in gas uptake, and ventilation was automatically adjusted to maintain a desired end-tidal PCO_2. These advantages make for a smoother and more rapid induction, simpler use of a closed-rebreathing circuit, enhanced decision making, and better $PaCO_2$ control.

REFERENCES
1. Boquet G, Bushman JA, and Davenport HT: The anaesthetic Machine--
   A Study of Function and Design. Br. J. Anaesth. (1980), 52, 61.
2. Drui AB, Belm RJ, and Martin WE. Predesign Investigation of the
   Anesthesia Operational Environment: (1973). Anesth Analg, 52, 584.
3. Cooper JB, Newbower RS, Moore JW, and Tautman ED. A New Anaesthesia
   Delivery System: (1978). Anesthesiology, 49, 310.
4. Westenskow DR, and Jordan WS. The Utah System: Computer Control
   of Fresh Gas Flows for Feedback Controlled Anesthesia Delivery:
   (1983) Contemporary Anesthesia Practice, Volume 8, In Press.
5. Westenskow DR, Jordan WS, Jordan Robert, and Gillmor ST. Evaluation
   of Oxygen Monitors for Use During Anesthesia: (1981) Anesthesia and
   Analgesia, 60, 53.
6. Westenskow DR, Johnson CC, Jordan WS, and Gehmlich DK. Instrumentation
   for Measuring Continuous Oxygen Consumption of Surgical Patients:
   (1977) Transaction on Biomedical Engineering, 24, 331.
7. Westenskow DR, Jordan WS, Gehmlich DS. Electronic Feedback
   Control and Measurement of Oxygen Consumption During Closed
   Circuit Anesthesia: Low Flow and Closed Circuit Anesthesia.
   Aldrete JA, Lowe HJ, Virtue RW (eds.). Grune & Stratton Publishers,
   (1979), page 135-146.
8. Lowe HJ. The Anesthetic Continuum. Low Flow and Closed Circuit
   Anesthesia. Aldrete JA, Lowe HJ, Virtue RW, (eds.), Grune &
   Stratton Publishers, (1979), page 11-37.
9. Westenskow DR, Jordan WS, Hayes JK. Feedback Control of Enflurane
   Delivery in Dogs: Inspired Compared to End-Tidaal Control: (1983)
   Anesth. Analg. (In Press).
10. Ohlson KB, Westenskow DR, Jordan WS. A Microprocessor Based Feed-
    back Controller for Mechanical Ventilation: (1982) Annals of Bio-
    medical Engineering, 10, 35.
11. East TD. A Microprocessor Based Differential Lung Ventilation System
    and Its Use to Evaluate a Variety of Differential Lung Ventilation
    Protocols: (1982) Ph.D. Thesis, Presented in the University of
    Utah Department of Bioengineering.
12. Dripps RD, Eckenhoff JE, Vandam LD. Introduction to Anesthesia:
    The Principles of Safe Practice. (5th ed.) Philadelphia: WB
    Saunders, 1977: 125-126.
13. Westenskow DR, Jordan WS, Hayes JK. Uptake of Enflurane: A Study
    of the Variability Between Patients: (1983) Brit. J. Anaesth. (In
    Press).
14. Chilcoat RT, Lunn JN, Blewett MC, and Khatib MT. Computer AAssistance
    in the Control of Depth of Anaesthesia: (1980), Brit. J. Anaesth.,
    52, 234P.
15. Cowles AL, Borgstedt HH, and Gillies AJ. Digital Computer Prediction
    of the Optimal Anaesthetic Inspired Concentration: (1972), Brit. J.
    Anaesth., 44, 420.
16. Eger EI. Anesthetic Uptake and Action: (1974). 1st ed. page 439.
    Baltimore: Williams aand Wilkins.
17. Chilcoat RT. An Adaptive Technique for Programmed Anaesthesia: (1973)
    Brit. J. Anaesth., 45, 1235.
18. Chilcoat RT. Servo Loops in the Control of Anesthetic Parameters:
    (1975). A Thesis, Presented in the Welsh Nat'l School of Medicine.
    University of Wales.
19. Westenskow DR, Houtchens BA, Franklin MG, Gehmlich DR, and Johnson CC.
    Dynamic Metabolic Response to Septic Shock in the Primate: Proceedings

278

30th ACEMB, Los Angeles, CA (1977).
20. Westenskow DR, and Jordan WS. Change in Oxygen Consumption Induced by Fentanyl and Thiopentone During Balanced Anaesthesia: (1978) Canad. Anaesth. Soc. J., 25, 18.
21. Westenskow DR, Huffaker JK, and Stanley TH. The Effect of Dopamine, Atropine, Phenylephrine and Cardiac Pacing on Oxygen Consumption During Fentanyl-Nitrous Oxide Anaesthesia in the Dog: (1981), Canad. Anaesth. Soc. J., 28, 121.
22. Westenskow DR, Jordan WS, Hodges MR, and Stanley TH. Correlation of Oxygen Uptake and Cardiovascular Dynamics During N_2O Fentanyl and N_2O-Thiopental Anesthesia in the Dog: (1978) Anesth Analg. 57:37.
23. Bursztein S, Glaser P, Trichet B, Taitebman U, and Nedey R. Utilization of Protein, Carbohydrate, and Fat in Fasting and Postabsorptive Subjects: (1980) Amer. Clin. Nutr., 33, 998.
24. Bursztein S, Saphar P, Glaser P, Taitelman U, De Myttenaere S, and Nedey R. Determination of Energy Metabolism From Respiratory Functions Alone: (1977) J. Appl. Physiol.: Respirat. Environ. Exercise Physiol., 42, 117.
25. Westenskow DR, and Jordan WS. Automatic Control of Closed Circuit Anesthesia and the Management of Enflurane N_2O and Oxygen Uptake: (May, 1982) Internationales Symposium, Institut fur Anasthesiologie. Dusseldor.

COMPUTER CONTROLLED ANAESTHESIA

J.M. EVANS, A. FRASER, C.C. WISE and W.L. DAVIES

1. INTRODUCTION

The development of microcomputers has allowed sophisticated computer techniques to be applied to many clinical procedures. The practice of clinical anaesthesia presents a wide field for computer systems - in a variety of functions from record keeping to life support systems.

The principal facilities offered by computers are as follows:

1. Rapid and complex data processing.
2. Extensive data storage.
3. Sophisticated analysis and display.
4. Compatibility with electronic monitors (i.e. input devices).
5. Compatibility with therapeutic systems, e.g. syringe pumps, infusion controllers, lung ventilators (i.e. output devices).

2. APPLICATIONS

It is clear that computers have considerable potential in clinical anaesthetic practice. The most obvious areas of application are:

2.1 Monitoring systems

The simpler biological signals e.g. ECG, blood pressure wave form, are easily and accurately recorded and displayed by hard-wired random logic. More complex signals e.g. EEG, EMG, or ocular microtremor, are more meaningfully interpreted when the signal has been processed e.g. by Fourier transformation. Such processing techniques have been available on main-frame and mini-computers for a long time, but on-line application in the operating room and intensive care is now possible with compact self contained monitors incorporating microprocessors.

2.2 Technological evolution

Many predominantly mechanical systems (e.g. lung ventilators and anaesthetic machines), despite great mechanical ingenuity, have severe practical design limitations. A marriage of mechanical systems, usually much simplified, with electronic controls and transducers can produce devices of great functional sophistication. Much of the elegance of such systems lies in the software and can be readily adapted or customised.

2.3 Applied control technology

Automated process control technology is highly developed and has many industrial and military applications. In the medical field it has been applied to the control of:

Systemic blood pressure	Analgesia
Muscle relaxation	Fluid balance
Pulmonary Ventilation	Diabetic therapy

Anaesthesia

The automated control of anaesthesia will be considered in further detail

3. AUTOMATED CONTROL OF ANAESTHESIA

A variety of control strategies have been used to date (see 1).

3.1 Open-loop control systems

An open-loop system can be compared to a "recipe" or a pre-programmed set of instructions with changes in anaesthetic drug administration occurring as preset events. Some variable elements are necessary to allow for factors such as patient weight and duration of operation.

The fundamental deficiency of an open-loop system is that it is unable to deal with individual patient variation. The magnitude of biological variation in response to anaesthetic agents, especially intravenous agents, is considerable - to the extent that open-loop systems cannot usefully control drug administration.

3.2 Hybrid systems

In an attempt to overcome the deficiencies of open-loop control additional information can be supplied to the control system to correct for drift.

Open-loop systems can be supplemented with a closed-loop feedback. In such an application it is clear that the feedback signal is itself of limited value only (i.e. it is not adequate feedback for a pure closed-loop) and is intended to correct the open-loop system. For example, the off-line analysis of blood drug levels could be used to provide some retrospective correction to a controlled intravenous infusion.

An open-loop system may also be supplemented with feed-forward control in certain circumstances. The uptake of inhalational agents is highly dependent upon alveolar ventilation. Thus prior knowledge of changes in alveolar ventilation can be fed-forward through the control system which can adjust the supply of the inhalational mixture. It can be seen that in this example the system is not "pure" in that the inhaled agent may change spontaneous alveolar ventilation and introduce an element of feedback.

3.3 Closed-loop systems

In a closed-loop system one or more output parameters are measured and compared to reference or "set" levels. The discrepancy between the measured and set levels gives rise to an "error" signal which can then be used to adjust the rate of drug administration so as to minimise the value of the error signal.

While this form of control is highly developed and reliable it is very dependent upon the measurement of meaningful output variables. Unfortunately the measurement of "depth" or "adequacy" of anaesthesia remains something of a Philosopher's Stone. We have to accept that the best we can do is to rely upon the measurement of physiological functions which provide an inferential guide to the adequacy of anaesthesia. A variety of physiological functions (see below) have been examined as suitable control system inputs.

The output of the control system used to control a drug-delivery device. During inhalational anaesthesia changes in drug level will be effected by changes in gas flow and vaporiser settings; to date such equipment is mostly experimental. During intravenous anaesthesia changes in the rate of drug administration can be achieved by direct electronic control of intravenous infusion devices.

4. PHYSIOLOGICAL VARIABLES/SYSTEM INPUTS

A variety of physiological variables have been used as a guide to the adequacy of anaesthesia.

4.1 Electroencephalography (EEG)

This has been used since the early 1950's by Bickford and others as a monitor of anaesthesia (2). Although the EEG is a measure of the principal target organ of anaesthesia - the Central Nervous System, its interpretation has created many problems. On crude examination of the EEG the most marked changes are produced by relatively large doses of anaesthetic drugs - several MAC multiples in the case of volatile agents. In routine clinical practice such doses are not used and the various cocktails of drugs commonly used may produce relatively subtle and specific changes in the EEG.

The development of more sophisticated signal processing, for instance power spectral analysis and spectral edge frequency (3) has re-aroused interest in the EEG. Although these forms of signal analysis enable relatively fine changes to be observed they are often agent specific, the effects produced by fentanyl for example differing from those produced by halothane.

4.2 Ocular-Microtremor (OMT)

OMT, usually measured by the application of an accelerometer to the conjunctiva, is the normal microscopic oscillation of the eyeball produced by the gaze control mechanism. OMT is changed in various disease states and has been shown to be suppressed by intravenous thiopentone.(4) Unfortunately it is readily suppressed by muscle relaxants and is thus of limited value in routine clinical practice.

4.3 Clinical signs

Individual clinical signs and measurements e.g. blood pressure or heart rate and spontaneous ventilation often show dramatic changes in magnitude as evidence of stress. Similarly, changes in sweating, tear formation and pupillary size can be observed during "light" anaesthesia. Attempts have been made to employ one or other of the traditional clinical signs as a controlled variable in a closed-loop control system. Suppan used the heart rate and the blood pressure for this purpose (5,6). Although attractive, such a simple approach has limitations; the heart rate alone cannot be relied upon as a patient output variable, anaesthetic agents and various adjuvant drugs such as muscle relaxants will disturb the rate as will events such as haemorrhage.

Despite their many limitations it cannot be denied that the great bulk of practical expertise in the use of anaesthetic drugs is based on clinical experience - the foundation of which is clinical monitoring.

4.4 Skeletal Muscle Activity

Skeletal muscle activity clearly indicates (for practical purposes) insufficient anaesthesia but is seldom associated with recall in the non-paralysed patient. Skeletal muscle relaxants clearly suppress this response.

It is interesting to note that in Guedel's classification of the stages of ether anaesthesia, measurements of blood pressure and heart rate are not considered. Furthermore, of the nine variables monitored only two (pupil size and tear formation) remain to be observed in the paralysed patient.
Tunstall has extended the scope for examining the potential of the skeletal muscle response by isolating the forearm from systemic muscle relaxants with a tourniquet (7). In suitably prepared patients he has been able to demonstrate

the integrity of auditory perception, voluntary control and coordination, and peripheral skeletal muscle response during anaesthesia for Caesarean sections. The widespread use of this technique outside of obstetrics for routine purposes presents many problems not the least of which is the fact that it can only be applied for a limited period of time (8).

The potency of inhalational agents is conventionally assessed by the minimum alveolar concentration (MAC) required to prevent a skeletal muscle response. General clinical experience and the observations of Tunstall using his isolated forearm technique, suggest that anaesthetic equivalence less than MAC is sufficient to produce adequate anaesthesia without recall but may not be sufficient to prevent some muscle response. In other words the amount of anaesthetic required to produce unconsciousness and lack of recall is in general likely to be less than that required to suppress skeletal muscle response to noxious stimuli.

4.5 Skin Resistance

Skin resistance or conductance has been examined by many workers. Although significant changes in skin resistance can be observed in response to stress, the pattern of response tends to be rather inconsistent (9).

Technical considerations such as electrode design, material, placement and current characteristics (AC/DC etc) have not been standardised so that results are seldom comparable in absolute terms.

4.6 Electromyogram (EMG)

Interest has been aroused in the use of the integrated EMG of the frontalis muscle. It has been proposed that the frontalis muscle is not as sensitive as other muscles to skeletal muscle relaxants (10). In turn it is argued that frowning, a function of the frontalis muscle, can be monitored as a sign of lightening anaesthesia by measurement of the frontalis EMG. (11). Changes in the frontalis EMG certainly appear to occur during anaesthesia and these can be seen to respond to further drug administration. It remains to be clarified to what extent the frontalis muscle can be relied upon especially during muscle relaxation. It is important that the monitoring system is able to discern the EMG signal from the frontal EEG signal to minimise crosstalk.

5. TWO NOVEL APPROACHES TO ANAESTHESIA MONITORING

As a development of our interest in anaesthetic monitoring and control we have examined and investigated two novel techniques for monitoring anaesthesia. These are:

1. Clinical scoring system.

2. Lower oesophageal contractility.

5.1. Clinical scoring system

With the evident deficiencies in using any single clinical sign or measurement as a patient output variable we considered that the summation of a number of individual clinical signs might prove to be more useful.

The following clinical signs/noninvasive measurements are generally available during anaesthesia:

1. Skeletal muscle activity.

2. Pupil size.

3. Blood pressure.

4. Heart rate.

5. Sweating.

6. Tear formation.

5.1.1. Skeletal muscle activity is of limited value. In the fully paralysed patient it is supressed: in the partially paralysed patient the absence of muscle activity may provide some reassurance that anaesthesia is adequate.

5.1.2. Pupil size can provide some guidance in certain circumstances. Guedel's description of changes in pupil size during ether anaesthesia is similarly observed with most volatile agents. In contrast intravenous agents and analgesics have a completely different effect. Most opioid analgesics produce a miosis which is often intense and persistant. Althesin (Glaxo) on the other hand produces a mydriasis in large doses; mydriasis is less marked as the infusion is reduced but may return during inadequate anaesthesia as a response to stress!

5.1.3 Blood pressure and 5.1.4.Heart rate are two related cardiovascular indices regularly recorded during anaesthesia. A rise in blood pressure or heart rate are both taken to indicate insufficient anaesthesia. Clearly these changes may be obscured by other events.

Haemorrhage will tend to lower the blood pressure and increase the heart rate. A variety of drugs will change the heart rate e.g. atropine, gallamine and pancuronium will tend to increase it while digoxin and beta-blockers will reduce it.

Changes in blood pressure may also be attenuated by beta-blockers, ganglion blocking drugs - including curare and alcuronium. Despite these limitations, changes in blood pressure and heart rate are often relied upon as evidence of insufficient anaesthesia.

5.1.5 <u>Sweating</u> is again a clinical sign generally acknowledged to indicate insufficient anaesthesia. The very earliest indication of sweating can be detected by electrical measurement of skin resistance. Clinicians have not been enthusiastic in making these measurements routinely and appear to rely upon their clinical acumen.

Sweating is under the control of the sympathetic nervous system but has cholinergic post-ganglionic fibres. Thus it may be reduced by anticholinergic drugs and will obviously be affected by ambient temperatures and humidity.

5.1.6 <u>Tear formation</u> An excess of tears is frequently observed during periods of insufficient anaesthesia. The exact mechanism of the response is a little uncertain - it probably has two components: in part it is due to pain and it is also part of a wider response to a foreign body (the endotracheal tube) in the airway.

The efferent neurological pathway is parasympathetic and thus anticholinergic drugs may attenuate the response.

In considering the clinical signs it is clear that the magnitude of the response may be altered by various drugs - notably those with autonomic effects. Similarly certain disease states will alter the response. Diseases involving the heart, peripheral vasculature, eyes, skin and autonomic nervous system may alter the pattern of clinical signs.

In order to collate these clinical signs and measurements into a single entity we have developed a scoring system. Four patient variables are examined:

Blood <u>P</u>ressure	P
Heart <u>R</u>ate	R
<u>S</u>weating	S
<u>T</u>ear Formation	T

This conveniently allows the score to be referred to as the PRST score. It is interesting to note that the P and R components predominantly involve a sympathetic response whereas the S and T components involve cholinergic mechanisms.

A score value of 0, 1 or 2 is attached to changes in each of the 4 indices.

Control values of Pressure and Rate are obtained preoperatively shortly before the induction of anaesthesia.

TABLE I

SYSTOLIC BLOOD	LESS THAN CONTROL + 15	0
PRESSURE	LESS THAN CONTROL + 30	1
(mm Hg)	MORE THAN CONTROL + 30	2
HEART RATE	LESS THAN CONTROL + 15	0
(beats/min)	LESS THAN CONTROL + 30	1
	MORE THAN CONTROL + 30	2
SWEAT	NIL	0
	SKIN MOIST TO TOUCH	1
	VISIBLE BEADS OF SWEAT	2
TEARS OR	NO EXCESS TEARS WITH EYELIDS OPEN	0
LACRIMATION	EXCESS TEARS VISIBLE WITH EYELIDS OPEN	1
	TEAR OVERFLOW FROM CLOSED EYELIDS	2

As anaesthetic drug administration is reduced, score values are seen to increase, conversely, an increasing anaesthetic administration decreases the score values. The score has no inherent objectivity - it is simply a means of standardising the expression or description of changes in these selected clinical signs. Thus the clinician will have to decide what level of score is acceptable. In making this judgement he will have to bear in mind factors that will foreseeably affect the score values e.g. the use of agents such as pancuronium may increase the scores of the PR components.

5.1.7 Application of PRST scores. We have used the scoring system in two ways.

5.1.7(a) Control of incremental drug administration. If the anaesthetic or adjuvant drug (e.g. fentanyl) is administered in increments, these can be given when a specified maximum score value (e.g. 2, 3 or 4) is obtained. Clinical indices are assessed regularly at intervals of approximately 5 minutes. It is usual to observe a fall in score value following the administration of the drug followed by a progressive rise towards the maximum acceptable score value.

5.1.7(b) Control of continuous drug administration. If the anaesthetic agent is continuously administered or infused then a form of closed-loop control can be employed. The clinician selects a desired score value (DSV) and monitors the clinical indices at regular intervals. The measured score value (MSV) can be compared to the DSV and an error signal generated to change the infusion rate accordingly.

A variety of control processes can be used but the following equation provides a very simple control facility if scores are assessed at regular intervals (5 minutes).

$$NDR = ODR (1 - kE)$$

where NDR = new drug rate,

     ODR = old drug rate,

       k = system/drug constant (e.g. 0.1)

       E = (DSV - MSV) i.e. error.

5.1.8 <u>Results</u>. The score control system employing the above control technique has been used in 3 groups of 10 patients to control infusions of fentanyl (as an adjuvant to nitrous oxide), Althesin/fentanyl mixture (exclusively intravenous) and etomidate/fentanyl mixture (exclusively intravenous).

The anaesthetic was infused by a digitally controlled syringe pump, manually set after a simple computer programme calculated the new drug rate from the clinical data entered. The control system was set to maintain a DSV of 3.

Over a period of an hour individual variations in the anaesthetic requirements soon became apparent. A ratio of high:low demand rates of 4:1 was seen in these groups of 10 patients.

No cases of recall were found and all patients awoke in a relatively short time.

Speed of recovery was assessed by measuring the time, from discontinuing anaesthesia and giving neostigmine/atropine, to "eyes open on command" - TEOC.The mean duration of anaesthesia and TEOC are shown in Table II.

TABLE II

ANAESTHETIC	DURATION (mean mins (SD))	TEOC (mean mins (SD))
Fentanyl/N_2O	108.4 (42.4)	3.9 (1.7)
Althesin/fentanyl	127.5 (79)	11.4 (14.8)
Etomidate/fentanyl	104.5 (47.6)	15.4 (15.5)

5.2 <u>Lower Oesophageal Contractility (LOC)</u>

The lower half of the human oesophagus is unusual in that it is composed of smooth muscle. Thus its contractile activity is not directly affected by skeletal muscle relaxants.

Oesophageal activity can be classified into 3 forms.

5.2.1 <u>Primary Peristaltic Activity</u>. This is the prime physiological function of the oesophagus - to convey a bolus of masticated food from the pharynx to the stomach. The primary peristaltic wave starts at the pharyngo-oesophageal junction and progresses over a period of about 5 seconds to the lower oesophagal sphincter. The passing constriction band can be observed by a balloon, catheter transducer system as a single contraction with a pressure amptitude of up to 100 mm.Hg.

5.2.2 <u>Secondary Peristaltic Activity</u>. This peristaltic activity which commences not at the top of the oesophagus but at some point along the body of the oesophagus. The secondary peristaltic wave is similar to the primary peristaltic wave except that it is usually triggered by a particle of food or other material lying in the oesophageal lumen. It fulfills the function of a "clearing up" process.

5.2.3 <u>Tertiary Oesophageal Activity</u>. This is a <u>non-peristaltic</u> contraction of the oesphagus which may involve the whole or isolated segments of the oesophagus.

It is an interesting form of oesophageal activity which has no obvious physiological function. It can be observed in fit subjects but is seen more frequently in association with oesophageal disease and old age.

A particularly interesting feature of the tertiary activity is its relationship to stress. An increase in activity can be induced by exposure of subject to stressful situations (12,13).

We have observed tertiary activity during general anaesthesia. If oesophageal pressure is monitored with a balloon/catheter/transducer system activity is seen as a contraction lasting between 2 and 5 seconds with a typical amplitude of 50mmHg. These spontaneous lower oesophageal contractions (SLOC) occur during light general anaesthesia. They are seldom seen during inhalational anaesthesia at 1.0 MAC but generally appear as anaesthesia is lightened, and may reach a rate of 4-5 contractions/min. during very "light" anaesthesia.

A technique has also been developed for examining the secondary peristaltic response. This is achieved by introducing a second balloon into the oesophagus. This is briefly inflated and may, during "light" anaesthesia, provoke a secondary peristaltic contraction which can be sensed by the monitoring balloon.

5.2.4 <u>Closed-loop control in anaesthesia</u>. In preliminary studies we have used SLOC as a patient output variable to control administration of

inhalational anaesthetics (enflurane, halothane) and intravenous anaesthetics
and adjuvants (Althesin, etomidate, fentanyl).

The control of fentanyl administration will be described in greater
detail.

5.2.5 <u>Method</u>. Oesophageal activity was monitored with a
balloon/catheter/transducer system. Contractions in excess of 25mmHg were
registered as a significant event (by an electronics discriminator) and a pulse
fed to a digitally controlled syringe pump. The pump was set to deliver an
increment of fentanyl intravenously (5 ug/70Kg).

Anaesthesia was induced with thiopentone, pancuronium and an initial
loading dose of fentanyl (1ug/kilo). Anaesthesia was maintained with nitrous
oxide:oxygen (70:30) using a non-rebreathing circuit and a minute volume of 8.4
1/70 kilo.

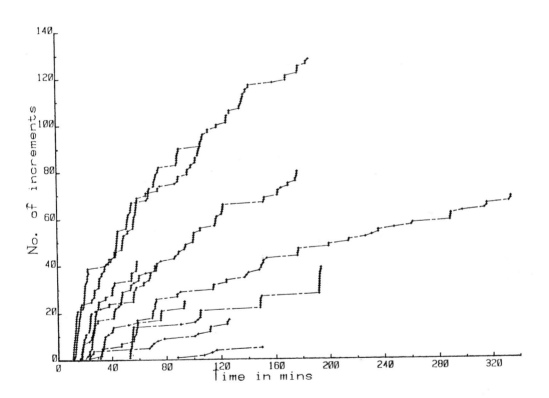

No other supplementation (other than extra doses of pancuronium as needed)
was required. At the end of surgery muscle relaxation was reversed with
atropine/neostigmine and anaesthetic administration stopped. The duration of
TEOC was recorded.

5.2.6 <u>Results</u>. Ten patients were included in this study. The mean duration
of anaesthesia was 123 (SD 60) minutes.

Eight anaesthetics lasted for more than 90 minutes and at this time the
lowest fentanyl uptake was 5 ug/70 kg while the highest was 445 ug/70 kg. The
highest total demand was 635 ug and the lowest 25 ug. Despite these wide
variations in dose all patients woke rapidly- the mean TEOC was 5.3 (SD 2.9)
minutes.

Anaesthesia was judged to be adequate and there were no cases of
postoperative recall.

The figure shows the uptake of fentanyl (1 increment=5 ug/70 Kg) against
time. The wide range of demand is obvious. It is interesting to note that a
high fentanyl demand rate is associated with an <u>early</u> first demand (following
the initial loading dose).

The majority of the uptake curves fit the following form of the equation

$$Uptake = a + bt + c \log t$$

where a = loading dose   b,c = constants   t = time

The best fit equation for the patient with the longest anaesthetic (335
minutes) takes the following form

$$Uptake = -53 + 0.08 \, t + 16.2 \log t \qquad\qquad (R^2 = .99)$$

The loading dose is shown as a negative intercept since it was not part of
the controlled dosage.

5.2.8 <u>Limitations of Lower Oesophageal Contractility monitoring</u>. It may
be subject to interference from a number of sources.

Smooth muscle relaxants such as sodium nitroprusside or nitroglycerine may
inhibit LOC. Inhibition may also be produced by ganglion blocking drugs and
large doses of intravenous anticholinergics.

Oesophageal disease or autonomic neuropathy may naturally inhibit
oesophageal contractility.

6. CONCLUSIONS

As an alternative to existing techniques we have examined the potential
value of two new methods of monitoring anaesthesia, clinical PRST scoring and
lower oesophageal contractility .

In preliminary studies, both methods were successful in maintaining satisfactory closed loop control of a variety of inhalational and intravenous anaesthetics. Lower oesophageal contractility may also prove to be a useful monitor to indicate "lightening" or insufficient anaesthesia.

REFERENCES

1. Chilcoat R.T.
    A review of the control of depth of anaesthesia.
    Trans.Inst.Meas.Cont. 2,38-45 1980
2. Faulconer A. and Bickford R.G.
    Electroencephalography in anaesthesiology.
    C.C.Thomas, Illinois, USA. 1960
3. Rampil I.J., Sasse F.J., Smith N.T., Hott B.H. and Flemming D.C.
    Spectral Edge Frequency - A new correlate of anaesthetic depth.
    A.S.A. Abstracts 53,3,Sept 1980
4. Coakley D., Thomas J.G. and Lunn J.N.
    The effect of anaesthesia on ocular microtremor.
    Brit.J.Anaesth. 48,1122-1123,1976
5. Suppan P.
    Feedback monitoring in anaesthesia II: Pulse rate control of halothane
    administration.
    Brit.J.Anaesth. 44,1263,1972
6. Suppan P.
    Feedback monitoring in anaesthesia IV: The indirect measurement of arterial
    pressure and its use for the control of halothane administration.
    Brit.J.Anaesth. 49,141-150,1977
7. Tunstall M.E.
    Detecting wakefullness during general anaesthesia for caesarian section.
    Brit.Med.J. 1,1321,1977
8. Breckenridge J. and Aitkenhead A.R.
    Isolated forearm technique for detection of wakefullness during general
    anaesthesia.
    Brit.Med.J.53,665P,1981
9. Goddard G.F.
    A pilot study of the changes of skin electrical conductance in patients
    undergoing general anaesthesia and surgery.
    Anaesthesia 37,408-415,1982
10. Smith S., Brown H.O.,Toman J.E.T. and Goodman L.S.
    Lack of cerebral effects of d-tubocurare.
    Anaesthesiology 8,1,1947
11. Harmel M., Kline F.F. and Davies D.A.
    EEMG - a practical index of cortical activity and muscular relaxation
    Acta Anaest.Scand.Suppl.70,97-102,1978
12. Rubin J., Nagler R., Spiro H.M. and Pilot M.L.
    Measuring the effect of emotions on esophageal motility
    Psychosomatic Medicine 24,2,1962
13. Stacher G., Schimierer G. and Landgraf M.
    Tertiary oesophageal contractions evoked by acoustical stimuli.
    Gastroenterology 77,49-53,1979

COMPUTER REGULATED SODIUM NITROPRUSSIDE INFUSION FOR BLOOD PRESSURE CONTROL

N.L. PACE, M.D.
D.R. WESTENSKOW, PH. D.

1. INTRODUCTION

The use of the fast-acting vasodilator sodium nitroprusside (SNP) for the control of blood pressure has been in practice for the last 20 years. Originally, the only indication for SNP therapy was management of hypertensive crises. Later, the use of this vasodilator for controlled hypotension became popular. Finally, within the last 10 years, the use of SNP for the management of myocardial dysfunction and ischemia has emerged. Computer, rather than manual, control of SNP infusion to control blood pressure will probably be the next step in the safer and even wider use of the drug.

In this paper we will briefly review the effects and uses of SNP, the control theory used to create computerized SNP infusors, and the literature on computer controlled SNP infusion. We will conclude with a listing of criteria for a good computer controller for the infusion of SNP for blood pressure regulation.

2. PHARMACOLOGY, PHARMACOLINETICS, AND TOXICOLOGY OF SODIUM NITROPRUSSIDE

Sodium nitroprusside (SNP) is a unique vasodilator.[1-3] Its structure has 5 cyanide (CN) molecules and a nitroso (NO) group covalently attached to one iron atom. On being metabolized, SNP releases the 5 CN and therein lies the toxic effect. Mechanistically, the drug causes a relaxation of the smooth muscle of the peripheral vasculature, both arterial and venous; this action is direct, not via autonomic or central nervous systems, explaining the rapid onset. Alpha and beta adrenergic receptors are free and available for other drug intervention if necessary.

The exact cellular mechanism is unknown. SNP binds to sulfhydryl groups; there is speculation that SNP ties up Ca^{++} intracellularly. An increase of intracellular cyclic GMP is also associated with SNP infusion.

SNP infusion produces a relatively balanced arteriolar and venular dilation, resulting in a reduction in both afterload and preload. This dilating occurs throughout in the body, including the coronary and cerebral vessels.

Within the heart, the decrease in preload and afterload associated with SNP infusion causes a significant reduction in myocardial oxygen consumption. This beneficial action of SNP is offset by the possible detrimental coronary "steal" effect caused by the arteriolar dilation of blood supply to normal myocardium. Therefore, although the heart needs less oxygen, the decrease in collateral flow caused by the "steal" might shunt blood supply from an already partially ischemic area of the heart, thereby creating total ischemia of that area of myocardium. This latter effect is still debated.

Within the brain, SNP initially causes vasodilation with increased cerebral blood flow and cerebral volume. When using SNP for neurosurgery, it has been suggested that one immediately decrease the MAP to 70% of control to avoid this complication. From this pressure on down, brain blood flow and volume correlate with the MAP.

Brain blood flow autoregulation is impaired when surgery has required hypotension for extended periods. Therefore, when one returns blood pressure to the control value, autoregulation does not immediately take over. Overperfusion of the brain can take place unless the patient is gradually taken off the SNP infusion.

Within the pulmonary system, SNP is noted to alter the ventilation-perfusion ratio, resulting in a decreased PaO_2. This shunt-like effect is thought to be caused by a vasodilation of the pulmonary system resulting in a reversal of the normal hypoxic pulmonary vasoconstriction mechanism which lowers blood flow to the unventilated or poorly ventilated alveoli. This could present problems in patients who already have a compromised oxygenation. It has been suggested that at least 40% O_2 be administered during controlled hypotension.

SNP is administered exclusively intravenously. Following a bolus injection, mean arterial pressure (MAP) falls in 40 to 90 sec, and peak effect is noted in 1 1/2 to 2 minutes. After about 5 minutes, drug effect is dissapated. As the elimination half-life of SNP is one to two hours, termination of drug effect is by redistribution. The short duration of action of SNP is thought to be the time for the drug to cross the red blood cell membrane where each SNP molecule quickly receives one electron from oxyhemoglobin to begin degradation.

After cessation of infusion, MAP returns to control values in about 4 minutes. Quite commonly, a "rebound phenomenon" is noted and thought to be caused by an increased activation of the Renin-Angiotension system (RAS). This rebound hypertension may be ameliorated by a slow, staged reduction in SNP infusion rate. Others have noted an increased activity of the norepine-phrine/epinephrine system (NES) during SNP infusion and consequently found that simultaneous administration of beta adrenergic blocking agents prevented rebound hypertension when terminating the hypotensive state. Furthermore, reducing the activity of the NES system reduces activity of the RAS system.

SNP is metabolized to thiocyanate (SCN), which is excreted principally via the kidneys. The half-life of thiocyanate is 4 hours and has a normal renal clearance of 2.2 ml/min.

Cyanide formation is thought to be directly dose-related. Once controlled-hypotension is achieved, it is imperative that one calculate the total amount to be infused (infusion rate X duration of induced hypotension). If this amount exceeds the recommended toxic limit (1.5 mg/kg within 2 1/2 hours), measures must be taken to prevent CN build up. Several suggestions include:

1) Increase the volatile anesthetic.
2) Change patient position to decrease venous return.
3) Switch hypotensive agents.
4) Administer an anti-cyanide agent concurrently (Sodium Thiosulfate).
Recommendations for maximum drug limits over longer periods are less well established.

Younger patients frequently require more SNP than the elderly. However, they are just as susceptable to dose-related CN toxicity as the elderly.

SNP is also noted to be an inhibitor of platelet aggregation and should be carefully administered to those with associated platelet dysfunction. The metabolic product (SCN) is noted to decrease iodine trapping and there-fore SNP should not be used with those in a hypothyroid condition. (SCN toxicity is manifest at blood levels of 8-10 mg % or greater).

If the SNP dose will be close to the maximum, symptoms of CN toxicity (metabolic acidosis, increased venous oxygen content, decreased venous-arterial oxygen content difference) should be checked frequently. If unexplained metabolic acidosis is noted, immediate cessation of SNP is indicated. The acidosis might need to be corrected by administering sodium bicarbonate. Anti-cyanide agents are administered to reduce the cyanide level (sodium thiosulfate).

1. THERAPEUTIC INDICATIONS

Probably the most accepted use of SNP is for the control of hypertensive crisis. Originally used for relief of such extreme cases as malignant hypertension and eclampsia, there are now many more indications. Possibly the most common is management of the postoperative cardiac patient. On emergence from anesthesia, catecholamine levels are dramatically increased due to pain, hypoxia, hypercarbia, shivering, and/or anxiety. The associated increased cardiac work may result in myocardial ischemia. Thus a reduction of elevated blood pressures to normal levels will decrease myocardial work and decrease the chance of myocardial ischemia. In addition, reduction in blood pressure will generally lower mediastinal blood loss postoperatively.

Generally the dose required is significantly lower than the toxic level and is needed for only the first 12-48 hours postoperatively. Nevertheless, short term use requires observation for possible cyanide toxicity; long term use also requires observation for both cyanide and thiocyanate toxicity.

Induced hypotension during surgery to prevent or reduce blood loss and to provide a clearer surgical field has been in use since WW II. SNP is helpful especially for neurosurgery because it also can shrink the brain once blood pressure has dropped. If necessary, very low MAP levels can be maintained with SNP for short intervals.

SNP induced hypotension is also helpful in reducing the amount of blood loss and can be used in the event of a blood bank deficit.

The most sensitive areas of the body to controlled hypotension include: cardiac, cerebral, and spinal areas. Careful monitoring of their condition (ECG, EEG, spinal reflexes, etc.) is vital.

An unwanted tachycardia is immediately seen in many instances of induced hypotension. Beta adrenergic blockers will prevent this reflex.

Use of SNP to ameliorate heart failure (HF) and low cardiac output states is now common. Vasodilators, in general, have become a third component in management of the patient with HF which also includes the use of positive inotropic drugs and diuretics.

Using SNP to improve CHF is not necessarily associated with tachycardia. The more impaired the cardiac function, the more the improvement (increased stroke volume and cardiac output) seen with SNP. The increased cardiac output produces increased renal blood flow and correspondingly increased urine flow, sodium excretion, and creatinine clearance. Catecholamine levels decrease with the increased cardiac efficiency.

Most recently Durrer et al[4] has reported a significant reduction in mortality when using SNP to reduce the infarction size. Use was within the first 5 hours after the initial myocardial infarction (MI) and continued for 24 hours.

Three beneficial actions of SNP therapy for acute MI were postulated.

1) A reduction in afterload, thereby reducing energy requirement of the jeopardized tissues.

2) An increased coronary blood flow, thereby supplying more oxygen to the jeopardized tissue even though perfusion pressures might be lowered

3) A reduction in the amount of myocardium irretrievably lost.

As is well known, there is a very wide range of effective infusion rates among patients. The dose required to drop blood pressure can vary over at least a 2 log range (0.1 ug/kg/min to 10 ug/kg/min). In addition, the sensitivity of a given patient can also vary enormously over very short time intervals (minutes), especially during anesthesia. The titration of SNP infusion rate is a tedious, highly labor intensive activity. Computer control, with proper safety restrictions, could alleviate this burden.

3. COMPUTER CONTROL OF SNP INFUSION

A SNP controller generally includes an automated infusion pump, a blood pressure monitor, and a computer (figure 1). The blood pressure is measured and compared with the desired pressure, the difference is used by the controller through some decison making routine to adjust the SNP infusion rate.

This type of feedback control is not new to medicine. It has been used to control blood volume,[5] blood pressure,[6-10] depth of anesthesia,[11,12] blood gases,[13-17] and blood glucose level.[18] These numerous applications indicate that computer control can be safe and reliable, and at times, extremely useful.

In designing a computer controller, the decision routine will determine the safety and the success of the system. Basically three types of routines have been proposed for sodium nitroprusside. The first category includes rule based or "wait-and-see" routines.[8,10,19] These initiate a step change in SNP infusion rate, then wait to observe the blood pressure response. The next step change in infusion rate depends on the previous response in blood pressure. This mimics current manual control. The size and frequency

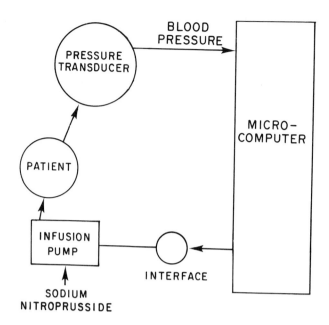

BLOOD PRESSURE

PRESSURE TRANSDUCER

MICRO-COMPUTER

PATIENT

INFUSION PUMP

INTERFACE

SODIUM NITROPRUSSIDE

FIGURE 1.

of the steps are determined empirically by each designer. These systems tend to have response times which are quite long; on the other hand, they have the advantage of providing stable, non-oscillatory control when delivering drugs with longtime constants.

The second category includes classical controllers of the proportional-integral-derivative (PID) type.[6,7,19] A PID controller tracks the difference between actual and desired pressure in 3 ways: the absolute value (proportional), the rate of change (derivative), and the accumulated error (integral). A weighted average of these 3 measurements is then used to control infusion rate. Because of their wide spread industrial application, numerous analytical techniques are available for optimization of PID Controllers.[20,21] An ICU in Birmingham, Alabama headed by L. Sheppard et al has used a modified PID controller for SNP for many years.[19] They have, in fact, documented that better control of blood pressure is provided by computer control than is provided manually. Recently, Slate et al and Smolen have developed techniques by which the parameters of these PID controllers are modified on-line, thus improving response time of these otherwise slow controllers.[22,23] This self-adaptation significantly improves the contollers performance and the desired pressure is achieved in 5 to 10 minutes.

The third category of controllers include those which use adaptive control theory.[22,24-26] Adaptive control is a scheme of simultaneous identification and control.[21,27,28] It combines an identification algorithm with the classical control procedure. The approach assumes that the patient can be described by a mathematical model in which the values of coefficients may be uncertain. Real time algorithms are used to estimate the coefficients and the resulting estimates affect a controller designed to match the assumed model.

Self-tuning control is possibly the simpliest possible adaptive control algorithm for sodium nitroprusside control.[27,28] It uses algorithms which are as simple as possible, it is of a form which can readily be implemented on available microcomputers, and theoretical results although incomplete, indicate the satisfactory stable performance can sometimes be expected. Successful applications of adaptive control have generally been self-tuning.

Model reference adaptive controllers use a model of the patient which is continually updated by an adaptive process.[27,28] Inputs to the model are determined which will cause the desired outputs. When the same inputs are applied to the patient, the patient will be closely controlled.

Successful applications with self-tuning or model reference controllers report response times on the order of 5 to 10 minutes. Adequate control has been shown in simulations and animal studies, however, patient data is still lacking.

Of the three catagories ("wait and see", PID, and adaptive) discussed, adaptive control has several advantages. By adjusting the system response to a particular patient, the adaptive controller is better optimized to that patient. Also, if the patient's circulatory system or sensitivity to sodium nitroprusside changes, an adaptive controller will change to compensate. In contrast, as conditions change, the classical controllers become less than optimum and may provide unsatisfactory control.

4. CRITERIA FOR SAFE, SUCCESSFUL COMPUTER CONTROL

As computer controlled infusion pumps become commercially available, by what standards should they be judged? These criteria should include standards of effectiveness, reliability, ease of use, safety and security. Our recommendations are the following:

The controller should be fast. (If a slower ascent or descent to a desired pressure is needed, several small step changes can be used.) After initializing a change in the setpoint (desired pressure), the step change should be accomplished within 2-3 minutes, with an overshot of no more than 10 mmHg. Once the setpoint is reached, actual blood pressure should vary no more than $\pm$ 5 mmHg. At all times, the controller should be adapting itself to possible changes in patient sensitivity to the drug. If there is a near catastrophic event (sudden massive blood loss, inadvertent bolus injection of SNP or vasopressor drug), the controller should restore MAP to the setpoint within 3 to 5 minutes.

During initializing of the controller, the following parmeters should be entered: setpoint, patient weight, lowest pressure allowed, maximum infusion rate, etc. Thus, possible safety checks that can be implemented in the system include:

1) limiting maximum dosage rate (8-10 mcg/kg/min)
2) limiting maximum total dose (1.5 mg/kg over 2 1/2 hours) and displaying the time when this limit will be reached
3) installing an alarm to detect unstable pressures that are beyond the controllers capability

Computer controlled infusion of SNP must distinguish changes in blood pressure due to body function from that due to care procedures. Common intraoperative and post-operative care procedures include:

1) sampling of blood from the arterial cannula
2) flushing the arterial line

In addition, damping of the pressure waveform by patient movement or line clotting must not destroy control stability.

For security reasons, changing the setpoint or other parameters of the controller should be easy, but not allow absent minded fiddling or uninformed trespassing.

5. CONCLUSION

Sodium Nitroprusside is a valuable drug for the managment of hypertension, control of hypotension and management of myocardial dysfunction and ischemia. Because of the range of patient sensitivities to the drug is so large and because sensitivity may change during its administration, the drug is difficult to deliver with manual adjustment of the infusion pump. Computer control of SNP infusion offers a means of overcoming this problem. A computer controller can adjust the infusion rate automatically to compensate for changes in patient sensitivity. A self adapting controller meeting the safety criteria listed may result in even more effective use of the drug and better control of the patient's blood pressure.

REFERENCES

1. Tinker JH, Michenfelder JD: Sodium nitroprusside: pharmacology, toxicology and therapeutics. Anesthesiology 45:340-354, 1976.
2. Ivankovitch AD (ed): Nitroprusside and Other Short-Acting Hypotensive Agents, 1978 International Anesthesiology Clinics. Little, Brown and Company, Boston, 1978, Volume 16, Number 2.
3. Cottrell JE, Gupta B, Turndorf H: Induced hypotension in Anesthesia and Neurosurgery, eds Cottrell JE and Turndorf H. The C.V. Mosby
4. Durrer JD, Lie KI, van Capelle FJL, Durrer D: Effect of sodium nitroprusside on mortality in acute myocardial infarction. N Engl J Med 306:11211128, 1982.
5. Sheppard LC, Kouchoukos NT: Automation of measurements and interventions in the systematic care of postoperative cardiac surgical patients. Med Instrum 11:296-301, 1977.
6. Jackson RV, Love JB, Parkin WG, Wahlqvist ML, Williams NS: Use of a microprocessor in the control of malignant hypertension with sodium nitroprusside. Aust NZ J Med 7:414-417, 1977.
7. McNally RT, Engelman K, Noordergraaf A, Edwards M: A device for the precise regulation of blood pressure in patients during surgery and hypertensive crisis. Proc San Diego Biomedical Symposium 16:419-424, 1977.
8. Hammond JJ, Kirkendall WM, Calfee RV: Hypertensive crisis managed by computer controlled infusion of sodium nitroprusside: a model for the closed loop administration of short acting vasoactive agents. Comput Biomed Res 12:97-108, 1979.
9. Sheppard LC: Computer control of the infusion of vasoactive drugs. Ann Biomed Eng 8:431-444, 1980.
10. Auer LM, Rodler H: Microprocessor-control of drug infusion for automatic blood-pressure control. Med Biol Eng Comput 19:171-174, 1981.
11. Chilcoat RT: An adaptive technique for programmed anaesthesia. Br J Anaesth 45:1235, 1973.
12. Mapleson WW, Chilcoat RT, Lunn JN, Blewett MC, Khatib MT, Willis BA: Computer assistance in the control of depth of anaesthesia. Br J Anaesth 52:234P, 1980.
13. Frumin MJ: Clinical use of a physiological respirator producing N_2O amnesiaanalgesia. Anesthesiology 18:290-299, 1957.
14. Hilberman M, Schill JP, Peters RM: On-line digital analysis of respiratory mechanics and the automation of respirator control. J Thorac Cardiovasc Surg 58:821-828, 1969.
15. Lampard DG, Coles JR, Brown WA: Computer control of respiration and anaesthesia. Aust J Exp Biol Med Sci 51:275-81, 1973.
16. Coon RL, Zuperku EL, Kampine JP: Systemic arterial blood pH servo-control of mechanical ventilation. Anesthesiology 49:201-204, 1978.
17. Demeester M, Grevisse PH, VanderVelde CH, et al: Real-time and interactive control of O_2-CO_2 transport in mechanically ventilated patients in ICU. IEEE Computers in Cardiology pp. 1-8, 1978.
18. Pfeiffer EF, Thum CH, Clemens AH: The artificial beta cell - A continuous control of blood sugar by external regulation of insulin infusion (glucose controlled insulin infusion system). Horm Metab Res 6:339-342, 1974.
19. Brown TK: A controller for automating vasoactive drug infusions to regulate hemodynamic variables. Twenty eighth ACEMB, New Orleans, Louisiana, September, 1975.

20. Eveleigh VW: Introduction to Control System Design. McGraw Hill, New York, 1972.
21. Isermann R: Digital Control Systems. Springer-Verlag, Heidelberg, 1981.
22. Smolen V, Barile R, Carr D: Design and operation of a system for automatic feedback - controlled administration of drugs. Med Dev Diag Indu 1:52-68, 1979.
23. Slate JB: Model-Based Design of a Controller for Infusing Sodium Nitroprusside during Postsurgical Hypotension, PhD Thesis. University of Wisconsin - Madison, 1980.
24. Koivo AJ, Larnard D, Gray R: Digital control of mean arterial blood pressure in dogs by injecting a vasodilator drug. Ann Biomed Eng 9:185-197, 1981.
25. Stern KS, Walker BK, Katona PG: Automated blood pressure control using a self-tuning regulator. IEEE 1981 Frontiers of Engineering in Health Care pp. 255-258, 1981.
26. Kaufman H, Roy R, Xu X: Model reference adaptive control of drug infusion rate. Sixth IFAC Symposium on Identification and System Parameter Estimation, Washington, D.C., 1982.
27. Harris CJ, Billings SA, Eds: Self-Tuning and Adaptive Control: Theory and Applications. IEE Press, London, 1981.
28. Arnsparger JM, McInnis BC, Glover JR Jr, Normann NA: Adaptive control of blood pressure. IEEE Trans Biomed Eng 30:168-176, 1983.

COMPUTER CONTROLLED INFUSION OF DRUGS DURING ANESTHESIA: METHODS OF MUSCLE RELAXANT AND NARCOTIC ADMINISTRATION

G. RITCHIE, J. SPAIN, J.G. REVES

INTRODUCTION

One of the anesthesiologist's tasks during surgery is controlling the effects of the drugs he administers. This is usually done by manually adjusting the dose so that the desired effect is achieved. Effects of IV drugs are usually controlled by administering them as a series of boluses, constant infusion, or some combination of the two.

The usual type of control can be classified as intermittent manual closed-loop control. Closed-loop control describes a system in which the output (in this case, the drug effect) and perhaps other system variables (such as temperature, heart rate, etc.) affect the control of the system. Current techniques may limit how finely the drug effect can be controlled. For bolus injections, the control action is extreme (high gain), and only intermittently applied. For constant infusion, the infusion rate may be intermittently adjusted. These features tend to make control imprecise.

One of the most promising uses of computers in anesthesia is in infusion systems that control a drug's effect. Such a system may be an automatic closed-loop control system where drug effect is monitored by a computer and infusion is automatically adjusted to bring the effect to the desired level. This type of system has been used to control blood pressure in post-operative cardiac patients with nitroprusside.[1] Another system has been reported that automatically controls thiopental anesthesia.[2]

Manual control of a drug's effect may also be improved by the use of computer-based infusion systems. In these systems, the computer can control the infusion of drug so that it is infused according to its pharmacokinetics. The drug effect can be more evenly controlled because constant plasma concentration of the drug is more closely achieved than with bolus injections or constant rate infusion. Drug effect can then be manually controlled by altering the desired equilibrium plasma concentration of the drug rather than injecting a bolus or changing the infusion rate.

Two computer-based infusion systems for the infusion of drugs during surgery have been developed at the University of Alabama in Birmingham. One system is an automatic closed-loop control system that controls muscle relaxation during surgery. The other is an infusion system that infuses a narcotic according to its pharmacokinetics.

AUTOMATIC CONTROL OF MUSCLE RELAXATION

In controlling muscle relaxation during surgery, one must balance two opposing problems. Enough muscle relaxant must be infused to provide adequate relaxation for the procedure and the infusion must be limited to avoid prolonged recovery of muscular function and to reduce the risk of impaired respiration in the recovery room. This task is complicated by the variabiliy in sensitivity to muscle relaxants among patients, making appropriate doses difficult to predict.

Automatic closed-loop control of muscle relaxation accounts for the patient's sensitivity to the drug by continuously monitoring the level of relaxation and adjusting the infusion rate of muscle relaxant accordingly. In this way, only as much drug as needed to induce and maintain the desired level of relaxation is infused.

Two systems for the control of neuromuscular blockade have been reported. One has been used to compare four non-depolarizing muscle relaxants in sheep.[3] The other has been used to maintain muscle relaxation in surgical patients with pancuronium.[4] In this system, relaxation was induced with an initial bolus of the drug. Both systems used the evoked, rectified and integrated electromyogram (EMG) as the feedback signal to control the infusion of drug.

We have developed a new system that induces and maintains the desired level of muscle paralysis. This computer-based control system uses the evoked, rectified and integrated EMG to control the infusion of succinylcholine.

System Description: A block diagram of the system is shown in figure 1. The controller triggers a Grass S48 stimulator (A) every 10 seconds. The stimulator delivers a 0.2 ms voltage pulse to the ulnar nerve through needle electrodes applied at the elbow or wrist. The stimulator is electrically isolated from the patient by a Grass SIU-5 isolation unit. The stimulation voltage is adjusted for supramaximal stimulation. The resulting EMG is then amplified, rectified, and integrated by an EMG signal processor (B) designed for this system. The processor begins integration 3 ms after the stimulus to avoid processing the stimulus artifact. The integration period is specified to be 16, 20, 24, or 32 ms, depending on the duration of the EMG. The EMG is simultaneously displayed on a storage oscilloscope so the quality of the signal can be visually checked and the integration period selected.

The output of the EMG processor is a voltage proportional to the rectified and integrated EMG. This voltage is converted to a numerical value by the controller (C). The controller is implemented on a Motorola EXORset microcomputer. Before the infusion of succinylcholine begins, the controller averages the processed EMG with the previous two to obtain a baseline value. Afterwards, the processed EMG is divided by its baseline value and multiplied by 100 to express the response as a percentage of the baseline. This value is subtracted from the desired level of relaxation (the setpoint) to give the error. The infusion rate is calculated as mg of succinylcholine/kg of patient weight/minute, then converted to ml/hr by multiplying it by the patient weight times 60 and dividing it by the drug concentration. This value is then communicated to an IMED 929 computer controlled infusion pump (E) which adjusts the infusion rate accordingly. This cycle is repeated every 10 seconds. The setpoint, patient mass, and drug concentration are entered into the controller before the infusion begins. The setpoint can be changed at any time. Infusion can be manually controlled on the IMED pump should it be desirable to bypass the controller.

The control algorithm holds the infusion rate constant at 0.1 mg/kg/min until the response is depressed to 90% of the baseline. Then the infusion rate is calculated according to the following equation:

infusion rate = (P x error) + (I x sum of the error) +

(D x difference between current error and previous error)

where P, I, and D are constants that govern controller performance. When the response is within 1% of the setpoint, the P and D terms are made zero in order to prevent the system from responding to small random variations in response. The maximum infusion rate is limited to 0.2 mg/kg/min.

An algorithm to detect for interference from the electrosurgical unit was included in the program. This interference usually caused the amplifiers on the EMG processor to saturate. Thus, when the rectified and integrated EMG was above a predetermined threshold, the controller assumed the signal was interference from the electrosurgical unit and ignored it.

System Evaluation: The system was evaluated on 12 surgical patients. Anesthesia was induced with thiopental (3-4 mg/kg) and maintained with an end-tidal concentration of 1% enflurane and 66% nitrous oxide in oxygen. Endotracheal intubation was performed without relaxants. Setpoint for the degree of relaxation was 20% of the baseline. The infusion was arbitrarily limited to 30 minutes to prevent Phase II response. After the infusion was terminated, the EMG response was monitored until it recovered.

The system successfully initiated and controlled the desired level of muscle relaxation in 10 of the 12 patients. A typical example of automatic control of muscle relaxation is shown on figure 2. Table 1 summarizes the results obtained from the automatic control of muscle relaxation in the 10 patients. The total dose administered for 30 minute infusion and 80% depression of the EMG ranged from 1.21 to 3.77 mg/kg (mean = 1.92, S.D. = 0.72). The mean ($\pm$ S.D.) time to reach the setpoint was 5.5 minutes ($\pm$ 1.87), and the mean time for 95% recovery was 5.4 minutes ($\pm$ 0.83). Two patients were relatively insensitive to the drug and the system was unable to control them.

PROGRAMMED INFUSION OF NARCOTIC

The administration of IV anesthetics usually involves the intermittent bolus administration of a drug whose elimination half-life exceeds the interval within which it is repeatedly administered. Figure 3 shows a hypothetical time course of the plasma concentration of a drug administered in this way. Not only does drug effect vary with the swings in plasma concentration but accumulation results from repeated injections of a drug at intervals shorter than its elimination half-life. Thus during a case of multiple IV bolus administrations of IV anesthetics (e.g., fentanyl, diazepam, etc.) the plasma level of these drugs will rise, and presumably the action will be prolonged. If as in Figure 3, a last administration is given to facilitate skin closure, the highest drug levels will occur at the end of operation causing a prolonged recovery.

A more rational method for infusion of anesthetic drugs may be based on knowledge of the particular drug's kinetics.[5] Plasma concentration of the drug can be made constant if the drug's kinetics in a particular patient are known. The amount of drug which is eliminated from the plasma per unit time is simply replaced. Figure 4 shows a hypothetical time course of the plasma concentration for a drug infused in this way. Unfortunately, drug kinetics vary among patients; nevertheless, constant plasma concentration can be more closely achieved with this technique using pharmacokinetic data obtained from other patients than with current techniques.

A computer which controls an infusion pump can be programmed with an infusion function designed to infuse drug at the rate it is eliminated from the plasma (central compartment). This type of system has been used to control the infusion of fentanyl, etomidate, and midazolam.[6,7] These systems enable the physician to more finely control the drug effect by changing the equilibrium plasma concentration rather than injecting a bolus of drug. It also provides a "background" effect of the desired drug which permits utilization of small amounts of other adjuvant anesthetics, e.g., halothane or enflurane.

We have designed a programmed infusion system that quickly achieves and maintains a constant plasma concentration of fentanyl. The desired plasma concentration is quickly established by rapid automatic injection of the drug. The concentration is maintained by infusing the drug according to the calculated amount of drug that is lost from the central compartment.

System Description: The system consists of an Apple II+ computer and an IMED 929 computer controlled infusion pump. A program written in PASCAL for the Apple computer controls the operation of the system. Before the infusion begins, the user enters the patient weight (in kg), the fentanyl concentration of the injectate (in mcg/ml), and the desired fentanyl concentration in the plasma (in ng/ml) into the computer. The computer calculates the amount of fentanyl needed to load the central compartment to the desired concentration, then infuses this amount at a rate of 1599 ml/hr. To achieve the desired therapeutic drug level at this rate usually takes less than 1 minute. Afterwards, the infusion rate is calculated according to the following equation:[5]

$$\dot{u}(t) = V_c C_1(0) \left(K_{10} + K_{12}e^{-K_{21}t} + K_{13}e^{-K_{31}t} \right)$$

where

$\dot{u}$ = infusion rate

t = time

V_c = volume of central compartment

$C_1(0)$ = concentration of drug in central compartment after loading

K_{10} = elimination rate constant from central compartment

K_{12} = transfer rate constant from compartment 1 to 2

K_{21} = transfer rate constant from compartment 2 to 1

K_{13} = transfer rate constant from compartment 1 to 3

K_{31} = transfer rate constant from compartment 3 to 1

This equation reflects the theoretical loss of fentanyl from the central compartment in a three compartment open model. The equation is based on the pharmacokinetics of fentanyl.[8] Every 15 seconds the computer calculates the infusion rate and communicates it to the IMED infusion pump. The user may stop the infusion at any time. An example of the infusion function is shown in figure 5 and cumulative dose is tabulated in Table 2. Ultimate design will permit the anesthesiologist to raise or lower the therapeutic blood level much as he regulates the inspired concentration of inhalation anesthetic by adjusting the vaporizer setting.

DISCUSSION

Computer-based infusion systems offer a number of advantages over manual methods of drug administration. The primary advantage is that control of the drug effect is more precise. Additional benefits include possible reduction in the amount of drug used, fewer side effects, and speedier recovery. A smooth anesthetic course can be obtained (Fig. 6) without the use of large "front end dosing".

Automatic closed-loop control can be especially useful for controlling the effects of drugs for which there is a large variability in sensitivity among patients. The control algorithm used in our muscle relaxation system was relatively simple. A more sophisticated algorithm will probably be more successful in controlling a higher percentage of patients. An adaptive control algorithm that adjusts itself to the patient sensitivity may be required for some drugs.

Not all drugs produce effects which are easily measured. The physician may use considerable judgement in adjusting the dose of these drugs. Automatic control of the effects produced by these drugs may be difficult to achieve. However, computer controlled infusion based on the anesthetic drug's pharmacokinetics offer significant advantages over the manual methods while retaining the physician's direct control over the drug's effect.

Computer controlled infusion systems show even greater promise for future drugs. The benefits of these systems are maximized with drugs that produce specific effects, have fast onset and recovery of effect, and have a high therapeutic index. These are precisely the design goals for new drugs being developed such as alfentanil.

SUMMARY
We have presented two systems of drug infusion for use in anesthetized patients. Both systems depend on computer assistance, and both have promise for widespread routine clinical application as well as immense clinical research value.

TABLE 1

PATIENT	SEX	AGE (YRS)	WT (KG)	TOTAL DOSE* (MG)	DOSE/WT* (MG/KG)	TIME TO SETPOINT (MIN)	TIME TO 95% RECOVERY (MIN)
1	F	27	59	91	1.55	3.9	5.2
2	F	30	43.6	68	1.55	4.0	4.4
3	F	22	65	114	1.75	4.7	4.4
4	M	56	78	149	1.91	5.2	5.8
5	F	51	69.5	84	1.21	4.3	6.1
6	F	57	87	165	1.90	7.6	5.6
7	M	36	85	120	1.41	3.8	5.2
8	M	36	67	154	2.30	6.2	5.1
9	F	39	63	118	1.87	5.4	5.0
10	M	33	70	264	2.77	9.6	7.2
MEAN		38.7	68.7	132.7	1.922	5.47	5.4
S.D.		+12.1	+12.8	+55.76	+0.72	+1.87	+0.83

Muscle relaxation characteristics obtained with the computer controlled system. In all patients the setpoint was 20% of the baseline. *For 30 minute infusion period.

TABLE 2

FENTANYL INFUSION DESIGNED TO MAINTAIN 5 ng/ml*

Elapsed Time (min)	V(ml)	mcg	mcg/kg	ml Fentanyl
1	18	180	2.0	3.6
3	33	330	3.7	6.6
5	42	420	4.7	8.4
10	62	620	6.8	12.4
15	78	780	8.6	15.6
20	92	920	10.2	18.4
25	104	1040	11.5	20.8
30	114	1140	12.6	22.8
40	133	1330	14.7	26.6
50	149	1490	16.5	29.8
60	163	1630	18.1	32.6
70	176	1760	19.5	35.2
80	187	1870	20.7	37.4

Patient's wgt = 90 kg. Where V = volume infused, mcg = mcg of fentanyl (cumulative dose), mcg/kg = cumulative dose in mcg/kg, ml Fentanyl = cumulative dose in ml of fentanyl (50 mcg/ml). (See figure 5)

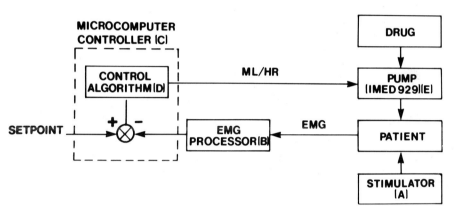

FIGURE 1: Block diagram of muscle relaxation controller (see explanation in text).

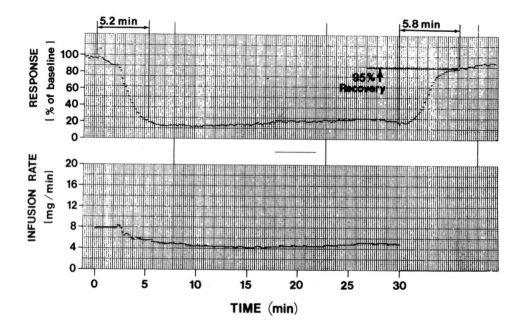

FIGURE 2. Example of automatic control of muscle relaxation (patient #4, see Table 1). The upper graph shows the response as percent of baseline. The lower graph shows the infusion rate. In this case, the setpoint was reached 5.2 minutes after infusion of succinylcholine began and recovery of 95% of muscular function occurred 5.8 minutes after the infusion was stopped. The setpoint was 20% of the baseline. Absolute recovery to the baseline was not achieved probably because of the peripheral effect of the enflurane.

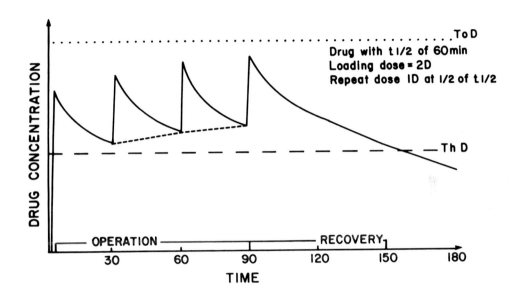

FIGURE 3. Hypothetical time course of the plasma concentration of an IV drug administered as a sequence of bolus injections. This graph shows how drug accumulation results from injections at intervals less than the elimination half-life. To D is the toxic dose and Th D is the therapeutic dose. (From ref #5 with permission of authors and publisher.)

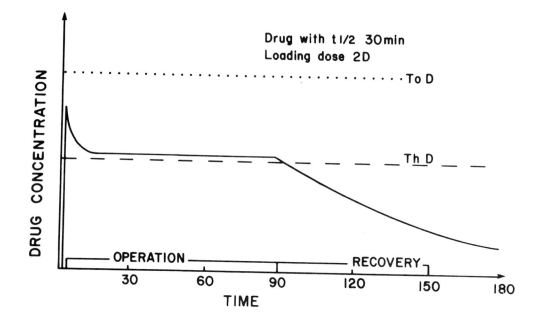

FIGURE 4. Hypothetical time course of the plasma concentration of a drug infused according to its pharmacokinetics to keep the plasma concentration constant. (From ref #5 with permission of authors and publisher.)

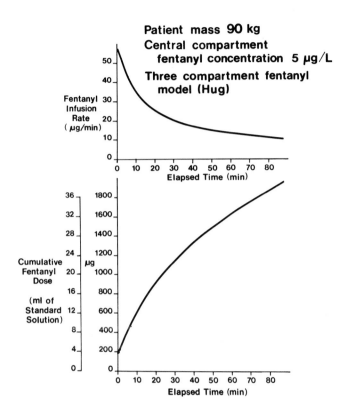

FIGURE 5. Fentanyl infusion rate and cumulative dose for 80 minutes of programmed infusion. The patient mass was 90 kg and the desired plasma concentration was 5 mcg/l.

314

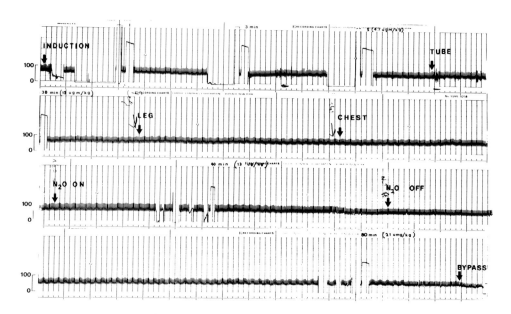

FIGURE 6. Blood pressure in a 90 kg man anesthetized with diazepam 0.3 mg/kg, pancuronium 0.1 mg/kg and a continuous infusion of fentanyl designed to maintain a plasma fentanyl level of 5 ng/ml. Note the stable blood pressure at all times, including induction (INDUCTION), tracheal intubation (TUBE), leg incision (LEG), chest incision (CHEST), with and without N2O 50:50 (N2O ON and N2O OFF).

REFERENCES

1. Sheppard LC: Computer control of the infusion of vasoactive drugs. Ann Biomed Eng 8:431-444, 1980

2. Cosgrove RJ, Smolen VF: Systems for automatic feedback-controlled administration of drugs: analog and digital optimal-adaptive control of thiopental and anesthesia. Proc San Diego Biomedical Symposium, North Hollywood, Western Publications, 1978:261-275

3. Cass NM, Lampard DG, Brown WA, Coles JR: Computer controlled muscle relaxation: a comparison of four muscle relaxants in the sheep. Anaesth Intensive Care 4:16-22, 1976

4. Brown BH, Asbury J, Linkens DA, Perks R, Anthony M: Closed-loop control of muscle relaxation during surgery. Clin Phys Physiol Meas 1:203-210, 1980

5. Reves JG, Greene ER Jr., MacKrell TN: Continuous infusion of intravenous anesthetics: automated IV anesthesia, a rational method of drug administration, New Anesthetic Agents, Devices and Monitoring Techniques. Edited by Stanley TH, Petty WC. Boston, Martinus Nijhoff Publishers, 1983, pp 196-203

6. Schwilden H: A general method for calculating the dosage scheme in linear pharmacokinetics. Eur J Clin Pharmacol 20:379-386, 1981

7. Hengstmann JH, Stoeckel H, Schuttler J: Infusion model for fentanyl based on pharmacokinetic analysis. Br J Anaesth 52:1021-1025, 1980

8. McClain DA, Hug CC: Intravenous fentanyl kinetics. Clin Pharmacol Ther 28:106-114, 1980

OXYGEN REQUIREMENTS DURING ANESTHESIA

STUART F. SULLIVAN

Department of Anesthesiology, UCLA School of Medicine, Los Angeles

1. INTRODUCTION

Oxygen requirements of the body during general anesthesia will vary with depth of narcosis. Whole-body oxygen consumption has been measured by closed and open-circuit methods. In the closed-circuit method, the subject breathes from a spirometer and returns the exhaled gas to the spirometer. Carbon dioxide is absorbed within the spirometer, and rebreathing of dead-space air is prevented by a series of one-way valves in the breathing circuit. Spirometer volume is decreased by an amount equal to the subject's oxygen consumption. The spirometer reservoir gas must be of sufficient volume to allow several minutes of rebreathing, and must, start with an enriched oxygen mixture to prevent hypoxia. Benedict, a pioneer investigator of human metabolism, was instrumental in developing and refining clinically useful closed-circuit spirometry.[1] Benedict's spirometer included the measurement of carbon dioxide production; Roth's modification eliminated this aspect, thereby measuring oxygen consumption exclusively. The Benedict-Roth apparatus has remained the most widely used closed-circuit spirometer, with small refinements adapted by individual investigators where applicable. The foundation for thinking that VO2 can be controlled by specific anesthetic agents begins in 1951, when Shackman, Graber and Redwood reported a 15% decrease in measured oxygen uptake in patients anesthetized with thiopental/nitrous oxide or thiopental/cylopropane.[2] A Benedict-Roth spirometer with CO2 absorber was used. Topkins and Artusio in 1955, demonstrated a significant increase in oxygen consumption during diethyl ether and during cylopropane anesthesia.[3] A similar experimental method was used. In these studies and in subsequent studies when the closed-circuit method is used, carbon dioxide production and RQ cannot be measured.

In the open-circuit method, a known inspired oxygen concentration (FIO2) is breathed from a reservoir, and exhaled gas is collected. A correction must be made for the difference between inspired and expired volumes. The combined measurement of VCO2, VO2, RQ and anesthetic gas has presented formidable methodological and technological barriers. Using new technology for simultaneous multiple gas analysis and on-line computation, it is now possible to measure minute-to-minute anesthetic and respiratory gas exchange reliably. The purpose of this work is to describe and demonstrate our approach to the measurement of total respiratory gas exchange during the uptake of inhalational anesthetics.

2. METHODS

2.1 Pulmonary Gas Exchange[4,5]

The volume of pulmonary gas uptake or elimination is:

$$\dot{V}_I F_{IX} - \dot{V}_E F_{EX} = \dot{V}_X \qquad \text{(Eq. 1)}$$

where

$\dot{V}_I$	=	Inspired gas volume/minute
$\dot{V}_E$	=	Mixed expired gas volume/minute
F_{IX}	=	Inspired fractional concentration of gas X
F_{EX}	=	Mixed expired fractional concentration of gas X
$\dot{V}_X$	=	Volume of gas X uptake or elimination/minute

Measurement of both inspired and expired volumes can be used by having the subject inspire from a large spirometer of known gas composition and exhale into another spirometer. This is an ideal system where all the variables are measured directly. Although this approach would be expected to yield the most reliable steady-state data, it is very cumbersome and rarely used.

More commonly only expired air volume is measured, requiring evaluation of steady-state conditions. When gas exchange is in a steady-state (implying that gas exchange at the tissues equals gas exchange measured at the mouth), then the volume of nitrogen (N_2) exchange is zero.

where

$$\dot{V}_{N_2} = \dot{V}_I F_{IN_2} - \dot{V}_E F_{EN_2} = 0 \qquad \text{(Eq. 2)}$$

and

$$\dot{V}_I F_{IN_2} = \dot{V}_E F_{EN_2} \qquad \text{(Eq. 3)}$$

and

$$\dot{V}_I = \dot{V}_E (F_{EN2}/F_{IN2}) \qquad \text{(Eq. 4)}$$

substituting Eq. 4 in Eq. 1

$$\dot{V}_X = \dot{V}_E \left[\left[F_{IX} (F_{EN_2}/F_{IN_2}) \right] - F_{EX} \right] \qquad \text{(Eq. 5)}$$

This equation for $\dot{V}_X$ may be used for the volumetric measurement of any gas (respiratory or anesthetic). The only conditions necessary are: (1) an inert gas is present in the inspired mixture (nitrogen, argon, or other); (2) a steady-state is present or closely approximated[6,7] (more discussion of non-steady-state errors to follow).

Using this approach, the equations of interest are:

$$\dot{V}_{CO_2} = \dot{V}_E \left[F_{ECO2} - \left[F_{ICO_2} \left(F_{EN_2}/F_{IN_2} \right) \right] \right]$$

$$\dot{V}_{O_2} = \dot{V}_E \left[\left[F_{IO_2} \left(F_{EN_2}/F_{IN_2} \right) \right] - F_{EO_2} \right]$$

$$\dot{V}_{ANES} = \dot{V}_E \left[\left[F_{I_{ANES}} \left(F_{EN_2}/F_{IN_2} \right) \right] - F_{E_{ANES}} \right]$$

The volume of exhaled air ($\dot{V}_{E_{APTS}}$) is measured at spirometer temperature, saturated with water vapor, and at ambient barometric pressure. This volume is reduced to standard conditions, i.e., $\dot{V}_{E_{STPD}}$ for the calculation of $\dot{V}_{X_{STPD}}$.

2.2 Instrumentation

The on-line gas exchange measurement system[8] is depicted schematically (Figure 1). Data acquisition, analog input, digital input/output, timing, computation, data storage and other functions are managed in a program run on a small digital computer (NOVA, Data General, Southboro, Mass). Inspired, mixed expired and calibration tank gas analyses are made for O2, CO2, N2 anesthetic using a multiple inlet Perkin-Elmer MGA-1100 gas analyz-

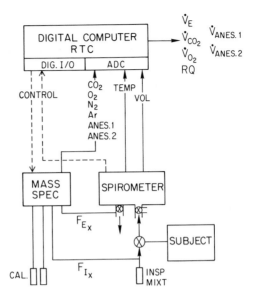

Figure 1.

ing mass spectrometer (Pomona, California). Exhaled air is collected in a modified, 10 liter, dry rolling seal, displacement spirometer (Cardiopulmonary Instruments Inc., Houston, Texas). Spirometer logic includes detection of (user preset) full volume and end-exhalation. Typically at completion of the collection cycle, the computer real time clock is read, together with the voltage representing spirometer position, the gas operated spirometer inlet valve closes (outlet valve opens), the collected exhaled air is dumped and analyzed for the gases of interest. Analysis of the entire collected sample is necessary as gas mixing in the spirometer is not always complete. During spirometer dumping and at the completion of current exhalation (flow sensor in external limb of spirometer inlet), the spirometer outlet valve closes (inlet valve opens). At this moment the clock is read, together with the voltage representing spirometer position. This is the start of a collection cycle. During the filling cycle both inspired gas and two calibration gas tanks are analyzed through alternate mass spectrometer inlets selected under computer program control. All of the required information, i.e., inspired gas concentrations, collected gas volume, spirometer temperature, collection time, and expired gas concentrations are available, each cycle to compute $\dot{V}CO2$, $\dot{V}O2$ and $\dot{V}ANES$.

2.3 Steady-State Evaluation

During transient conditions the validity of open-circuit gas exchange equations were examined to determine the magnitude of errors that may exist.[9] Open-circuit measurement of O2 uptake requires that net N2 exchange be zero ($\dot{V}N2=0$). Increasing FIO2 necessarily decreases FIN2 resulting in adjustments of body O2 and N2 stores. Since $\dot{V}N2$ is non-zero during these transients, open-circuit measurement of $\dot{V}O2$ is not valid. A dynamic model of body N2 stores was developed to predict: (1) the time required to re-establish zero net N2 gas exchange, and (2) the error magnitude in transient state values of open-circuit $\dot{V}O2$. Since the open-circuit $\dot{V}O2$ equation is invalid during transient conditions, a second equation is needed, transient $\dot{V}O2$ ($T\dot{V}O2$), which describes O2 uptake during periods of non-equilibrated N2 stores.

$$T\dot{V}O_2 = \dot{V}_{O_2} + (\dot{V}N_2 FIO_2/FIN_2)$$

The error term, ($\dot{V}N2FIO2/FIN2$), is simulated by the model and provides magnitude and time course error information in transient state open-circuit $\dot{V}O2$ values. It is clear that at the moment of change in FIO2, the two functions produce significantly different values of oxygen consumption rate. The larger the step change in FIO2, the greater the initial value error. As FIO2 changes, FEO2 changes to adjust to inspired conditions. The greater the inspired O2 change, the greater the displacement of N2 and thus a larger value of $\dot{V}N2$.

For example, during eucapnic ventilation, when increasing FIO2 from 0.21 to 0.40, the model predicts a 10% and 1% relative difference between open-circuit $\dot{V}O2$ and $T\dot{V}O2$ at 0.55 and 1.44 minutes respectively, following initial FIO2 change. For a change in FIO2 from 0.21 to 0.80, the 10% and 1% times are predicted to be 0.9 and 1.70 minutes. The results provide a method to estimate transient values of $\dot{V}O2$ and to predict the earliest time of O2 equilibration following a step change in FIO2.

2.4 System Reliability

The reliability of the system over a 2-hour period has been measured using a model with constant ventilation and constant inspired and expired gas concentration. Individual variation in gas concentration measurement is minimal. for example, FIO2 (%) is measured at 20.94 $\pm$ 0.0113 (X $\pm$ S.E.), FEO2 (%) 15.75 $\pm$ 0.0064, $\dot{V}E$(L/min) at 7.16 $\pm$ 0.0023, and $\dot{V}O2$ (ml/min) at 332.9 $\pm$ 0.81. A coefficient variation for $\dot{V}O2$ is 2.9%. In a similar analysis, the coefficient of variation for $\dot{V}$HAL was 1.7%. This variability is the summation of contributions from all aspects of measurement (spirometer, mass spirometer, and computer).[10,11]

3. RESULTS

3.1 Laboratory Studies

Oxygen uptake during halothane anesthesia[9] was measured in seven dogs, average 23.5 kg, given pentobarbital, 30 mg/kg intravenously, intubated, and ventilated artificially. Pancuronium 0.1 mg/kg/hr provided muscle paralysis. Arterial (femoral artery) and mixed venous (right ventricle) blood samples were analyzed for pH, PO_2, PCO_2, and hematocrit using a blood gas electrode system (I.L. 313). Cardiac Index (C.I.) was computed from $\dot{V}O_2$ and a-v O_2 content difference. Ventilation was adjusted to provide normal pH and $PaCO_2$. $\dot{V}E$, $\dot{V}CO_2$, $\dot{V}O_2$, and RQ were measured on a minute-to-minute basis. Following 2 hours of constant ventilation with air, halothane 1% was added to the inspired mixture. Halothane uptake ($\dot{V}$HAL) was measured for 2 hours (See Figure 2). In addition to the continuous gas exchange measurements, other relevant measurements were made at 5, 10,

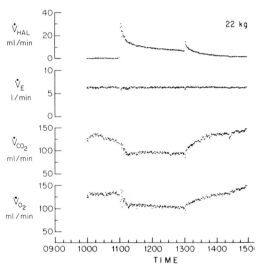

Figure 2. Halothane Uptake and Washout with Measured $\dot{V}CO_2$ and $\dot{V}O_2$

15, 30, 60, 90, and 120 minutes. During this 2 hour period, $\dot{V}O_2$ (ml/m²/min) decreased from 151 ± 5 (mean ± S.E.) to 118 ± 6 (P < 0.002), heart rate decreased from 179 ± 9 to 132 ± 4. Systemic blood pressure reached a minimum value at 30 minutes and then began to return toward initial values. The rate of decrease of oxygen consumption and cardiac output (half-time = 5 minutes) had a high degree of correlation with the initial phase of anesthetic uptake. The decrease in metabolic rate of the body, as measured by oxygen uptake and cardiac output, parallels the initial rapid phase of halothane uptake.

322

3.2 Intraoperative Studies

On-line $\dot{V}O2$ during halothane anesthesia was studied in twelve patients undergoing cardiac surgery.[12] The purpose of this study was to define sequential changes in respiratory gas exchange during inhalation anesthesia in man. Following premedication with lorazepam (0.05 mg/kg IM) anesthesia was induced with thiopental (3-5 mg/kg) and maintained with halothane (0.8%) in 50% O2, balance N2; endotracheal intubation was facilitated with pancuronium (0.1 mg/kg). Induction to intubation period varied from 15 to 20 minutes. Data collection began following intubation; the Engstrom ECS 2000 ventilator provided constant inspired gas concentration and tidal volume. PCO2 was maintained at 33 ± 2 torr. $\dot{V}E$, $\dot{V}CO2$, $\dot{V}O2$, and RQ were computed at approximately once a minute. Data were grouped at 10, 20, 30, 40, 50, and 60 minutes post-intubation for statistical analyses (See Figure 3). $\dot{V}O2$ did not change significantly during the entire period of measurement, ranging from 96-100 ml/m^2/min (25% below basal $\dot{V}O2$ of 130 ml/m^{2}min). $\dot{V}CO2$ did change significantly (p < 0.005), decreasing to a steady-state level after 30 minutes. RQ decreased in the same manner during this period. Body temperature decreased significantly (p < 0.005) from 36.1 °C to 35.0 °C. The decrease in $\dot{V}O2$ seen in these patients is due to both a decrease in body temperature and the effect of halothane anesthesia. A drop of 2 °C in body temperature can account for 12% decrease in $\dot{V}O2$. The metabolic depres-

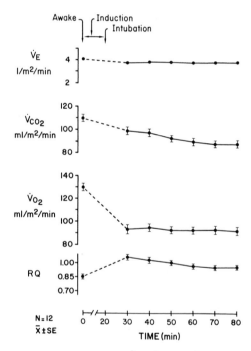

Figure 3. Plot of $\dot{V}_E$, $\dot{V}_{CO_2}$, $\dot{V}_{O_2}$, RQ
During Halothane Anesthesia

sion of VO2 by halothane anesthesia is very rapid, with a new steady level of $\dot{V}O2$ seen within 20 minutes. The change in $\dot{V}CO2$ is slower than that of $\dot{V}O2$ due to the larger reservoir of CO2 in the body, thus a longer period is required to reach a new equilibrium. In our study, changes in $\dot{V}CO2$ and RQ require up to 30 minutes dependant upon the magnitude of alveolar ventilation. The RQ remains well within the expected range off 0.7-1.0.

3.3 Postoperative Studies

Oxygen uptake during anesthetic washout was studied in twelve postoperative patients.[13] Anesthesia consisted of thiopental (3-5 mg/kg), N2O/O2 (50/50), enflurane (0.5-1.5%) and muscle relaxation was provided by either dimethyl tubocurarine or pancuronium chloride. Moderate hypothermia (28-30 °C) and enflurane in O2 were used during cardiopulmonary bypass. Ventilation ($\dot{V}E$) was controlled throughout. Anesthetic concentrations were maintained into the recovery room. In the recovery room, the patients were ventilated with O2-N2 mixtures through a volume cycled ventilator (Engstrom ECS 2000). $\dot{V}E$ and FIO2 were matched to those during anesthesia. $\dot{V}O2$, $\dot{V}CO2$, anesthetic washout ($\dot{V}N2O$ and $\dot{V}ENF$) were measured. Measurements were taken at 5, 10, 15, 30, 45, 60, 90, 120, 150, and 180 minutes postoperatively (See Figure 4). Rectal temperature was monitored

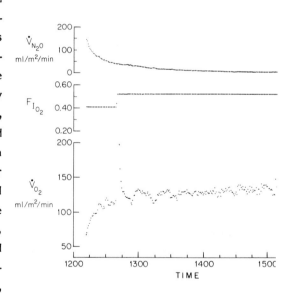

Figure 4. Postoperative $\dot{V}O_2$ During Anesthetic Washout. Adjustment in F_{IO_2} Demonstrates Transient Effect on Measured $\dot{V}O_2$

continuously. During the study period, the patients were sedated with morphine sulfate as required (4-14 mg/3 hours) and the mean arterial blood pressure was maintained between 80 and 90 Torr with Nitroprusside. Average body temperature was 35.5 °C on arrival in the recovery room and 36.5 °C at the end of 3 hours. $\dot{V}O2$ and $\dot{V}CO2$ increased following the cessation of anesthesia.

The increase in $\dot{V}O2$ was proportionally larger than that of $\dot{V}CO2$ initially, this resulted in a gradual decrease in respiratory quotient (RQ); finally approaching steady-state at 60 minutes. The $\dot{V}O2$ also reached a new level after 60 minutes and showed a maximum of 118 $ml/m^2/min$ after 3 hours and at that time the PaCO2 and pHa averaged 32 Torr and 7.43. The low value of $\dot{V}O2$ at the end of general anesthesia is not unexpected and is due to both the depressant effects of enflurane and that of hypothermia. Post-bypass hypothermia is well recognized, and at 35.5 °C can cause a 10% decrease in $\dot{V}O2$. The postoperative rise of $\dot{V}O2$ is rapid and correlates well with the rapid washout of anesthetic. In our series of patients, postoperative $\dot{V}O2$ is minimized by sedation and mechanical ventilation, thus the $\dot{V}O2$ after 3 hours is relatively low. The first hour of emergence is the time of the greatest metabolic change.

4. DISCUSSION

Multiple reliable measurements of whole body oxygen consumption are a prime requisite of our studies. With a view to clinical use, we also desired to develop a non-invasive method using expired respiratory gas analysis. Some of our early studies delineated the barriers, both in techniques and interpretation. Typical of such a problem is that, conceptually, a change in cellular metabolic rate is expected to effect changes in the circulation and in gas exchange within the lung which will be reflected by a change in expired gas concentrations. However, the gas stores of the body act as a volume buffer, so that tissue or circulatory changes are not immediately reflected in the expired gas. Breath to breath respiratory oscillations in normal man at rest cause a continual change in the distribution of lung ventilation to perfusion ratios, further reducing the accuracy of intermittent sampling of expired gases or of blood gases to determine $\dot{V}O2$. We also demonstrated the need for on-line data availability. This preliminary work led to the development of our system of continuous collection of expired gas in an automated spirometer, its analysis by respiratory gas mass spectrometer and subsequent processing by an on-line computer system. To measure oxygen consumption of patients in the perioperative period in the recovery room and in the ICU, we require a continuous analysis of $\dot{V}O2$ showing the trends and asymptotes, as well as an indication of steady-state gas exchange conditions defined as a constant ratio of CO2 production to O2 consumption (RQ), or alternatively, a constant ratio of inert gas exchange (ratio of expired to inspired nitrogen, FEN2/FIN2).

The fundamental aim of general anesthesia is to provide reversible unconsciousness without limiting oxygen-dependent processes. Oxygen availability during anesthesia has been traditionally considered as primarily a problem of pulmonary ventilation, controllable to a variable degree, but whose distribution as well as the remainder of the pathway (alveolar/capillary gas transfer, mass transfer by the circulation, tissue utilization) was essentially a sequence of passive uncontrolled dependent variables. Tissue metabolism, i.e., oxygen requirements, determines circulatory and respiratory function and viewed from this aspect, various interdependent relationships appear which are potentially subject to modification or disruption by disease, surgical intervention, anesthetic agents and techniques.

OXYGEN TRANSPORT MODEL

The oxygen content of the body is constant (steady-state) when volume of oxygen uptake via the lungs equals oxygen consumption of the body. CaO_2 depends upon $Cc'O_2$, Qs/Qt, $\dot{V}O_2$ and QT.[14] Oxygen delivery $(QT \cdot CaO_2)$ in turn depends upon CaO_2 and QT. It is apparent that in the presence of a shunt, an increase in oxygen consumption produces a decrease in arterial oxygen content and initiates a potentially vicious cycle if compensation by changes in QT are restricted.

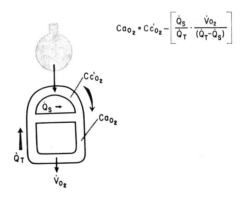

$$Ca_{O_2} = Cc'_{O_2} - \left[\frac{\dot{Q}_S}{\dot{Q}_T} \cdot \frac{\dot{V}_{O_2}}{(\dot{Q}_T - \dot{Q}_S)} \right]$$

Figure 5. Oxygen Transport Model

The overall equation relating arterial O2 content (CaO2) or oxygen availability to tissue is:

$$C_aO_2\ (S_aO_2,\ P_aO_2) = Cc'O_2 - \left[\frac{Qs}{QT} \cdot \frac{\dot{V}O_2}{(QT-QS)} \right]$$

To further illustrate the role of $\dot{V}O_2$: when both sides of the above equation are multiplied by QT the following results:

$$CaO_2 \cdot QT = C\dot{c}O_2 \cdot QT - \left[\frac{QS}{(QT-QS)} \cdot \dot{V}O_2 \right]$$

| Total O2 available | Maximum O2 for a given QT and Hb | Term decrementing available O2 as QS and/or $\dot{V}O_2$ increase |

This emphasizes the functional interrelationships between four major physiological entities involved in the delivery of oxygen: (1) cardiac output (QT), (2) body O2 consumption ($\dot{V}O_2$), (3) the fraction of venous blood not being ventilated in the lung (QS/QT), and (4) the oxygen content in the pulmonary capillaries ($C\dot{c}O_2$), and with a contribution from V/Q inequalities this may be represented by mixed end capillary O2 content ($C\dot{c}O_2$).

There are a significant number of conditions which will increase $\dot{V}O_2$ (hyperthermia, alkalosis, anesthetic emergence, work of breathing, et alia) and adversely alter O2 delivery in the critically ill patient. Control of oxygen consumption can be beneficial to patient welfare. For example, mechanical ventilation is used to combat respiratory insufficiency and hypoxemia following major abdominal, thoracic, and cardiac surgery. Adverse alterations in both lung volume and mechanics of breathing occur during the immediate postoperative period, especially when associated with preoperative impairment in pulmonary function. Increased expenditure of energy for breathing will increase the oxygen cost of breathing, or in the amount of oxygen utilized by the respiratory muscles during spontaneous respiration. The increase in whole-body O2 consumption secondary to the addition of the oxygen cost of breathing is undesirable in the immediate postoperative period.

5. CONCLUSION

Measurement of oxygen uptake during anesthesia has not been used to guide clinical care, primarily because of the difficulty in measurement. Crucial to the success of our studies is the ability to continuously measure body oxygen uptake so that transient changes in oxygen stores of the body or transient changes in respiratory gas exchange are not misinterpreted as being of significance. Conventional methods of sampling expired air, with gas analysis at a later time does not provide the real-time information needed to assess steady-state conditions during the actual data collection. Our approach has resolved these barriers. Using portable equipment in the operating room (spirometer, gas analyzing mass spectrometer, and digital computer), it is now possible to reliably quantitate respiratory and anesthetic gas exchange in the anesthetized patient.

REFERENCES

1. Benedict, F.G. A portable respiration apparatus for clinical use. Boston Med. Surg. J. 178:667-678, 1918.
2. Shackman, R., Graber, G.I., and Redwood, C. Oxygen consumption and anaesthesia. Clin. Sci. 10:219-228, 1951.
3. Topkins, M.J., Artusio, J.F. The effect of cyclopropane and ether on oxygen consumption in the unpremedicated surgical patient. Anesth. Analg. 35:350-356, 1956.
4. Fenn, W.O., Rahn, H., and Otis, A.B. A theoretical study of the composition of the alveolar air at altitude. Am. J. Physiol. 146:637-653, 1946.
5. Rahn, H., Fenn, W.O. A graphical analysis of the respiratory gas exchange. The O2-CO2 diagram. Washington, D.C. Am. Physiol. Soc., 1955.
6. Farhi, L.E., Olszowka, A.J. Analysis of alveolar gas exchange in the presence of soluble inert gases. Resp. Physiol. 5:53-56, 1968.
7. Scrimshire, D.A., Tomlin, P.J. Gas exchange during initial stages of N2O uptake and elimination in a lung model. J. Appl. Physiol. 34:775-789, 1973.
8. Sullivan, S.F., Patterson, R.W., Smith, R.T., and Ricker, S.M. Quantitative respiratory gas exchange during halothane induction. In Proc. Low Flow and Closed System Anesthesia Sympos., Aldrete, J.A., ed., pp. 85-97, Grune and Stratton, 1979.
9. Nowakowski, V.A., Sullivan, S.F., and Campfield. A dynamic model of nitrogen storage in man. Proc. Ann. Conf. Eng. Med. Biol. 19:22, 1977.
10. Smith, R.T., Sullivan, S.F., and Patterson, R.W. On-line measurement of oxygen consumption; clinical feasibility and application. Proc. San Diego Biomed. Sympos. 16:11-16, 1977.
11. Smith, R.T., Sullivan, S.F., Patterson, R.W., and Ricker, S.M. Quantitative on-line measurement of anesthetic gas exchange. Proc. San Diego Biomed. Sympos. 17:287-291, 1978.
12. Huang, D.H., Shigezawa, G.Y., and Sullivan, S.F. On-line VO2 during halothane anesthesia. Abstr. Sci. Papers 1982 Int'l Sympos. Computing in Anesth., p 21.
13. Huang, D.H., Shigezawa, G.Y., Gilbert, M., Viljoen, J.F., and Sullivan, S.F. Oxygen uptake during anesthetic washout. Anesthesiology 53:S256, 1980.
14. Sullivan, S.F. Oxygen transport. Anesthesiology 37:140, 1972.

REAL TIME OXIMETRY

Mark Yelderman, M.D.

James Corenmen

The foremost responsibility of the physician in the care of
the anesthetized or critically ill patient is to provide assurance
of oxygen delivery to vital organs. State of the art monitoring
extends to following indirect parameters of oxygen transport such
as heart rate via EKG or plethsthymograph, blood pressure
invasively or non invasively, and cardiac output in very selected
and isolated situations. Earlier attempts to directly monitor
tissue oxygenation by measuring transcutaneous oxygen tension
using Clark electrodes has seen limited success in adults (34).
The commercial availability of solid state components such as the
microprocessor, light emitting diodes, and miniaturized photo-
detectors has made possible the application of classical
spectrophotometric techniques of measuring oxygen saturation to
the development of a monitor to accurately and precisely in real
time, on a beat by beat basis to measure arterial blood oxygen
saturation.

Oxygen transport depends heavily upon the ability of hemoglobin to reversible load and unload large quantities of oxygen at
physiological oxygen tensions. This relationship between oxygen
tension and the oxygen binding is explified in the well known
classical oxyhemoglobin dissociation curve. The sigmoid shape is
crucial for physiologic oxygen transport. During circulation
through the lungs, blood is nearly fully saturated with oxygen
over a fairly large range of oxygen tensions (pO_2) and during
flow through systemic capillaries a relatively large amount of
oxygen is unloaded with a relatively small drop in oxygen tension.
This allows oxygen to be released into the plasma at sufficiently
high concentration to provide an adequate gradient for diffusion
into the interior of cells.

The sigmoid shape of the oxyhemoglobin dissociation curve is due to the 'heme-heme' interaction. The hemoglobin protein contains four subunits, each containing a heme moiety capable of binding with one oxygen molecule. In heme the iron atom occupies the center of a porphyrin ring. The shift of iron in and out of the plane of the porphyrin ring with oxygenation and deoxygenation results in the marked alteration in the quanternary structure of hemoglobin. The salt bonds holding the molecule in its tense conformation represent a considerable amount of potential energy. With oxygen binding to successive heme groups, the small shift in the heme iron is amplified into much larger conformational changes as the salt bonds are ruptured. As the successive oxygens bind to the hemoglobin molecule at one stage, the hemoglobin molecule snaps into the relaxed or 'oxy' conformation. The remaining un-bound heme groups of this intermediate then have an increased affinity for oxygen (7).

The affinity of oxygen for hemoglobin can be conveniently expressed by the term P50, the oxygen tension at which hemoglobin is half saturated. The higher the affinity of hemoglobin for oxygen, the lower the P50 and visa versa. Thus P50 is inversely related to oxygen affinity. Oxygen affinity varies inversely with pH and varies inversely with temperature. The P50 tends lower with decreasing pH and increasing temperature. The P50 for human blood at physiologic pH (7.4) and temperature (37 C) is 26 mmHg. The P50 of whole blood increases directly with 2,3-DPG, the prime determinant of whole blood oxygen affinity, by directly binding to a specific site on hemoglobin and by effectively lowering intracellular pH due to its high charged impermeant anion. Carbon dioxide has a dual effect on the oxygen affinity of hemoglobin. First, CO_2 binds directly to hemoglobin, forming carbamino com-pounds. Second, there is the indirect but quantitatively more important effect of pCO_2 on pH. An organism can be considered to bind and unload oxygen and CO_2 reciprocally:oxygen is picked up by the lungs as CO_2 is expelled. In the tissues, the reverse process occurs. CO_2 exchange facilitates oxygen exchange. This phenomenon is a direct corollary of the dependence of oxygen affinity on pH.

It is important to realize that the saturation or oxygen content of hemoglobin is independent of P50 and the factors which determine it. The P50 is an indication of the tissue oxygen tension necessary for oxygen unloading of hemoglobin to occur, not of the amount of oxygen available (24).

The oxygen carrying capacity of blood is expressed quantitatively in the Fick equation:

$$VO_2 = 0.139 * Q * Hb * (SaO_2-SvO_2)$$

where VO_2 is the amount of oxygen released (1/min), 1.39 is the amount in milliliters of O_2 bound by 1 gram of fully saturated hemoglobin, Q is blood flow (1/min) and SaO_2 and SvO_2 are arterial and mixed venous oxygen saturation (%). The term (SaO_2-SvO_2) is a quantitative expression of the fractional unloading of oxygen from hemoglobin during the flow of blood from artery to vein. This parameter is dependent upon the blood oxy-hemoglobin dissociation curve, which determines the amount of oxygen the blood can release for a given decrement in pO_2.

It has long been appreciated that oxyhemoglobin is red and reduced hemoglobin is blue. A technique which measures color changes allows determination of degree of hemoglobin oxygenation or saturation. Since color changes are due to difference in selective light absorption, similar results can be obtained by using one monochromatic light source and noting the amount of absorption. For a given wavelength, red oxyhemoglobin will have a different absorption than blue reduced hemoglobin. This spectrophotometric technique, known mathematically as 'Beers' Law, applies to a large number of other 'simple solutions' (9-14,16-21,35,39,40,46-49).

Beers's law assumes (1) that the light source is monochromatic, (2) that the light is all parallel and directed perpendicular to the test chamber, (3) that the unknown sample is in a non interfering solution, (4) that the test chamber can be compared to a blank with suspending solution only for comparison, (5) that only one unknown solution is present, (6) that the solution is clear with no turbidity, and (7) that no luminescence

nor phosophorences occurs. For each substance and for each
discrete wavelength, there exist a unique amount of light
absorption included in Beers's law as the molecular extinction
coefficient.

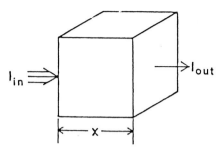

$$I_{out} = I_{in} \, exp^{(-\beta_\lambda *C*X)}$$

where I_{in} is the incident light to the test chamber
I_{out} is the transmitted light from the test chamber
X is the length of the test chamber
C is the concentration of the species sample
β_λ is the molecular extinction coefficient for the
species sample.

Since the molecular extinction coefficients are both wavelength and species dependent, it would be expected there would be
great variability among hemoglobin species as seen in figure 1.
(46)

If the test chamber were filled with oxyhemoglobin and a
wavelength of 660ηm were used, the molecular extinction coefficient (β_λ^o) would be 92 thus allow solving for any one of the
four variables if the other three are known.

To know the degree of saturation implies that the sample
contains a mixture of both reduced and oxyhemoglobin. It can be
assumed that all the oxyhemoglobin can be put into saturation
fraction (S) of the test chamber and the reduced hemoglobin put
in the remaining fraction (1-S). The light would be directed
trough both compartments sequentially.

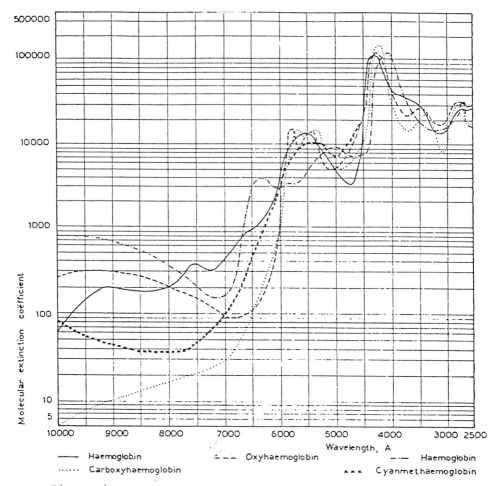

Figure 1

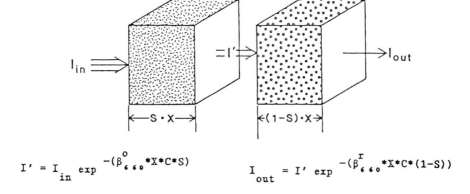

$$I' = I_{in} \exp^{-(\beta^o_{660}*X*C*S)}$$

$$I_{out} = I' \exp^{-(\beta^r_{660}*X*C*(1-S))}$$

where β_λ^o is the molecular extinction coeffficient for oxyhemoglobin and β_λ^r is the extinction coefficient for reduced hemoglobin at a specific wave length λ. Note that β_λ^o and β_λ^r do not have the same value.

Combining the two into one unit, one has

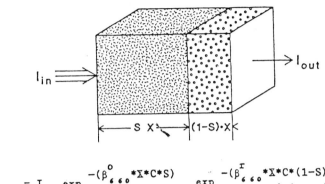

$$I_{out} = I_{in} \exp^{-(\beta_{660}^o *X*C*S)} \exp^{-(\beta_{660}^r *X*C*(1-S))}$$

This then becomes

$$\log[\, I_{out}/I_{in} \,]_{660} = -(\beta_{660}^o *X*C*S + \beta_{660}^r *X*C*(1-S))$$

from which saturation, S, can be calculated if 'X' and 'C' are known.

$\log[\, I_{out}/I_{in}]$ is often referred to as optical density.

This approach assumes that purified hemoglobin, not red blood cells, is present, that only two species of hemoglobin are present and works quite well in laboratory instruments. However, it must be modified to work invivo. Vetebrate hemoglobins in general have identical absorption spectra in visible light because of the uniformity of the heme moiety (7). Differences in globin structure accounts for the various differences in the function properties such as P50 in various hemoglobin such as A1, A2,A3,F,H. There is excellent agreement between spectrophotometric and gasometric measurements of oxygen binding to vetebrate hemoglobins(7,13).

Early invivo oximeters utilize ear arterial vasculature. Single wavelength models obtain a reference or calibration point

by allowing the subject to first breath 100 percent oxygen (26).
Such instruments can only trend saturation. Dual wavelengths models
use mechanical pressure to first 'avascularize' the tissue bed to
obtain a 'tissue' baseline(5,41-43). 'Arterialization' is achieved
by heat or chemical treatment. Since it is virtually impossible
to solve the two simultaneous Beer equations in real time using
analogue circuitry, the calculation must be simplified. By
requiring one wavelength to be at the isobestic wavelength, the
point where the extinction coefficient for two hemoglobin species
is the same (805 ηm), the two equations degenerate into only one.
However, this complicates the manufacture of the instrument since
it is likewise difficult to produce a stable wavelength at exactly
the isobestic wavelength (15,27,32,37).

Numerous factors introduce errors into the values derived
by these early oximeters. The values obtained are not real
arterial saturation since some venous blood always remains in the
'arterialized' vasculature bed. Ambient light causes some interference. The tenuous pressure relationship between ear tissue and
the transducer light source, detector, and heater allows significant error secondary to motion.

The principles of operation of the early oximeters are based
on Beer's law which had been developed using hemolyzed hemoglobin
in very controlled test chambers. Invivo oximetry uses whole blood
and is subject to light scattering secondary to red blood cells,
surrounding tissue, etc. Light no longer follows parallel beams
nor Beer's law. Extensive studies have been made on errors
occuring with invivo oxygen saturation measurements. Numerous
researchers have attempted to describe invivo whole blood
absorption, but not sufficiently well to make it useful clinically.
Consequently, such oximeters utilize an empirical calibration
based on a manometric method of determining saturation (1-4,22,
23,30,31,33).

Whole blood contains not only reduced and oxyhemoglobin, but
frequently several dyshemoglobins such as carboxyhemoglobin and
methemoglobin. The actual 'oxyhemoglobin' value displayed by the
oximeter may be in error depending upon the treatment of the
dyshemoglobins (6,28,36). A wavelength is required to measure

each hemoglobin species assuming total hemoglobin is known or
remains constant. Four wavelengths are needed to measure reduced
hemoglobin, oxyhemoglobin, carboxyhemoglobin, and methemoglobin.
If fewer wavelengths are used, some error will be introduced, the
degree of which depends upon the number and characteristics of
wavelengths actually used. Other compounds such as bilirubin
have the potential to introduce errors if certain wavelength
ranges are used.

The definition of hemoglobin saturation depends upon the
treatment of the various hemoglobin species present. Hemoglobin
may be unbound, may be bound to oxygen, or may be functionally
inert. Saturation can be defined as the ratio of oxyhemoglobin
to the sum of dyshemoglobin and reduced hemoglobin, (functional
or reversible saturation) or alternatively as the ratio of oxyhemoglobin to the sum of all hemoglobin species present, whether
available or not for reversible binding to oxygen (total
saturation). Hemoglobin not available for reversible oxygen
binding is effectively removed from the functional hemoglobin
pool and appears inert with changes in oxygen partial pressure.
Excluding such dyshemoglobin species from the definition of
saturation provides a more physiologic indication of arterial
oxygen content versus oxygen saturation. However, the two
definitions are interrelated mathematically(6).

It is desirable to greatly reduce or eliminate the error
due to venous blood and tissue. This is accomplished by
realizing that arterial blood pulsates whereas other optical
components such as venous blood and tissue do not. The pulsating
arterial bed by expanding and relaxing will modify the amount of
light detected. The increase in absorption with onset of systole
is due primarily to inflow of arterial blood. Thus measuring the
difference in absorption or the amplitude of the increase in
absorption from the non-flow baseline will reflect absorption of
arterial blood. The amplitude of the arterial pulse change is
dependent upon all the components of Beer's las, that is (1)
pulse amplitude, (2) wavelength of light, (3) and saturation of
hemoglobin(44,45). Again two wavelengths are required to calculate
saturation of arterial blood. Modifying the model to calculate

saturation, the optical path length now is X at diastole and
X+ΔX at systole. The equations are then rewritten to look at
saturation only in the ΔX segment.

The equations then become

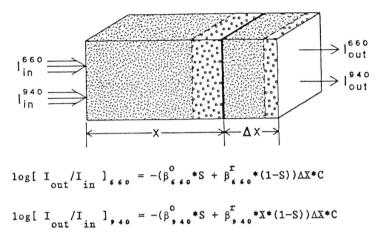

$$\log[\ I_{out}/I_{in}\ ]_{660} = -(\beta^o_{660}*S + \beta^r_{660}*(1-S))\Delta X*C$$

$$\log[\ I_{out}/I_{in}\ ]_{940} = -(\beta^o_{940}*S + \beta^r_{940}*\overline{X}*(1-S))\Delta X*C$$

from which arterial saturation can be calculated (44,45).

The microprocessor based real time oximeter contains several
hardware/software modules. The transduces consists of two light
emitting diodes (LED's), one in the visible red (660 ηm) and one
in the infrared (940 ηm) and a photodiode. The three components
are mounted in a finger receptacle which supports them and
maintains them in contact with finger tissue. The LED's more
or less transilluminate the finger permitting the photodiode to
receive a combination of a transmitted and backscattered light
from the finger vascular bed. The LED drivers and photodiode
amplifiers are coupled to the microprocessor via D/A and A/D
converters. Final levels are monitored by software control. Each
LED alternates through an on/off state such that the photodiode
detects the light from only one LED at a time. Because no part of
the transducer phase is temperature dependent nor temperature
sensitive, no heating nor temperature sensing elements are
required.

The microprocessor executes an algorithm to determine the
pulse amplitude associated with each wavelength. The baseline is

followed until thresholds are exceeded. If criteria for a pulse
are then met, the maximum pulse amplitude for each wavelength
is calculated. Criteria for acceptable pulses are based upon
present data and weighted historical data thus allowing some
adaptability to the artifact rejection alogrithm. Saturation is
calculated using the ratio of the two wave amplitudes. The
average of the last 5-7 values is then displayed. Heart rate is
calculated by using time between beats and the average of 5-7
values are displayed.

Front panel LED's under microprocessor control display
saturation and heart rate results, alarm limits, and pulse
amplitude. The amplitude of the detected pulse is portrayed
using a vertical sixteen segment LED post: the apparent lighted
height of the post rises with increase in pulse amplitude and
visa versa. Alarms for low and high heart rate and low saturation
are provided and default to initial values at power on: (1) Low
Saturation at 85 (2) Low Heart Rate at 55 and (3) Hight Heart
Rate at 140. Limits are user altered by depressing the
appropriately designated button. The active limit is displayed
and can be increased or decreased by turning the front panel
control knob.

Information on heart rate and saturation is provided using
audible tones. A beep is heard with each pulse and the pitch of
the beep tone is changed with the saturation value. As saturation
goes down, the pitch goes down and visa versa. When alarm limits
are exceeded, a continuous tone is heard. The loudness of each
beep is adjustable using the control knob. The user can know
heart rate and arterial saturation by listening only and with no
visual contact with the instrument.
Failure to achieve a reliable signal for calculation of heart
rate and saturation is revealed in several modes. If the transducer receptacle loses finger contact, the pulse amplitude post
indicates a no amplitude and the saturation and heart rate display
likewise show O. A panel indicator light illuminates indicating
no pulse can be found. If the pulse amplitude is present, but
weak, the amplitude post will indicate a very small pulse
amplitude.

No calibration of the instrument is required! The finger receptacle LED's are fixed wavelength devices and do not change with time. The change in absorption of hemoglobin with saturation does not vary with any known physiological phenomenon (pH, temperature, 2,3-DPG, hemoglobin species). Tissue effects are eliminated automatically by using ratios of arterial pulse amplitudes and by using automatic LED amplitude control. Since the measurement is absolute, no calibration is required.

Because pulse oximetry utilizes light absorption changes produced by arterial pulsation, any event which significantly reduces vascular pulsations will greatly reduce the instrument's ability to calculate saturation. Adequate finger pulsation is generally lost with (1) significant hypothermia, (2) hypotension (mean blood pressure less than about 50 mmHg.), (3) infusion of vasoconstrictive drugs, and (4) direct arterial compression. Pulsation of the nasal septal anterior enthmoid artery (supplied by the internal carotid) persists under greater extremes that the finger pulse. A special nasal sensor may be used in these circumstances.

Skin pigmentation is not a limitation since saturation is calculated on relative pulse amplitude ratios and not on absolute absorption (8).

The pulse oximeter has been clinically evaluated and found to have saturation error of 1-2% compared to simultaneously obtained invasive measurements over the range of 60-100% saturation (44). A IL282 Co-Oximeter was used as a standard. The pulse oximeter offers significant clinical utility by providing continuous, accurate, and precise measurement of patient arterial blood saturation (6,25,38,50). Such continuous real time information allows better assessment of patient status and allows immediate detection of sudden deleterious changes. Primary areas of operation are the operating room and intensive care environments.

REFERENCES

1. Anderson NM, Sekelj P. Studies on the light transmission of nonhemolyzed whole blood. Determination of oxygen saturation. J Lab Clin Med 65:153-166, 1965.
2. Anderson NM, Sekelj P. Light-absorbing and scattering properties of nonhaemolysed blood. Phys Med Biol 12(2):173-184, 1967.
3. Anderson NM, Sekelj P. Reflection and transmission of light by thin films of nonhaemolysed blood. Phys Med Biol 12(2): 185-192, 1967.
4. Anderson NM, Sekelj P. Studies on the determination of dye concentration in nonhemolyzed blood. J Lab Clin Med, 72(4): 705-713, 1968.
5. Brinkman R, Zylstra WG. Determination and continuous registration of the percentage of oxygen saturation in clinical conditions. Archirum Chirurgicum Neerlandicum 1:177-183, 1949.
6. Brown LJ. A new instument for the simulatneous measurement of total hemoglobin, % oxyhemoglobin, % Carboxyhemoglobin, % methemoglobin, and Oxygenm content in whole blood. IEEE Transactions on Biomedical Eng, 27(3):132-138, 1980.
7. Bunn HF, Forget BG, Ranney HM. Human Hemoglobins. Saunders, Philadelphia, 1977.
8. Comroe JH, Botelho S. The unreliability of cyanosis in the recognition of arterial anoxemia. Am J Med Sci 214:1-6, 1947.
9. Drabkin DL, Austin JH. Spectrophotometric studies. Preparation from washed blood cells: nitric oxide hemoglobin and sulf-hemoglobin. J Biol Chem 112:51-65, 1935.
10. Drabkin DL, Austin JH. Spectrophotometric studies: A technique for the analysis of undiluted blood and concentrated hemoglobin solutions. J Biol Cehm 112:105-115, 1935.
11. Drabkin DL, Singer RB. Spectrophotometric studies: A study of the absorption spectra of non-hemolized erthrocytes and of scattering of light by suspensions of particles, with a note upon the spectrophotometric determinations of the pH within the erythrocye. J Biol Chem 129:739, 1939.
12. Drabkin DL, Austin JH. Spectrophotometric studies. J Biol Chem 140:387, 1941.
13. Drabkin DL. Spectrophotometric studies. The crystallographic and optical properties of the hemoglobin on man in comparison with those of other species. J Biol Chem 164:703-723, 1946.
14. Drabkin DL. Spectroscope: Photometry spectrophotometry, Medical Physics Vol II, Year Book Publishers, Chicago, p1039-1089, 1950.
15. Enson Y, Briscoe WA, Polanyi ML, Cournand A. In vivo studies with an intravascular and intracardiac reflection oximeter. J Appl Physiol 17:552-558, 1962.
16. Gordy E, Drabkin DL. Spectrophotometric studies: Determination of the oxygen saturation of blood by a simplified technique, applicable to standard equipment. J Biol Chem 227:285-299, 1957.
17. Heilmeyer L. Spectrophotometer in medicine. Adam Hilger, London, 1943.

340

18. Hicks CS, Holden HF. The absorption of ultra-violet light by oxyhaemoglobin and by some of its derivatives. Aust J Exp Biol Med Sci 6:175-186, 1929.
19. Hill DW. Physics applied to anaesthesia: Physical optics, photometry and spectrophotometry. Brit J Anaesth 38:964, 1966.
20. Holden HF, Hicks CS. The absorption of ultra-viloet radiation by haemoglobin and some of its derivatives. Aust J Exp Biol Med Sci 10:219-223, 1932.
21. Horecker BL. The absorption spectra of hemoglobin and its derivatives in the visible and near infra-red regions. J Biol Chem 148:173-182, 1943.
22. Kramer K. Elam JO, Saxton GA, Elam WN. Influence of oxygen saturation, erthrocyte concentration and optical depth upon the red and near-infrared light transmittance of whole blood. Am J Physiol 165:229-246, 1951.
23. Loewinger E, Gordon A, Weinreb A, Gross J. Analysis of a micromethod for transmission oximetry of whole blood. J Appl Physiol 19:1179-1184, 1964.
24. Martin WE, Cheney FW, Dillard DH, Johnson C, Wong KC. Oxygen saturation versus oxygen tension. J Thoracic and Caridio-vascular Sur 65(3):409-414, 1973.
25. Mass AHJ, Hamelink ML, De Leeuw RJM. An evaluation of the spectrophotometric determination of HbO2 and Hb in blood with the co-oximeter IL 182. Clin Chim Acta 29:303-309, 1970.
26. Millikan GA. Physical instruments for the biologist: the oximeter, an instrument for measuring continuously the oxygen saturation of arterial blood in man. Rev Scient Inst 13:434, 1942.
27. Mook GA, Osypka P, Sturm RE, Wood EH. Fibre optic reflection photometry on blood. Cardiovasc Res 2:199-209, 1968.
28. Mook GA, Van Assendelft OW. Wavelength dependency of the spectrophotometric determination of blood oxygen saturation. Clin Chim Acta 26:170-173, 1969.
29. Naeraa N. The variation of blood oxygen dissiciation curves in patients. Scandinav J Clin Lab Investigation 16:630-634, 1964.
30. Pittman RN, Duling BR. A new method for the measurement of percent oxyhemoglobin. J Appl Physiol 38(2):315-320, 1975.
31. Pittman RN, Duling BR. Measurement of percent oxyhemoglobin in the microvasculature. J Apple Physiol 38(2):321-327, 1975.
32. Polanyi ML, Hehir RM. New reflection oximeter. Rev Sci Instr 31(4):401-403, 1960.
33. Refsum HE. Influence of hemolysis and temperature on the spectrophotometric determination of hemoglobin oxygen saturation in hemolyzed whole blood. Scandinav J Clin Lab Investigation 9:85-88, 1957.
34. Shoemaker WC. Physiological and clinical significance of PtcO$_2$ and PtcCO$_2$ measurements. Crit Care Med 9(10):689-690, 1980.
35. Sidwell AE, Munch RH, Barron ESG, Hogness TR. The salt effect on the hemoglobin-oxygen equilbrium. J Biol Chem 123:335-350, 1938.
36. Siggaard-Anderson O, Norgaard-Pedersen B, Rem J. Hemoglobin pigments. Spectrophotometric determination of oxy-, carboxy-, met-, and suflhemoglobin in capillary blood. Clinica Chimica

Acta 42:85-100, 1972.
37. Tait GR, Sekelj P. An analog computer for ear oximetry. Med Biol Engng, 5:463-471, 1967.
38. Theye RA. Calculation of blood O_2 content from optically determined Hb and HbO_2. Anesthesiology 33(6):653-657, 1970.
39. Van Assendelft. Spectrophotometry of haemoglobin derivatives. Thomas, Springfield, Ill., 1970.
40. Van Kampen EJ, Zijlstra WG. Determination of hemoglobin and its derivatives. Advan Clin Chem 8:141-187, 1965.
41. Wood EH, Geraci JE. Photoelectric determination of arterial oxygen in man. J Lab Clin Med 34:387-401, 1949.
42. Wood EH. Oximetry. Medical Physics 2:664-679, 1950.
43. Wood EH, Sutterer WF, Cronin L. Oximetry. Medical Physics 3:416-445, 1960.
44. Yelderman ML, New W. Evaluation of Pulse Oximetry. Anesthesiology, in press.
45. Yoshiya I, Shimada Y, Tanaka K. Spectrophotometric monitoring of arterial oxygen saturation in the fingertip. Med Biol Eng β Comput 18:27-32, 1980.
46. Zijlstra WG. Fundamentals and Applications of Clinical Oximetry. Van Gorcum, Assen, Netherlands, 1953.
47. Zijlstra WG. A Manual of Reflection Oximetry. Van Gorcum's Medical Library, N.R. 152, Assen, Netherlands, 1958.
48. Zijlstra WG, Mook GA. Medical reflection photometry. Van Gorcum Assen, 1952.
49. Zijlstra WG. Muller CJ. Spectrophotometry of solutions containing three components, with special reference to the simultaneous determination of carboxyhemoglobin and methemoglobin in human blood. Clinica Chimica Acta 2:237-245, 1957.
50. Zwart A, Buursma A, Osesburg B, Zijlstra WG. Determination of hemoglobin derivatives with the IL 282 co-oximeter as compared with a manual spectrophotometric five-wavelength method. Clin Chem, 27(11):1903, 1981.

Graphic Presentation of blood gas data

Osswald PM, Bernauer J, Bender HJ, Hartung HJ

In the practise of anaesthesiology and intensive medicine,
acid-base disturbances are everyday occurrences. Especially
in this field, one frequently meets problems of breath insufficiency and metabolic derangements, and one is forced to
intervene in partial functions of the organism. Often the
task arises here of taking over externally defunct control
functions, in order to maintain the acid-base homeostasis.
Disturbances in the acid-base content and gas exchange are
frequently to be found in the perioperative patient care of
a large hospital. Whilst during an operation, disturbances
of a respiratory kind as a consequence of an inadequate respiration pattern are more common, and post operative, the
respiratory acidosis is more to the fore, due to anaesthesia
overhang, or when breathing is limited because of pain, during
the intensive therapeutic treatment, the whole spectrum of
acid-base disturbances can be observed. Apart from restrictive
and obstructive lung changes, it is above all, inhomogenous
ventilation-perfusion conditions through atelectatic lung
areas or diffusion disturbances which are responsible for the
infringements of the gas exchange of the lungs. They go hand
in hand with an increase of the intrapulmonary shunt volume,
before lung changes can be detected by means of stethoscope
or x-rays. A pre-requisite of the precise interpretation of
blood gas data is an understanding of the complex physiological processes which acid-base disturbances induce in the
organism, and it is an unalterable condition for their specific treatment. The beginner especially often has difficulties
in the interpretation of the acid-base derangements and their
underlying mechanisms.

Interpretation of acid-base disturbances

The clinical symptoms of disturbances in the acid-base content
are often unspecific and sparse, especially for only moderate
pH changes. For their exact interpretation one is therefor
dependant on an arterial blood gas analysis, which apart
from the analysis of the actual blood gases CO_2 and O_2, also
contains the pH value and the bicarbonate concentration. As
a rule in blood gas laboratories or automatic analysis
equipment, the pH, pCO_2 and pO_2 parameters are measured by
specific electrodes and the bicarbonate or standard bicarbonate or the base excess are deduced from these. Here the
influence on the measurement of the temperature of the blood
sample is to be watched. If the adjustment to body temperature is not made directly in the equipment or laboratory,
then the relevant corrections must subsequently be made with
a temperature factor, by means of nomograms. This temperature
adjustment has a special significance in operations where
controlled hypothermia or fever conditions occur. The interpretation of blood gas data involves the task of defining the
extent of respiratory and metabolic components of a disturbance, distinguishing primary from secondary processes, and
evaluating compensation effects. This can only happen in the
context of the whole clinical situation of the patient,
whereby the basic illness and a possible medication must be
taken into consideration. The respiratory share of a disturbance can be obtained simply from the pCO_2 value of an arterial blood gas analysis. Its normal sphere lies between 36
and 44 mmHg. In the past, many efforts were made to find a
measure for the non-respiratory components of a disturbance.
Here there ist a choice of basically two opposing methods:
the standard bicarbonate and base-excess concept of Astrup
and Siggaard-Andersen (3), and the pH/pCO_2 concept of
Schwartz (18). Criticism of the Astrup concept is directed
at the assumption that the parameters gained in such a way
from isolated blood apply to the conditions of the whole
organism, and are equivalent in their in vivo and in vitro

titration curves. However, the case of acute hypercarbia
shows that the bicarbonate increase to be expected after the
buffer reaction is smaller in in vivo than in in vitro, since
a part of the newly formed bicarbonate diffuses into the
interstice (diag. 1). This discrepancy between the in vivo and
in vitro behaviour of the buffer bases is the basis of the
theoretical objection to the parameters of the Astrup method
as a measure of the metabolic components of acid-base disturbances. Howorth describes a fatal practical effect. He shows
the widely used formula for the corrective calculation of the
base deficit $NaHCO_3$ (mmol) = BE x 0,3 x body weight, can lead
to overestimations of the dose of up to 50 % in the case of
acute respiratory acidosis (14).
As a better solution Severinghaus suggests the new parameter
BE_3 as in vivo base excess.   On the assumption   theoretically and empirically proven, that the extracellular space as
a whole behaves in the sense of the buffer equilibrium in
such a way, as if it had an Hb concentration of 3 mg/100ml,
this parameter can be obtained from the nomogram of Siggaard-
Andersen for Hb=3, or can be calculated with an approximation.

Experiments were made in various ways into the in vivo behaviour of the buffer bases in isolated acid-base disturbances, and the expected reaction between pH and $PaCO_2$ in 95 %
confidence bands was described. Such bands are known for the
acute respiratory acidosis and alkalosis (2,7), for the
chronically respiratory acidosis (8) and for the chronically
metabolic cases (1,12). They can be depicted in semilogarith-
mic pH/pCO_2 coordinates in a linear plot and are summarized
in a diagram (diag. 2). For the interpretation of the diagram
it is important that the confidence bands not only statically
identify the expectal areas of isolated disturbances, but
also define dynamically the direction of their development.
There the bands of the acute disturbances can be interpreted
as vectors in a two-dimensional vector space, which allows
the division of an acid-base status into its respiratory and
metabolic components (diag. 3).

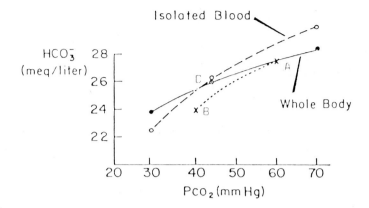

Diagram 1: Comparison of the effects of pCO_2-changes to the bicarbonate-concentration in vivo (whole body) and in vitro (isolated blood).

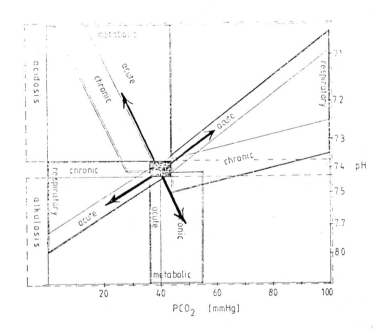

Diagram 3: The respiratory and metabolic vectors.

346

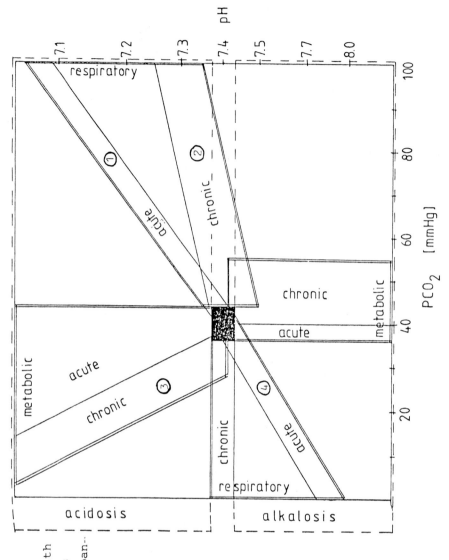

Diagram 2:

Acid-base diagram with
95%-confidence bands
for isolated disturban-
ces.

In this way disturbances situations can, by means of the
confidence bands, be illustrated in their pathophysiological
development, which Flenley has already pointed out (10).
In the interpretation of acid-base disturbances, the confidence bands give safe decision criteria in the evaluation of
the degree of compensation, and the distinction between simple
and mixed disturbances. The acute bands limit the conditions
to be expected for uncompensated disturbances, the chronic
bands respresent maximum compensation. Values outside these
bands point to the overlapping of respiratory and metabolic
components and suggest, if they cannot be explained by compensation, a mixed disturbance.

Computer-based interpretation of blood gas data

The exact interpretation of blood gas analysis is important
for the diagnosis of disturbances in the acid-base content
and for their suitable treatment. In view of the complexity
of the acid-base physiology this is not always straight for-
ward. In the past, computer programs for the interpretation
of blood gas data were written in various ways. In their
assessment of acid-base disturbances they are based partly
on the Astrup-method (9,17) partly on the concept of the
confidence bands of isolated disturbances (5,6,11), whereby
the electrolyte conditions in the serum and urine can additionally be taken into consideration (6).
How far the evaluation of blood gas analysis, which are
carried out routinely in the framework of the perioperative
patient care of a large surgical hospital, can be supported
by the use of computers, was tested with the development and
realisation of two program systems of the Institute for
Anaesthesiology. One program system was conceived as an
interactive information system, the other as a graphic
system for the pictorial representation of the course of
disturbances.

Information System

Assessment of the disturbance mechanism

In order to be able to undertake, for a given acid-base status,
the selection by a computer program of the disturbance mechanism relevant to the situation, rules of decision had to be
formulated. This happened in the form of binary decision
chains, which were defined, sectorwise, by means of simple
exclusion criteria.   The decision chains are stored
in the information system as a control basis. They form the
basis for short dialogues with the operator in the interactive evaluation of blood gas data, and after a few steps
they show the type of disturbance which most probably under-
lies an acid-base disturbance. To each disturbance possible
clinical causes are differential-diagnostically assigned, as
are measures for their therapeutic treatment. At the same
time the treatment reccomendations were applied overall, and
not made dependant on the extent of an acid-base derangement
or its course.

For the programming of the information system a command-
oriented programming language was used with the PASCAL system,
implemented by the Institute's own computer system, using a
conventional programming technic with the flow-diagram method.
In this respect the system is comparable to that of Bleich
and Goldberg (5,6,11). Such a technic forces the programmer
right at the beginning to consider all possible combinations
of input data and to take account of these in the program.
With goal directed software technics, as they are possible
with LISP-similar symbolic manipulation languages, the difficulties mentioned can be more easily overcome (13). Such
languages make no formal distinction between data and programs. On this same foundation, computer-based advisory
systems of a quite different structure have very recently
been developed under the term "expert systems". Examples of
medical expert systems are MYCIN (19), a program system for
the differential diagnosis of infectional illness for anti-
biotic treatment, PUFF (15), a system for lung function

diagnosis, or INTERNIST-I (16), which allows complex diagnoses of internal medicine. These systems have the capacity to be able to make their own logical deductions from a basis of stored facts, whereby the programming technics they have allow the moulding of complex medicinal associations in a much more comfortable way than is possible with PASCAL-similar languages.

Assessment of the virtual shunt

Disturbances in the gas exchange of the lungs can be led back to obstructive or restrictive ventilation disturbances, to a misproportion between ventilation and perfusion in individual lung sectors, or to an infringement in the diffusion in the alveolar membrane. Especially disturbances of the ventilation/perfusion condition and of the diffusion are manifested in an increase of the intrapulmonary (venous) shunt volume, and can be identified by a low arterial oxygen tension, relative to the inspiratory oxygen concentration (FIO_2). In order to be able to evaluate this relationship with a computer, the virtual shunt concept of Benatar and Nunn was consulted (4). In this concept, iso-shunt-lines are defined on the assumption of a fixed arterial venous O_2-difference ($avDO_2$) of 5 %. They are valid within a relatively broad pCO_2 area between 25 and 40 mmHg, and haemoglobin values between 10 and 14 mg/ml. Since the calculation of the venous admixture, amongst other things, assumes a knowledge of the present $avDO_2$ value, the shunt volume, definable by means of the iso-shunt-lines, is only a virtual shunt, based on an $avDO_2$ value of 5 %. However, by means of the virtual shunt volume, relative changes of the gas exchange conditions can be defined, even with changing FIO_2 factors. These iso-shunt-lines are implemented in the information system. On the basis of these, the virtual shunt volumes in artificial respiration situations are calculated and issued by the computer. This makes possible a qualitative orientation during the anaesthesia.

With the iso-shunt-lines predictions of the expected pO_2
with a changed FIO_2 are also possible. They are also suitable,
therefor, for the control of the oxygen treatment, and for
the avoidance of toxically higher oxygen tensions. The virtual character of the shunt lines, however, must be taken
into consideration for all applications of the shunt diagram.
In all cases shunt changes are to be regarded critically
when there are inconstant circulation conditions, or when
ventilation/perfusion disturbances exist.

Graphicsystem

Parallel to the information system, a program system was
constructed on a graphic computer (Tectronix 4051) for the
pictorial representation of the course of disturbances. It
allows the consecutive representation of blood gas data on
the acid-base and shunt diagrams, and explains their interpretation by means of an inclosed text. The program system
was written in the BASIC-programming language, whereby the
graphic functions of the computer were used for the diagrams
(20). It is stored in several segments on a cassette tape,
and from this it can be loaded into the work store of the
computer. This store, with 8 Kbytes, is relatively small.

In its basic form the operator has the choice of the available functions. The results of blood gas analyses of up to
5 people can be fed in and stored at any one time. pH, pCO_2,
pO_2 and FIO_2 are provided as input parameters. At the same
time incorrect inputs can be erased again by means of a
separate function. As a control, the values stored in the
computer can be listed for each patient.
In the course presentation the acid-base diagrams and/or the
iso-shunt-lines are drawn in on the screen, and the data of
a selected patient is listed in the sequence of its input.
For documentation purposes, the possibility exists of copying
the contents of the screen onto paper by means of a hardcopy
unit. For the explanation of the diagrams and the concepts

lying behind them, a short text with an index of reference literature was stored. It can be printed out via a separate function.

Conclusions

In the routine application of the graphic program, it has been seen that the presentation of the results of consecutive blood gas analyses on acid-bases and shunt diagrams is much clearer and more informative than their mere writing up in the anaesthesia protocol or the medical record of patient data.
Both systems are used in the evaluation of blood gas analyses, which are carried out in the perioperative therapy control. The experiences gained up till now show benefits both from a didactic and a diagnostically therapeutic point of view.

352

LITERATUR

1. Albert MS, Dell RB, Winters RW (1967) Quantitative displacement of acid-base equilibrium in metabolic acidosis.
Ann Intern Med 66:312.

2. Arbus GG, Hebert LA, Levesque PR, Etsten BE, Schwartz WB (1969) Characterisation and clinical application of the "significance band" for acute respiratory alkalosis.
N Engl J Med 280:117.

3. Astrup P, Siggaard-Andersen O, Jorgensen K, Engel K (1960) The acid-base metabolism, a new approach.
Lancet 278:1035.

4. Benatar SR, Hewlett AM, Nunn JF (1973) The use of the iso-shunt-lines for control of oxygen-therapie.
Brit J Anaesth 45:711.

5. Bleich HL (1972) Computer-based consultation: Elektrolytes and acid-base disorders. Am J Med 53:285.

6. Bleich HL (1969) Computer evaluation of acid-base disorders. J Clin Invest 48:1689.

7. Brackett NC, Cohen JJ, Schwartz WB (1965) Carbon dioxide titration curve of normal man. N Engl J Med 272:6.

8. Brackett NC, Wingo CF, Murren A (1969) Acid-base response to chronic hypercapnia in man. N Engl J Med 280:124.

9. Cohen MC (1969) A computer program for the interpretation of blood gas analysis. Comp Biomed Res 2:549.

10. Flenley DC (1971) Another non-logarithmic acid-base diagram? Lancet 1:961.

11. Goldberg M, Green SB, Moss ML, Marbach CB, Garfinkel D (1973) Computer-based instruction and diagnosis of acid-base disorders. JAMA 223:269.

12. Goldring RM, Cannon PJ, Heinermann HO, Fishman AP (1968) Respiratory adjustment to chronic metabolic alkalosis in man. J Clin Invest 47:188.

13. Hamann CM (1982) Einführung in das Programmieren in LISP. de Gruyter, Berlin.

14. Howorth PJN (1974) RIpH revisited. Lancet 1:253.

15. Kunz, Fallat, McClung, Osborn JJ (1980) Automated interpretation of pulmonary function test results. In: Nair S (1980) Computers in critical care and pulmonary medicine. Plenum Press, New York.

16. Miller RA, Pople HE, Myers JD (1982) Internist-I, an experimental computer-based diagnostic consultant for general internal medicine. N Engl J Med 307:468.

17. Möhr JR, Hartmann W, Fabel H (1973) Computerunterstützung für klinische Entscheidungen: Automatische Interpretation von Ergebnissen der Blutgasanalyse. In: Lange HJ, Wagner G (1973) Computerunterstützte ärztliche Diagnostik. Schattauer Verlag.

18. Schwartz WB, Relman AS (1963) A critique of the parameters used in the evaluation of acid-base disorders. N Engl J Med 268:1382.

19. Shortliffe EH (1976) Computer-based medical consultations: MYCIN. Elsevier Publ Comp, New York.

20. Tectronix (1976) Plot 50, Introduction to programming in BASIC, Texas.

TEACHING THE INTERPRETATION OF ACID-BASE AND BLOOD GAS PARAMETERS BY COMPUTER APPLICATION

E.VOIGT

INTRODUCTION

Management of acute disturbances of acid-base equilibrium and blood gases requires rapid and detailed information. In addition to measured values of pH, pCO_2, pO_2; derived parameters and additional parameters of pulmonary function and gas exchange must be available for evaluation of the severity of presenting disorders and for deciding on subsequent therapy, especially in patients undergoing open-heart surgery or those with severe thoracic or polytraumatic injuries.

Supplementation of alphanumerical printout of the various variables with graphical representation (17,18,19) offers many advantages for better teaching and understanding of the pathophysiological mechanisms.

Computer application is a valuable method (4,16) towards this end, because the task of tedious evaluation of different parameters using slide rules (12) or nomograms (13,15) can be performed more exactly and much faster. The time for processing and feedback of measured and computed data can be reduced even further by using data lines for electronic data transmission.

A complex system for measurement, computation, electronic data transmission, and graphical demonstration of the various parameters is described in the present paper.

INSTRUMENTATION

Analysis of pO_2, pCO_2, and pH is performed using a manually controlled GAS-CHECK-AVL[+] operating at 310 K (37°C). The pO_2

[+] AVL GmbH, Dietigheimer Str.3, D-3680 Bad Homburg v.d.H.

and pCO_2 electrodes are calibrated with two gases, whereas
the pH electrode is calibrated with buffer solutions. The
System is checked daily using Acid-Basol® test solutions.
The three measured values are fed "off-line" to a desktop
calculator (HP 9825A[++]). An "on-line" mode can be installed
if desired.

Parallel to this step (i.e. during the equilibration period
of the analyzer) the hematocrit; hemoglobin concentration; and,
if needed, oxygen saturation are determined and fed to the
calculator via keyboard. Furthermore, patient data such as
name, birth date, time and body temperature must be entered
(Fig.1).

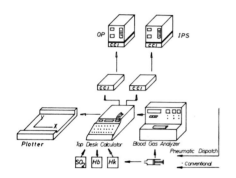

Fig.1
Equipment of the central bood
gas laboratory. Due to
substantial transmission
distance, two common carrier
interfaces per line are
necessary.

Temperature correction of the measured values, as well as
computation of acid-base equilibrium parameters and oxygen
dissociation curve are based on specifications in the literature
(4,12,16).

When all of the data has been entered, the program is
initiated and the measured and derived data are printed
together with a computer diagnosis of the acid-base status (14)
on a thermal printer at a velocity of 190 lines/minute.

[++]Hewlett-Packard, Herrenberger Str. 110, D-7030 Böblingen

Transmission to the external printers (HP 5150A) via the two
data lines is accomplished with a single "continue" step.
Transmission and printing of all data requires only 6 seconds
(Fig.2).

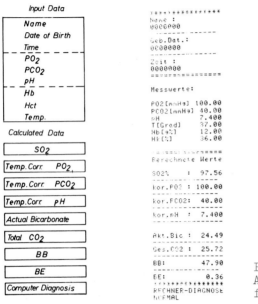

Fig.2
Acid-base status printout
for rapid information

A four-color X-Y plotter is connected in parallel for graphical representation.

The numerous programs are written in HPL (Hewlett-Packard
Language) and stored on a high speed cartridge (max. capacity
250kbytes) with 225 cm/s search and rewind speed. When needed
the program can be read into the calculator memory (6,844 bytes)
at a speed of 14,300 bytes/s.

COMPUTER INTERPRETATION

Interpretation of data indicating disturbances of the
acid-base equilibrium requires knowledge of basic principles
of respiratory and renal physiology. In many cases, such
interpretation is quite difficult for the beginner because the
complex phenomena are described by only three variables

(pCO_2, pH or $[H^+]$, and $[HCO_3^-]$) which are combined in the
Henderson-Hasselbalch equation. For initial help, 12 diagnoses
(14) can be printed out. The programed decision criteria are
the nonrespiratory hydrogen ion concentration nrH^+, the actual
hydrogen ion concentration H^+ and the actual pCO_2. This is
shown in the flow diagram (Fig.3).

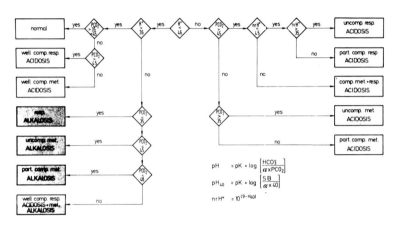

Fig.3   Flow diagram for computer diagnosis. nrH^+ = non-
respiratory hydrogen ion concentration, H^+ = actual hydrogen
ion concentration, pCO_2 = partial pressure of CO_2, SB = standard
bicarbonate (at pH 7.4, pCO_2 40 mmHg, 37°C, fully oxygenated
hemoglobin).

GRAPHICAL REPRESENTATION
Acid-base nomogram

The graphical representation of the Henderson-Hasselbalch
equation in a pH/HCO_3^- nomogram has distinctive advantages in
clinical practice (3). The actual situation is marked by only
a single point derived from the actual pH and pCO_2. The
disturbance of the acid-base equilibrium is obvious and the
direction of compensation towards pH 7.4 can be easily seen
because metabolic deviations cause a shift parallel to the
pCO_2 isobars, whereas endogenic or exogenic compensatory
mechanisms cause a shift parallel to the bicarbonate binding
curve.

358

Respiratory deviations proceed parallel to the bicarbonate
binding curve, and compensatory mechanisms (towards pH 7.4)
cause a shift parallel to the pCO_2 isobars (Fig.4). The
respective compensatory mechanisms are plotted starting from
the actual state and moving towards pH 7.4. The final points
of compensation are printed together with the computer diagnosis, beneath the nomogram.

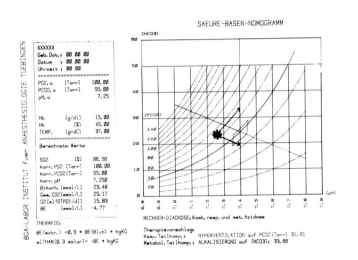

Fig.4   Four-colored acid-base nomogram with numerical printout of the measured, corrected and derived parameters; the
actual state (star) in relation to normal condition (square
area); computer diagnosis; and directions of compensatory
mechanisms.

Most cases reveal a combined disorder; due to the dynamic run
of events the therapeutic procedure should be adjusted to the
clinical condition and the patient's history.

  Temperature correction of measured data (at $37^{o}C$) to actual
patient conditions (5,12) is essential for accurate assessment
in extraordinary situations (severe hypothermia or hyperthermia).
Under closed-system conditions (8,9), the alpha-stat theory
calls for shifting of normal values to a new origin (Fig.5).
All disorders at a given temperature must be examined in
relation to the new origin at that temperature.

For example, pH 7.6 is a normal value at a body temperature
of 25°C (not unlikely during extracorporal circulation).

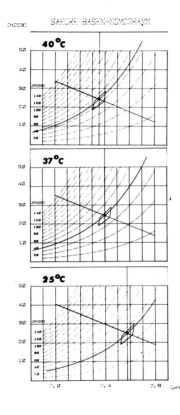

Fig.5
Normal acid-base values at
different body temperature as
indicated by the alpha-stat
theory.

Oxygen dissociation curve

   When oxygen saturation is not measured it can be computed
using a modified (16) Kelman fit (4) of the standard oxygen
dissociation curve (12). In addition to direct estimation
of actual saturation, the algorithm is also required for
computation of the whole curve which in turn, is required
for several program steps. Deviation of this curve from the
standard dissociation curve is only 0.7 % saturation in the
middle and lower ranges. Appropiate corrections for changes
in pH, pCO_2 and temperature are also made (16).

   Because the standard dissociation curve is based on
normal hemoglobin A in the presence of a normal amount of

2,3-DPG, all changes in these substances can influence the
shape of the curve. A different algorithm should therefore
be used in the presence of fetal hemoglobin (11).

   The plotting of the oxygen dissociation curve (Fig.6) has
many advantages in clinical practice (18). Deviations from
normal conditions become obvious not only from the $pO_{2,0.5}$
but also the shape of the curve - especially when the curve
is plotted as the relationship between the pO_2 and O_2 content.
If arterial and central venous blood are sampled simultaneously
- normally no problem with patients in an intensive care unit -
the arteriovenous oxygen difference can also be shown.

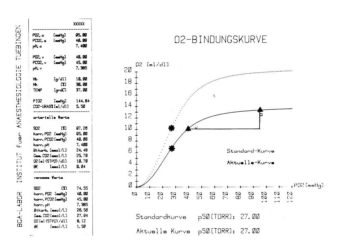

Fig.6   Original plot of the arteriovenous acid-base state,
and standard (dotted line) and actual oxygen dissociation
curve, a = arterial, v = central venous.

Estimation of unsatisfactory peripheral oxygenation is simplified (Fig.7). The major disturbances, e.g. "hypoxic anoxia",
"ischemic anoxia" and "anemic anoxia", as well as intermediate
situations are clearly documented.

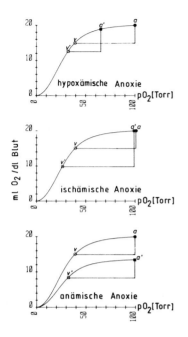

Fig.7
Classification of unsatisfactory
peripheral oxygen availability.
a – v = normal
a′ – v′ = pathological arteriovenous
oxygen difference.

O_2-CO_2 diagram and isoshunt line

Respiratory therapy of critically ill patients must
maintain sufficient oxygen tension for adequate tissue
oxygenation. It is also important to avoid unnecessarily
high inspiratory oxygen concentrations, which may lead to
absorption atelectasis or may even damage pulmonary tissue
secondary to oxygen toxicity (2).

Arterial hypoxemia is most commonly caused (hypoventilation
excluded) by pulmonary venous admixture ($\dot{Q}s/\dot{Q}t$), dead space
ventilation ($\dot{V}_D/\dot{V}_T$) and disturbed ventilation/perfusion ratios
(V_A/Q). Assessment of the influence of these factors on
pulmonary gas exchange and therapeutic planning is greatly
facilitated by the O_2-CO_2 diagram (7,10,22) and isoshunt lines
(1), although the complexity of the relationships necessitates
extensive computation (6,21).

The ventilation/perfusion ratio from zero to infinity

characterizes the possible intraalveolar gas concentrations between the mixed venous point (Pv), and the inspiratory point (PI). The basic assumption in the underlying program is that the respiratory quotient (RQ) in the gas phase equals that in the capillary blood during steady state conditions.

Because of such pecularities of the O_2 and CO_2 dissociation curves as the Bohr and Haldane effects, the equation for RQ cannot be solved algebraically for pO_2 and pCO_2. This can only be done graphically or with the aid of an iteration procedure (19).

The isoshunt line describes the relationship between inspired O_2 concentration (FIO_2) and arterial oxygen tension (paO_2). The relationship of these two variables is nonlinear and depends on five factors:

1. venous admixture in the lungs ($\dot{Q}s/\dot{Q}t$)
2. arteriovenous oxygen difference ($a - v - DO_2$)
3. hemoglobin concentration (Hb)
4. arterial CO_2 tension ($paCO_2$)
5. shifts of the oxygen dissociation curve ($pO_{2,0.5}$)

The initial values required for computation and plotting of the O_2-CO_2 diagram, the isoshunt line and other parameters of the acid-base state are:

1. simultaneously collected arterial and central venous blood sample
2. hemoglobin concentration
3. patient temperature
4. barometric pressure for conversion of vol % into partial pressure
5. inspiratory oxygen concentration (FIO_2)
6. endexpiratory CO_2 concentration ($FECO_2$)

With all these values the complex four-colored picture (Fig.8) can be plotted within 6 minutes.

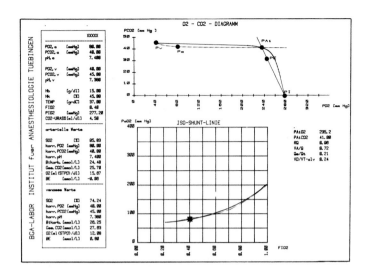

Fig.8   Original plot of the arteriovenous acid-base state,
the O_2-CO_2-diagram and isoshunt line.
Pv = venous point, Pa = arterial point, PAi = "ideal" alveolar
point, PE = endexpiratory point, PI = inspiratory point.

The basic underlying assumption, which should be kept in mind,
is that there are no diffusion gradients and that the alveolar
pO_2 equals the pulmonary capillary pO_2. Furthermore, steady
state conditions must exist and the respiratory quotient in
the blood phase must equal that in the gas phase. The global
ventilation/perfusion ratio is indicated by the "ideal"
alveolar point (PAi). Widely scattered VA/Q inhomogeneities
can only be detected using a more sophisticated method (20).

Changes in venous admixture are indicated by a shift of
the arterial point (Pa) on the blood RQ line. The venous
admixture (Qs/Qt) derived from this diagram is the sum of
desaturated blood bypassed to arterial blood in the lung,
and consists of the true shunt and so called "shunt-like"
effects due to disturbances of the ventilation/perfusion or
ventilation/diffusion ratios . An improvement can be achieved
by application of a positive endexpiratory pressure (PEEP)
during arteficial ventilation. This respiratory regime runs

364

the risk of partly overinflating apical alveolar areas,
especially in hypovolemic situations, thus leading to increased
dead space ventilation. The amount of dead space ventilation
is indicated by the endexpiratory point (PE) on the gas RQ
line.

Under such conditions, the O_2-CO_2 diagram and the isoshunt
lines provide a valuable aid for adjustment of respiratory
parameters (tidal volume, respiratory frequency, PEEP, time
ratio) so as to achieve minimal venous admixture, dead space
ventilation, and inspiratory oxygen concentration required
for satisfactory oxygenation.

Though some simplifications are inherent and a mixed venous
blood sample from the pulmonary artery is required, the above
graphical representation of analytical findings of acid-base
equilibrium and blood gases has proved beneficial in our ICU.
It has been an aid both in the management of arteficial
ventilation in critically ill patients with disturbed pulmonary
function as well as in training our junior medical and nursing
staff.

REFERENCES
1. Benatar SR, Hewlett AM, Nunn JF. 1973. The use of iso-shunt
   lines for control of oxygen therapy. Brit J Anaesth. 45:711
2. Clark JM, Lambertsen CJ. 1971. Pulmonary oxygen toxicity:
   a review. Pharmacol Rev. 23:37
3. Heisler N, Schorer R. 1970. Eine graphische Darstellungs-
   weise des Säure-Basen-Haushaltes zur qualitativen Therapie
   seiner Störungen. Anästhesist. 19:39
4. Kelman GR. 1966. Digital computer subroutine for the
   conversion of oxygen tension into saturation. J Appl
   Physio . 21:1375
5. Nunn JF, Bergmann NA, Bunatyan A, Coleman AJ. 1965. J Appl
   Physiol. 20:23
6. Olszowska AJ, Fahri LE. 1969. A digital computer program
   for constructing ventilation perfusion lines. J Appl
   Physiol. 26:141
7. Rahn H. 1949. A concept of mean alveolar air and the
   ventilation blood flow relationship during pulmonary gas
   exchange. Am J Physiol. 158:21
8. Rahn H, Reeves RB. 1982. Hydrogen ion regulation during
   hypothermia: from the amazon to the operating room. In:
   Applied physiology in clinical respiratory care.Prakash
   (ed).Martinus Nijhoff, The Hague Boston London. p.1

9. Reeves RB, 1976. Role of body temperature in determining the acid-base state in vertebrates. Fed Proc. 28:1204
10. Riley RL,Cournand A. 1949. "Ideal" a veolar air and the analysis of ventilation perfusion relationships in the lung. J Appl Physiol. 1:85
11. Ruiz BC, Tucker WK, Kirby RR. 1979. A program for calculation of intrapulmonary shunts, blood gas and acid base values with a programmable calculator. Anesthesiology. 42:88
12. Severinghaus JW. 1966. Blood gas calculator.J Appl Physiol. 21:1108
13. Siggaard-Andersen O. 1963. Blood acid-base alignment nomogram. Scand J Clin Lab Invest. 12:211
14. Suero JT. 1970. Computer interpretation of acid-base data. Clin Biochem. 3:151
15. Thews G. 1971. Nomogramme zum Säure-Basen-Status des Blutes und zum Atemgastransport. Anästhesie u. Wiederbelebung, Bd 53. Springer Heidelberg NewYork Berlin
16. Thomas LJ jr. 1972. Algorithms for selected blood acid-base and blood gas calculations. J Appl Physiol. 33:154
17. Voigt E. 1978. Enlarged acid-base and blood gas calculations by electrical data computing in the blood gas laboratory. Med Prog Technol. 5:179
18. Voigt E. 1981. Die Sauerstoffbindungskurve zur Differenzierung einer peripheren Anoxie. Anästh Intensivth Notfallmed. 15:47
19. Voigt E. vanDeyk K,Münch F. 1982. O_2-CO_2 diagram and iso-shunt lines for assessment of pulmonary gas exchange during arteficial respiration. Intensive Care Med. 8:125
2o. Wagner PD, Saltzman HA, West JB. 1974. Measurement of continuous distributions of ventilation-perfusion ratios: theory. J Appl Physiol. 36:588
21. Wagner PD, West JB. 1980. Ventilation-perfusion relationships In: West JB (ed). Pulmonary gas exchange.VolI Chapt 7. Academic Press NewYork London Toronto Sydney San Francisco
22. West JB. 1974. Blood flow to the lung and gas exchange. Anesthesiology. 41:124

VISUAL EVOKED POTENTIALS DURING CARDIAC SURGERY, BASIC CONSIDERATIONS.

W. RUSS, D. KLING, B. VON BORMANN, G. HEMPELMANN

Abteilung für Anaesthesiologie und operative Intensiv-
medizin am Klinikum der Justus Liebig-Universität Gieße
(Leiter: Prof. Dr. med. G. Hempelmann)

1. Introduction

Moderate and deep hypothermia are often applicated in cardiovascular surgery. Studies on physiologic/patho-physiologic changes have led to the development of monitoring techniques for the cardiovascular system (1), gas exchange, kidney function, oxygen supply of several tissues, and brain function (2,3). Continuous monitoring devices may provide the possibility for prompt and effective reaction to any adverse development in organ function during anesthesia, operation and recovery period. In order to reduce complications for the brain like severe hypoperfusion intraoperative and postoperative monitoring of brain parameters is mandatory. Various methods and aspects of monitoring the central nervous system during and after open-heart surgery have been described (7,8). Invasive monitoring of direct parameters like cerebral perfusion pressure (CPP), cerebral blood flow (CBF) and intracranial pressure (ICP) usually is not avaiable during surgery. Indirect measures base on the evaluation of cerebral funcition and use noninvasive electroencephalographic techniques in a computerized form (4,5,6). Sensory evoked potentials are being used increasingly to monitor brain funcition (9). Evoked potentials are an objective measure of cerebral function and integrity; they depend on the integrity of cortical flow and are specific for certain cerebral regions and afferent systems (10).

In neurosurgery visual evoked potentials (VEP) are used for monitoring optic nerve function during pituary gland - and aneurysm-surgery in the anterior cranial fossa (11);

brainstem auditory evoked responses (BAER) are detected during posterior fossa surgery (12). Somatosensory evoked potentials (SSEP) are monitored during spinal operations when cord's function may be impaired (13).

Evoked cortical potentials may be recorded when the afferent systems are in danger or the brain itself may be damaged by hypoperfusion (14). Like electroencephalography evoked potentials, particularly those of cortical origin, can be altered by anesthetic agents (15,16) premedication (17) or by other factors under the control of the anesthesiologists. Some of these factors are: temperature, arterial blood pressure and p_aCO_2. The effect and the extent of these potentially interacting veriables has to be known, when evoked potentials are monitored intraoperatively.

In our study we tried to get information about the effects of neuroleptanalgesia, etomidate, p_aCO_2 and temperature on visual evoked potentials enabling us in drawing conclusions about the feasibility of this method.

2. Method and materials

115 patients have been investigated, all of them being older than 18 years. Patients with preexisting psychic, neurological or visual deficits were excluded from the study.

2.1 In 35 urological patients VEP were recorded intraoperatively during steady-state neuroleptanalgesia with fentanyl and droperidol. Control measurements were made prior to induction of anesthesia.

2.2 In 10 patients undergoing abdominal surgery VEP were measured at different $p_a CO_2$ tensions (in the range from 20-50 mmHg).

2.3 In 31 patients the effects of etomidate on VEP were studied.

2.3.1 20 patients received a bolus injection of 0,3 mg/kg bw etomidate within 30 seconds. VEP were elicited before, 1, 2, 3 and 10 minutes after injection.

2.3.2 In 11 patients VEP were recorded before and after an infusion of 1 mg/kg/h.

These measurements were made during a basic neuroleptanalgesia, patients were normoventilated, body temperature was kept constant at 36°C by means of warming blankets.

2.4 39 patients were studied during surgery for coronary artery bypass grafting. After premedication with 0,02 mg/kg bw flunitrazepam i.m. 60 min. prior to induction of anesthesia a modified opiate analgesia with etomidate, fentanyl and pancuronium was performed. The management of extracorporeal circulation (ECC) has been standardized with a pump-flow of 2,4 l/min x m²; arterial pressure during ECC was kept between 50-100 mmHg with a perfusion pressure $(p_{art} - p_{ven})$ being always above 40 mmHg. Arterial pressure and nasopharyngeal temperature were recorded and monitored continuously. Recordings were made during steady-state opiate analgesia: first at 35°C, then at different temperatures during cooling (31°C, 29°C, 27°C, 25°C), during rewarming (27°C, 29°C, 31°C, 33°C, 38°C) and 1 h after ECC. The rapidity of cooling (°C/min) was measured for each patient.

Parameters and Equipment for Intraoperative Recording of VEP

Stimulus: biocular flash through closed eyelids

rate: 1,1/s

duration: 200 ms

intensity: not measured, depending on eyelid thickness

transducer: 3 arrows of 5 light emitting diodes

wavelength: 630 nmm

Recording Channels: O_z (-), C_z (+)

reference: A_1 or A_2

filters: 1-100 Hz

number of averages: 100 or more

analyse time: 500 ms

Electrodes: silver EEG cup electrodes, diameter 9,5 mm

                          interelectrode impedance less than 1 kΩ

skin preparation: conductive, abrasive, adhaesive paste

Equipment: NIC L.E.D. Eyepieces

                          HGA 100 Physiological Amplifier

                          CAL 200 Calibrator

                          NIC CA 1000

                          X-Y-Plotter

In order to ascertain that evoked responses were related to
the visual stimulus and not to artefacts the eyepieces were
removed from the patients while computer averaging continued,

being synchronized with the flash. The components n_2 and p_2 immediately disappeared after removal. Further information to the method can be taken from the Literature (18,19).

In groups 2.1 - 2.3 Student-t-test has been applied for statistical evaluation; in group 2.4 in addition analysis of variance and covariance for temperatture (as a dependent variable) has been performed (20).

3. Results

3.1 Major negative (n_2) and positive (p_2) peaks of the visual evoked potential increased during neuroleptanalgesia:
n_2 from 80,0 ms to 89,4 ms, p_2 from 100,3 ms to 110,1 ms, amplitude between n_2 and p_2 remained relatively constant.

Mean. S.D. Δ % for latencies and amplitude:

		n_2 (ms)	p_2 (ms)	$n_2 p_2$ (μV)
prior to NLA:	mean	80,0	100,3	10,8
	S.D	8,8	12,0	7,1
during NLA:	mean	89,4	110,1	8,43
	S.D	7,8	18,0	4,45
	p	0,005	0,025	n.s.
	Δ %	+11,7	+10,1	-22

3.2 Changes in $p_a CO_2$ in the range from 20-50 mmHg did not alter latencies or amplitude.

3.3.1 After injection of 0,3 mg/kg bw etomidate latencies of n_2 and p_2 increased. 10 minutes later the preinjection values were reached again (fig. 1)

3.3.2 Etomidate (1 mg/kg bw/h) caused a 9,6% latency increase for n_2 from 93,9 ms to 102,95 ms and a suppression of afterdischarge during the infusion period.

3.4 Mean latencies of n_2 and p_2 at different temperatures during cooling and rewarming are listed in fig. 2
With decreasing temperature latencies of n_2 and p_2 increased continuously. Mean latencies of n_2 were 97,1 $\pm$ 8,0 ms at 35°C, at 31°C 119,6 $\pm$ 9,2 ms, at 29°C 134,7 $\pm$ 12,8 ms, at 27°C 148,5 $\pm$ 15,8 ms, at 25°C 184,1 $\pm$ 27,0 ms, with respect to p_2 at 35°C 121 $\pm$ 10 ms, at 31°C 146,4 $\pm$ 13,4 ms, at 29°C 166,7 $\pm$ 17,9 ms, at 27°C 192,4 $\pm$ 26,5 ms, at 25°C 235,5 $\pm$ 49,8 ms.

Changes in latencies were significant for n_2: F = 106,9 (p= 0,001) and for p_2: F = 47,6 (p = 0,001).

At 31°C during cooling depression of aterdischarge occured.

After initiation of ECC nasopharyngeal temperature was falling continuously with 0,36°C $\pm$ 0,13°C per minute.

Depending on the rapidity of cooling visual evoked potentials disappeared at different temperatures:

Cooling with 0,6°C/min: VEP disappeared at 27°C (fig. 3).

Cooling with 0,25°C/min: VEP disappeard at 25°C or were detectable at lower temperatures (fig. 4).

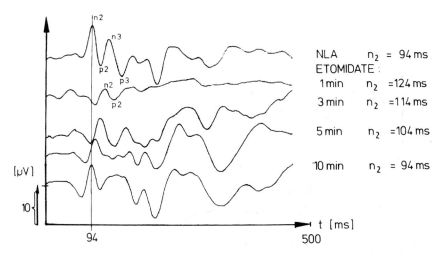

figure 1: The visual evoked potential after a bolus injection
of o,3 mg/kg bw etomidate: Latencies of n_2 and p_2
increase for some minutes. The traces 1,3 and 5
min after injection show the latency return for
n_2. 10 min after injection the pre-injection values
are reachieved.

Temperature (°C)	mean latency (ms), S.D. and % of n_2			mean latency (ms), S.D. and % of p_2		
before ECC	mean	S.D.	%	mean	S.D.	%
35	97,1	8,0	100	121	10,0	100
31	119,6	9,2	123	146,4	13,4	121
29	134,7	12,8	139	166,7	17,9	138
27	148,5	15,8	153	192,4	26,5	159
25	184,1	27,0	189	235,5	49,8	195
27	128,7	12,8	133	163,1	11,9	135
29	120,0	14,0	124	149,8	15,0	124
31	108,9	11,5	112	134,7	14,2	111
33	99,2	10,8	102	120,5	14,2	100
38	87,5	9,4	90	106,4	9,7	88
1 h after ECC 36	91,2	8,4	94	111,8	10,4	92,4

figure 2: Mean latencies and standard deviations of the major
negative (n_2) and positive (p_2) peak at different
temperatures during cooling and rewarming.

374

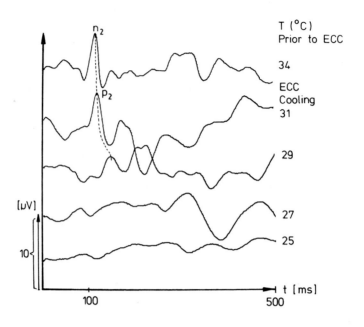

figure 3: Visual evoked potentials when cooling was performed
with o,6°C/min: The VEP disappears at 27°C.

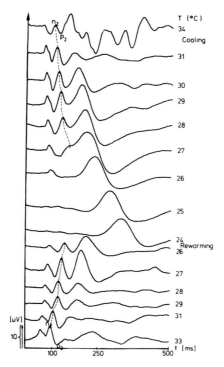

figure 4: The visual evoked potential is detectable during the whole time, even at the minimal temperature of 24°C. Cooling was performed with o,25°C/min. n_2 is marked with a dotted line.

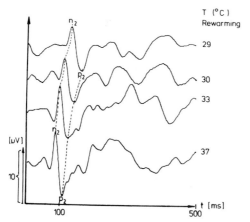

figure 5: Same patient as in figure 3, with increasing temperature latencies decrease, n_2 and p_2 are marked with a dotted line.

During rewarming an immediate recovery of latencies could be demonstrated (fig. 5).

With increasing temperature latencies decreased:
At 27°C mean latency for n_2 was 128,7 $\pm$ 12,8 ms, at 29°C 120,0 $\pm$ 14,0 ms, at 31°C 108,9 $\pm$ 11,5 ms, at 33°C 99,2 $\pm$ 10,8 ms, at 38°C 87,5 $\pm$ 9,4 ms, with respect to p_2 at 27°C 163,1 $\pm$ 11,9 ms, at 29°C 149,8 $\pm$ 15,0 ms, at 31°C 134,7 $\pm$ 14,2 ms, at 33°C 120,5 $\pm$ 14,2 ms, at 38°C 106,4 $\pm$ 9,7 ms.

At 33°C during rewarming the pre-ECC-values were reached again, then latencies become shorter in comparison to the pre-ECC-period. When perfusion pressure was kept above 40 mmHg no alteration in VEP wave form, except in correlation to temperature changes, was noticed.

4. Discussion

The human visual evoked potentials generally consist of five or more waves with defined amplitude an latency (19). Waves are subdivided in those with short latencies (primary response), which are not widely used in clinical work, latencies appearing between 70 and 250 ms (secondary response) and waves with latencies later than 250 ms (afterdischarge). The early waves are of subcortical origin and do not vary during anesthesia (15).

The most important peak appears at about 100 ms after the end of stimulus onset, thus it is called p_{100} or in our nomenclature p_2 (18). p_{100} is generally used when VEP are applied in ophthalmological or neurological diagnosis and for monitoring devices (21). For the appearence of p_2 the

integrity of visual pthways and of the occipital cortex is
necessary.

P_{100} and other peaks of the secondary response can be altered
by anesthetic agents (22, 23, 24, 25, 28, 29) or by premedication (26, 27):

Influence of anesthetics on visual evoked potentials

	latency	amplitude	afterdischarge
Thiopental (Ciganek,1961)	↑	—	↓
N₂O (Domino,1967)	—	↑	?
Promethazin (Corssen,1964)	—	↓	?
Diazepam (Bergamasco,1967)	—	↓	?
Halothane (Uhl,1980)	↑	—	—
Neuroleptanalgesia (Russ,1982)	↑	—	—
Sufentanil (Bovill,1982)	↑	?	?
Na-gammahydroxybutyrate (Desbordes,1982)	↑	?	?
Etomidate (Russ,1982)	↑	↓	↓

= increase of latency or amplitude

= decrease of latency, amplitude or afterdischarge

= no changes reported

= not investigated

Neuroleptanalgesia with fentanyl and droperidol causes a latency
increase of about 10 %; an increase of the same amount was
reported by Bovill (23) for sufentanil anesthesia.

Standard deviations in our patients often exceeded 10 %
of the mean. This leads to a general problem illuminating
difficulties with VEP during surgery:Under general anesthesia
only flash stimulation is feasable, interindividual and
intraindividual variability is larger than with pattern-
reversal stimulation (30), which is usually employed for
diagnostic procedures. Therefore each patient has to be
his own control when VEP are changing during surgery.
Nevertheless evoked potentials can easily be obtained
when electrodes are fixed accurately and skin has been
prepared.

To increase reliability VEP should be reproducable any
time under identical pharmacological conditions. The effect
of a bolus injection of a hypnotic agent like etomidate
causes short acting changes which could lead to misinter-
pretation and would reduce validity of the method. During
monitoring periods, when perfusion pressure is falling to
a critical level or when thoracic aorta is opened and air
embolism might happen, a constant pharmacological (with
respect to hypnotics) or physiological state (with respect
to temperature) should be maintained. From this point of
view a continuous infusion of anesthetic agents can help
to minimize the interferences of bolus injections. When
etomidate is given continuously a stable waveform results:
Etomidate causes a 9,6 % increase in n_2-latency and a
persisting depression of afterdischarge. These results
demonstrate that the effects of etomidate infusion on VEP-

latencies are less (only 50 %), than a temperature decrease
to 31°C, afterdischarge suppression is comparable. This
might add to our information on etomidate and its possible
effects in cerebral protection. Some workers (31) use a
continuous infusion of barbiturates or etomidate for brain
protection during ECC, the effects of this therapeutic procedure on evoked potentials should be known.

Alterations in VEP during hypothermia have been described
by various authors in different animal species. Wolin (32)
in cats and pigs, Aunon (33) in dogs and Boakes (34) in
rats found a latency increase of about 100 % at rectal
temperatures of 24-25°C. It is known that hypothermia
decreases generally body metabolism, this decreased metabolism appears to be a reflection of the general reduction
in rate of chemical reactions at reduced temperatures.
The amount of this reduction seems to be the same in animals
and humans.

In 1982 Bovill reported on VEP changes during sufentanil
anesthesia in six patients (23). Onset latency at 26°C
tympanal increased between 40-75 ms, during rewarming he
found a linear return of onset latency to normal (4-5 ms/°C).
This return of latencies correlates well with our findings
during rewarming: In our patients latency return was larger
at temperatures between 25-27°C and smaller in the range
from 33 to 38°C. Latency return was about 2ms/°C for n_2
and 3ms/°C for p_2. These differences can be explained with
varying temperatures in the heart-lung-machine and a different
rapidity of rewarming.

With systematic cooling latency of all components increased. In some cases early components disappered at higher temperatures than late components (fig.6, 7).This is in contrast to results reported by Stejskal (35), who investigated 8 epileptic patients during systemic and local cooling of the brain. After perfusion of brain ventricles with cold saline he found pronounced differences between early and late components: latency of early components increased slightly, while late components diminished.

In this study SSEP were evaluated, temperature reduction was performed by surface cooling or by local cooling of the brain. These differences may be explained with unequal cooling of brain structures. In our patients the different reaction of early and late components could be related with an insufficient perfusion of the brain. But none of these patients suffered from neurologic sequelae after operation. We could not find patterns of visual evoked potentials that correlate with insufficient cerebral blood flow and post-operative neurological deficits. In one patient we did not obtain VEP after rewarming. This patient suffered from circulatory arrest during induction of anesthesia and from cardiopulmonary problems during ECC.

Perfusion pressure could not be kept above 40 mmHg in this case. At the end of the operation this patient had dilated pupils and died during extracorporeal circulation. In all other patients VEP changed as described already. Latency decreases and increases in a certain range. This normal

range has to be defined for each temperature step and
for a defined rapidity of cooling and rewarming. A
depression of VEP at temperatures where they usually
are present and latency increases outside of normal
range may be signs of inadequate perfusion of the brain.
To verify this, further investigations in patients,
where postoperative neurologic dysfunction is aggravated,
are necessary.

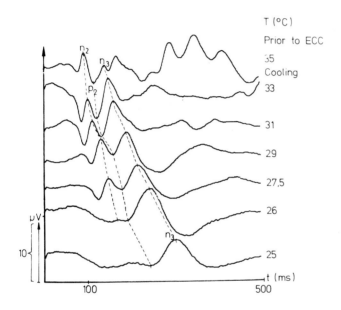

figure 6: VEP recordings of a patient where n_2 disappears
at 26°C while n_3 is detectable during the whole
cooling period.

382

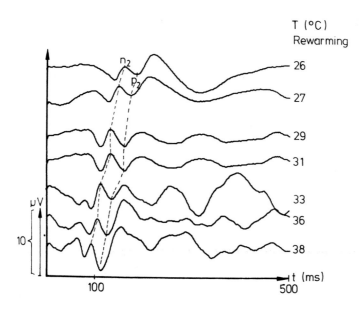

figure 7: Same patient as in figure 6, after rewarming an
immediate recovery latencies is demonstrated.

References:

1. Piepenbrock S, Hempelmann G (1976): Intraoperative and
   Postoperative Monitoring of Cardiocirculatory Function
   in Pediatric and Adult Cardiosurgical Patients.
   In: Anesthesia for Open-Heart Surgery. V. Wiechamn (ed.)
   International Anesthesiology Clinics 14:41-62

2. Mc Dowall G (1976): Monitoring the Brain.
   Anesthesiology 45:117-134

3. Levy WJ, Shapiro HM, Maruchak G, Meathe E (1980): Automated EEG Processing for Intraoperative Monitoring.
   Anesthesiology 53:223-236

4. Müller-Busch HC, Eberlein HJ, Hess W, Tarnow J (1981):
   Überwachung der elektrischen Hirnaktivität bei kardio-
   chirurgischen Patienten. Anästhesist 30:284-289

5. Volgyesi GA (1978): A Brain Function Monitor for Use during
   Anaesthesia.
   Canad. Anaesth. Soc. J. 25:427-430

6. Silvay G, Weinreich A, Owitz S, Mindich B, Litwak RS (1978):
   The cerebral function monitor during open-heart surgery.
   Herz 3:270-275

7. Hicks RG, Poole JL (1981): Electroencephalographic changes
   with hypothermia and cardiopulmonary bypass in children.
   J. Thorac Cardiovasc Surg: 781-786

8. Reilly EL, Brunberg JA, Doty DB (1974): The effect of deep
   hypothermia and total circulatory arrest on the electroencephalogram in children.
   Electroencephalogr Clin Neurophysiol 36:661-667

9. Grundy BL (1983): Intraoperative Monitoring of Sensory-
   evoked Potentials. Anesthesiology 58:72-87

10. Barber C (1980): Evoked potentials. Lancaster, MTP Press
    Limited.

11. Allen A, Starr A, Nudleman K (1981): Assesment of sensory
    function in the operating room utilizing cerebral evoked
    potentials.
    Clin Neurosurg 28:457-481

384

12. Raudzens PA (1982): Intraoperative monitoring of evoked potentials.
    Ann NY Acad Sci 388:308-326

13. Engler GL, Spielholz NI, Bernhard WN, Danziger F, Merkin H, Wolff T (1978): Somatosensory potentials during Harrington instrumentation for scoliosis.
    J Bone Joint Surg 60:528

14. Grundy BL, Heros RC, Tung AS, Doyle E (1981): Intraoperative Hypoxia Detected by Evoked Potential Monitoring.
    Anesthesia and Analgesia 60:437-439

15. Clark DL, Burton S, Rosner PhD (1973): Neurophysiologic Effects of General Anesthetics: I. The electroencephalogram and Sensory Evoked Responses in Man.
    Anesthesiology 38:564-582

16. Rosner S, Clard DL (1973): Neurophysiologic Effects of General Anesthetics: II. Sequential Regional Actions in the Brain.
    Anesthesiology 39:59-81

17. Domino EF (1967): Effects of Preanesthetic and Anesthetic Drugs on Visually Evoked Responses.
    Anesthesiology 28:184-191

18. Harding GFA (1974): The Visual-Evoked Response.
    Adv Ophthal 28:2-28

19. Desmedt JE (1977): Visual evoked potentials in man: new developments.
    Clarendon Press, Oxford

20. Kreyszig E (1975): Statistische Methoden und ihre Anwendungen.
    Göttingen, Vandenhoeck und Ruprecht: pp 239-257

21. Stöhr, M, Dichgans J, Diener HC, Buettner UW (1982): Evozierte Potentiale. Springer Verlag, Berlin, Heidelberg, New York: 233-323

22. Uhl RR, Squires KC, Bruce DL, Starr A (1980): Effect of Halothane Anesthesia on the Human Cortical Visual Evoked Response.
    Anesthesiology 53:273-276

23. Bovill JG, Sebel PS (1982): Visual evoked responses during sufentanil anesthesia and hypothermia.
Anesthesia, Volume of Summaries, 6th European Congress of Anesthesiology: 155-156

24. Ciganek L (1961): The EEG response (evoked potential) to light stimulus in man.
Electroencephalogr Clin Neurophysiol 13:165-172

25. Desbordes JM, Marillaud A, Roualdès G, Badouraly MJ (1982): Le gamma hydroxybutyrate de sodium. Action sur les potentiels évokés visuelles obtenues par flash.
Ann Fr Anesth Réanim 1:147-151

26. Corrsen G, Domino EF (1964): Visual Evoked Responses in Man: A Method for Measuring Cerebral Effects of Preanesthetic Medication.
Anesthesiology 25_330-341

27. Bergamasco B (1967): Modifications of cortical responsiveness in humans induced by drugs acting on the central nervous system.
Electroenceph Clin Neurophysiol 23:186-192

28. Russ W, Lüben V, Hempelmann G (1982): Der Einfluß der Neuroleptanalgesie auf das visuelle evozierte Potential (VEP) des Menschen.
Anästhesist 31:575-578

29. Russ W, Lüben V (1982): Der Einfluß von Etomidat in hypnotischer Dosis auf das visuelle evozierte Potential (VEP).
Anästhesist 31:483:484

30. Perry NW, Childers DG (1969): The Human Visual Evoked Response.
Springfield, Charles C Thomas

31. Michenfelder JD, Theye RA (1973): Cerebral protection by thiopental during hypoxia.
Anesthesiology 39:510

32. Wolin LR, Massopust LC, Meder J (1964): Electroencephalogram and Cortical Evoked Potentials Under Hypothermia.
Arch Ophthal 72:521-524

33. Aunon JI, Weinrich, WE, Nyholm (1977): Effects of
    Hypothermia on the Visual-Evoked Brain Potential
    in Dogs.
    Ann J Vet Res 38:383-385

34. Boakes RJ, Kerkut GA, Munday KA (1967): Effect of
    Hypothermia on Cortical Evoked Potentials.
    Life Sciences 6:457-459

35. Stejskal L, Travnicek V, Sourek K, Kredba J (1980):
    Somatosensory evoked potentials in deep hypothermia.
    Appl Neurophysiol 43:1-7

Phosphorus Nuclear Magnetic Resonance (^{31}P NMR):
A Computer Based Instrument for Studying Brain Hypoxia.

M Hilberman, V. Harihara Subramanian, L Gyulai, B Chance
Departments of Anesthesia, Biochemistry and Biophysics
University of Pennsylvania, Philadelphia, PA 19104

Introduction

The brain is a critical organ for human function, yet techniques for quantifying brain function or predicting outcome following acute injury remain poorly developed, particularly by comparison with the heart. The wealth of information and the limitations in existing data regarding brain energy metabolism and brain protection from ischemic and/or hypoxic injury have recently been reviewed (Siesjo, 1978; Myers, 1979; Hossman, 1982). Inability to quantify intracellular bioenergetic state in a non-destructive manner is one reason for the conflicting conclusions which exist regarding the minimum blood pressure adequate for cerebral perfusion. Thus, studies in higher mammals and man have suggested that permanent brain damage may be caused if mean arterial blood pressure (MABP) falls below 50 mmHg (Stockard, et al., 1974; Michenfelder & Theye, 1977). Other investigators have found that hypovolemic hypotension in monkeys to a level at or below 25 mmHg was required to produce permanent brain damage (Selkoe & Myers, 1979). Trimethaphan induced hypotension in dogs failed to produce permanent brain damage even though MABP fell to 15-25 mmHg (Dong, et al., 1983). The relevance of these low pressures to humans is emphasized by recent observations in patients undergoing cardiopulmonary bypass, which indicate that perfusion pressures of 30-50 mmHg are well-tolerated (Kolkka & Hilberman, 1980; Ellis, et al., 1980).

Further examples of the difficulty in differentiating between normal and necessary may be found in the literature on cerebral blood flow and neurophysiological function. Harper (1966) demonstrated that cerebral blood flow (CBF) was maintained at approximately 80 ml/100gm/min until mean arterial pressure fell below 70 mmHg, and that an arterial pressure of approximately 30 mmHg still maintained CBF at 30 ml/100gm/min. The levels of CBF at which injury occurs are apparently still lower. Thus, in their review of data relating neurophysiological changes and damage to CBF, Morawetz, et al. (1979) and Hossman (1982) indicate the CBF falls below 20 ml/100gm/min before electroencephalographic silence ensues, and that evoked potentials disappear at about 15 ml/100gm/min. Loss of cellular integrity and permanent damage occurs below these extremely low values.

Reconciliation of these observations, and understanding the relationship of these extremes to norms for clinical decision-making is important and requires precise methods for quantifying bioenergetic and functional state in a sequential and non-destructive manner.

^{31}P NMR spectroscopy is the best method available for the non-destructive quantification of tissue bioenergetic state and the functional integrity of the mitochondrial redox system. As such, we believe it the linchpin requisite for understanding the relationship between various hypoxic or ischemic insults, function, permanent tissue damage, and protection. The correlation of changes in brain bioenergetics, measured by ^{31}P NMR, with detailed and quantified neurophysiologic measurements promises fundamentally important insights into these latter, inherently more portable, measurements. Finally, important experimental observations obtained with ^{31}P NMR in animals, can provide scientific information during controlled acute pathophysiological perturbations, not ethical in man, thereby enhancing knowledge and therapeutic capability.

Such studies are inherently computer dependent, and offer an excellent example of how advances in computer technology permit advances in the scientific basis of anesthesia not possible otherwise.

Technical Description of ^{31}P NMR Spectoscopy

NMR spectroscopy is based on the fact that nuclei such as ^{1}H, ^{13}C and ^{31}P, etc., possess magnetic moments due to their non-zero spin angular momentum. In the presence of an applied d.c. magnetic field B_0, the nuclear magnetic moment tends to align itself along B_0. Since the nuclear spin angular momentum is quantized, this process leads to a set of energy levels. NMR spectroscopy is a method used to study the transitions induced between these energy levels by an applied electromagnetic field B_1 of the correct frequency. Since different nuclei have different magnetic moments, they have very different B_1 resonant frequencies at a given B_0 thus permitting study of a single isotope without interference from other elements. For each element, the NMR resonant frequency of a particular nucleus depends on its chemical environment. Thus, the spectrum of a molecule consists of several lines, one for each chemical group. The intensity of the signal at a given resonant frequency is linearly proportional to the total number of absorbing nuclei in the sample in that chemical environment. At present, in vivo ^{31}P NMR distinguishes 7 peaks: sugar phosphates (SP), inorganic phosphate (Pi), phosphodiesters (PD), phosphocreatine (PCr), and adenosine triphosphate (ATP, 3 peaks). The theory of NMR methods and relevant experimental techniques are more fully discussed in several monographs, e.g., Gadian (1982); Fukushima and Roeder (1981). We would like to discuss some practical aspects of in vivo ^{31}P NMR spectroscopy.

The most important component of an NMR spectrometer is the magnet producing B_0. Since chemical shifts are of the order of a few parts per million (ppm), the magnetic field, B_0, must be homogeneous to less than 1 ppm over the sample volume. Since the theoretical sensitivity of NMR depends on the strength of B_0, one would like to have large B_0 values (typically 1.5 to 2 Tesla (T), where 1 Tesla is 10,000 times the earth's magnetic field). The use of NMR for in vivo tissue study further requires wide-bore magnets so that the whole animal (or human limb) can be inserted in the magnet. These considerations make it imperative that one use superconducting magnets for in vivo NMR spectroscopy studies.

The observation of NMR requires radio-frequency electronics. Most of the modern spectrometers are pulsed Fourier Transform NMR spectrometers. The nuclear spins are excited by a short radio frequency (rf) pulse and one "listens" to the response of the spin system following the pulse; this signal is called a free induction decay (FID). The spectrometer is coupled to a minicomputer which performs the function of control as well as data processing. A simplified block diagram of our experimental set up is given in Figure 1.

Since one normally uses the NMR signal from tissue water protons to adjust the homogeneity of the B_0 field around the specimen, our NMR spectrometer system can be used either at 60.1 MHz for proton NMR, or at 24.3 MHz for ^{31}P NMR. We use a single coil transmit/receive system for in vivo NMR. Most of our NMR coils are "surface coils" (Chance, et. al., 1980; Ackerman, et al., 1980).

Fig 1 Simplified Block Diagram of the NMR Spectometer

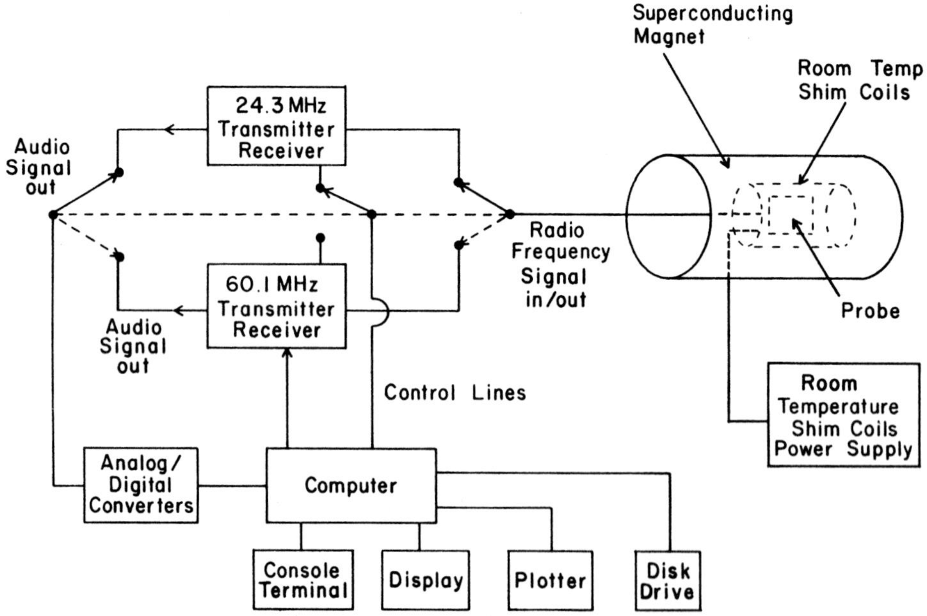

The basic process of obtaining ^{31}P NMR spectra can be represented by the flow chart in Figure 2. This process can be split into 3 stages.

Fig 2   Process of Obtaining NMR Spectra

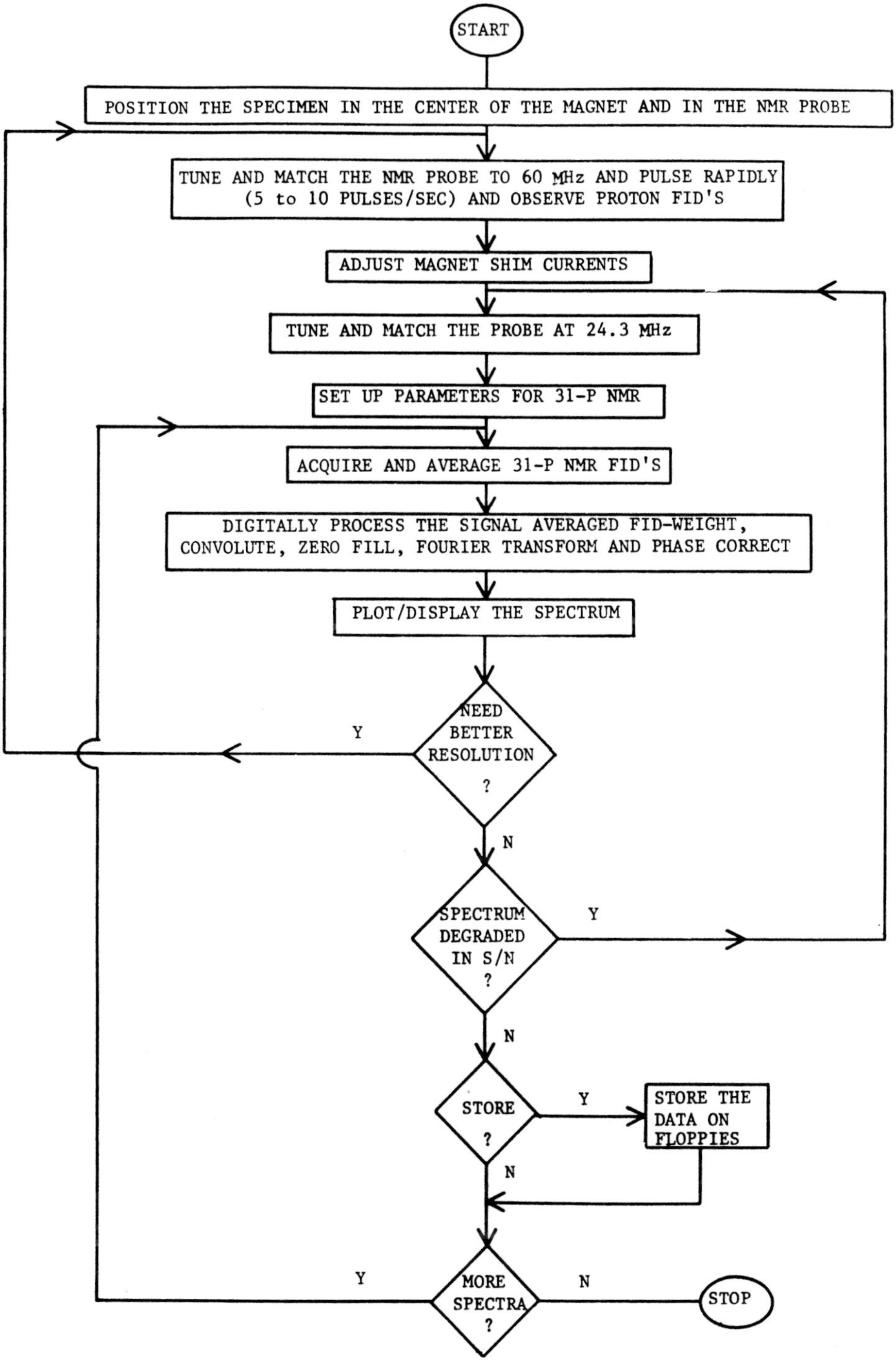

First, is the set up stage in which the specimen is positioned inside the homogeneous volume of the magnet and the magnet homogeneity is adjusted (shimmed) using the proton NMR signal from the tissue. The pulse parameters are set up for acquiring ^{31}P NMR spectra. The parameters that are important are 1) the pulse width, 2) the waiting time between pulses, and 3) the acquisition time. Next, is the acquisition stage. Sequential rf pulses generate FID's which are acquired and coherently added to improve S/N ratios. The third stage is the digital processing of the signal averaged FID. The final ^{31}P NMR spectrum is plotted on paper, the data may be stored on floppy discs. If the probe is being used for the first time, the correct set of parameters must be determined experimentally. If the resolution is unsatisfactory, the process must be repeated.

The currently implemented steps in the digital processing of the NMR data are illustrated and explained in Figure 3. The extent to which the data are dependent upon this mathematical processing is evident therein. Beyond the steps shown, the large PD peak evident in the dog (and human) ^{31}P NMR brain spectra (see Figs 4-7) has made precise quantification of these peaks difficult. Therefore, we are in the process of developing and validating curve fitting routines which will permit such quantification, further automate the process, and enhance our ability to modify experimental perturbations based upon the brain's bioenergetic response measured in more or less real time.

Animal Experiments

Studies in cats demonstrated the feasibility of combining the electroencephalogram (EEG) with ^{31}P NMR data. However consistent high quality spectra were difficult to obtain, and the scan times required for good spectra (16-32 mins) were unsatisfactory for the study of a number of interesting pathophysiological problems in which rapid changes in brain bioenergetic state may be expected. Since September of 1982, we have focused our efforts on improving the time resolution and consistency of the brain ^{31}P NMR spectra. We can now routinely obtain high quality spectra in 4 minutes, and 1 minute spectra may be used to study rapidly changing events. In addition, shielding and filtering of

Fig 3   Data Processing of the FID to Obtain the ^{31}P NMR Spectrum

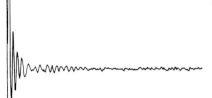

RAW FID: The time-dependent response of the ^{31}P nuclear spins.

$Y^1(t)$

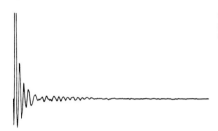

WEIGHTED FID: Weighting reduces the noise contribution from the tail of $Y^1(t)$.

$$Y^2(t) = Y^1(t) * e^{-(\pi * LW * t)}$$
$$LW = 10$$

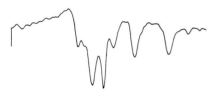

FID WITH CONVOLUTION DIFFERENCE: This removes noise from the initial portion of the FID.

$$Y^3(t) = Y^2(t) - FA * e^{-(\pi * L2 * t)}$$
$$\text{with } L2 = 100, \ FA = 1.0,$$

SPECTRUM WITH NO PHASE CORRECTION: The real part of the Fourier Transform of $Y^3(t)$. Instrument limitations delay FID acquisition from the true time origin of the FID, introducing phase errors into the spectrum.

$$s(\nu) = \int_0^t Y^3(t) \, e^{-i2\pi\nu t} \, dt \qquad Y^4(\nu) = \text{Re}\left[s(\nu)\right]$$

SPECTRUM WITH PHASE CORRECTION: $Y^5(\nu)$ the phase errors can be corrected using a phase angle ϕ, and making a linear combination of the real and imaginary parts of $s(\nu)$.

$$Y^5(\nu) = \left[\text{Re}\left\{s(\nu)\right\}\right] * \cos\phi +$$
$$\left[\text{Im}\left\{s(\nu)\right\}\right] * \sin\phi$$

scale: 1 cm = 3 ppm

the leads from amplifier to skull have permitted us to obtain electroencephalographic data without degrading the NMR signal. The factors responsible for this improvement include:

1. Revision of the animal holder to permit reproducible centering of the brain in the homogeneous field. In addition, shielding of the animal's hind quarters, which protrude from the magnet, has been greatly simplified by the new holder and a bolt of conducting fabric.

2. Increasing the amount of phosphorus compound detected in the homogeneous field was achieved by switching from cat to dog, and increasing coil diameter.

3. Improvement in surface coil performance. Our best results have been obtained with a simple single turn, 4 cm diameter coil made of ¼" copper tubing. Further coil work is needed to define optimum size and improve fit to the irregular surface of the dog's skull.

Figure 4 illustrates selected 4 minute brain NMR spectra, electroencephalographic, hemodynamic and arterial blood gas data, from a dog subjected to severe hypoxia (PaO_2 < 20 mmHg for 45 minutes). The initial scan (A) at PaO_2 = 96 mmHg is normal. The dog responded to the hypoxic stress by hypertension and tachycardia, which for 10-15 minutes succeeded in maintaining cerebral perfusion by EEG and ^{31}P NMR criteria. At 18-22 minutes (scan B) a distinct decline in PCr and increase in Pi is evident; the EEG, recorded at 5mm/sec, shows slowing, loss of amplitude and bursting. At 26-30 minutes, the blood pressure has declined and a further decline of PCr is evident, as is marked slowing of the EEG (scan C). Of extreme interest, the Pi peak has shifted to the right and disappeared into the PD peak. This result differs from that seen in the next data set and may reflect a distinct pH shift from the more extreme brain lactic acidosis in this animal due to: a) Prolonged sustained hypoxia and, b) potential hyperglycemia from continuous dextrose infusion (Rehncrona, et al., 1981; Myers and

Yamaguchi, 1976). By 42–46 minutes (scan D), systemic arterial pH declined to 6.8, MABP declined to 85 mmHg, and the EEG was flat, despite normal brain ATP levels. Scan D also shows a further decline in PCr and a suggestion that Pi has moved further into the phosphodiester peak. Finally, at 46–50 minutes, during extreme hypotension and bradycardia, deterioration of brain ATP levels is evident and the development of a single phosphorus peak is seen (scan E).

Fig 4. Dog brain response to systemic hypoxia
created by decreasing the inspired oxygen concentration.

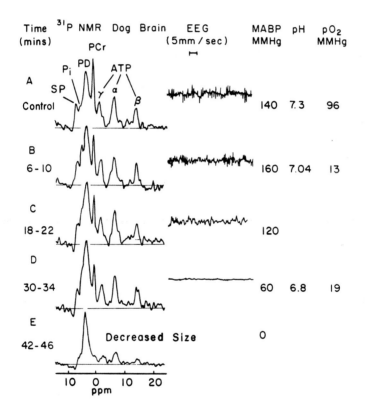

Figure 5 illustrates a second graded hypoxia experiment in which a lesser degree of hypoxia (PaO_2 = 35 mmHg) was reasonably well tolerated for an hour; thereafter, gradual undetected hemmorhage from the operative site superimposed hypovolemia on more profound hypoxemic stress. These data differ from those above in showing less systemic acidosis (pH just prior to death = 7.0 vs. 6.8) and less shift in the Pi peak, which remains distinct from the phosphodiester peak until the onset of death. The EEG was recorded at 25 mm/sec and no glucose was administered. Scan A control. Scan B, 58-62 minutes, shows a slight increase in the height of the Pi peak and loss of high frequency activity on the EEG. Scan C, 12 minutes later, shows a sharp decline in PCr, and increase in Pi associated with further slowing and flattening of the EEG. The subsequent 4 minute scan (D) shows progression of the PCr and Pi changes. Again, the EEG is nearly silent prior to the onset of ATP depletion and the loss of the "background hump" associated with the development of a single phosphorus peak (beginning in E). The EEG is flat.

Fig 5. Dog brain response to systemic hypoxia created by decreasing the inspired oxygen concentration.

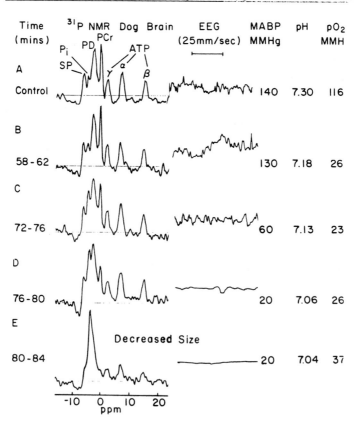

High repetition rates cause saturation (decreased intensity) in all P-compounds, especially Pi and PCr (Shoubridge, et al., 1982), our data indicate this is severe below 3 second intervals. Nonetheless, for certain insults, rapid repetitions and short scans allow useful data to be obtained. Figure 6 illustrates the consequence of a respiratory arrest in the dog brain ^{31}P NMR acquired at a repetition rate of 2/sec, pulse width 50 microseconds, for one minute each. No difference was detectable between the first and second and between the third and fourth scans, and these were averaged to simplify the illustration. Similarly, scans beyond seven minutes showed no change and were deleted.

Fig 6. Time resolved
^{31}P NMR: Respiratory Arrest

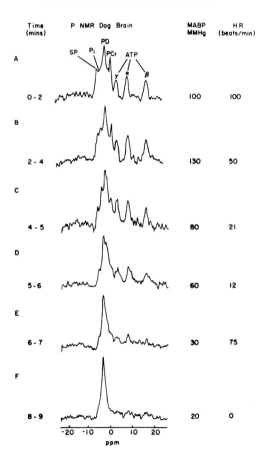

At 2-4 minutes, the animal became hypertensive, Pi increased, PCr decreased, and the ATP peaks remain unchanged. Further decrease in PCr and increase in Pi is evident at 4-5 minutes, the beta-ATP peak may be somewhat diminished by this time. Profound depression of creatine phosphate is evident before significant ATP depletion takes place (5-6 minutes). Beyond 6 minutes, a single peak progressively dominates in the area of the original PD peak, presumably, this represents a composite Pi and PD peak with Pi right shifted by intracellular acidosis. Detailed analytical biochemical and high resolution NMR studies will be required to fully characterize the changes shown in Figures 4-6. (See Glonek et al., 1982).

A human brain ^{31}P NMR spectra obtained from a neonate with fetal alcohol syndrome is shown in Figure 7. The high sugar phosphate peak, low phosphocreatine peak, and prominent phosphodiester peak are characteristic. While pertubation protocols in humans are not now justified, we believe our animal studies will greatly facilitate interpretation of these spectra.

DISCUSSION

In these spectra (Figures 4-7) quantification of SP, Pi, PD, and PCr is complicated by limited resolution which results in overlap of the

Fig 7. ^{31}P NMR spectrum of human neonatal brain.

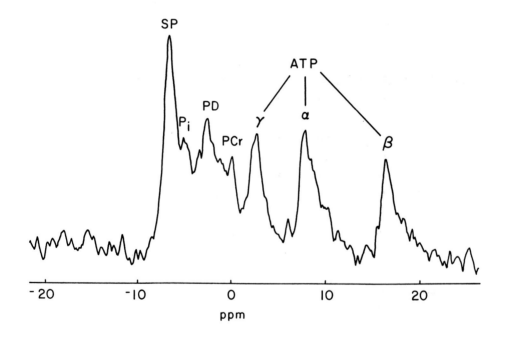

bases of the spectral peaks with creation of a background hump (which disappears after death). The "phosphodiester" peak we have observed in the human and dog brain ^{31}P NMR spectra is higher than in the rabbit (Delpy, et al., 1982), and little PD is evident in rat (Ackerman, et al., 1980; Shoubridge, et al., 1982) or gerbil brain (Thulborn, et al., 1982). These results also differ from those obtained in rodents in showing better time resolution, better signal to noise ratio, and simultaneous neurophysiological, blood gas, and hemodynamic data.

We find these preliminary data exciting. They demonstrate the increasing time resolution of ^{31}P NMR and the power and potential of combining in vivo brain phosphorus biochemistry with measurement of neurophysiological function. Furthermore, they suggest that in the brain, as in muscle (Chance, et al., 1981), loss of PCr limits work (measured here by the spontaneous EEG) prior to ATP depletion. Further observations with more complete physiological control and quantification of spontaneous EEG and evoked potential measurement is needed to fully characterize and validate these initial observations.

Finally, we believe this example important to the purposes of this conference. both the NMR measurements and the appropriately quantified measurement of brain electroencephalographic and evoked potentials which are being incorporated into our measurement system are inconceivable without the application of contemporary computing power. Thus, in this application computing power is being applied to develop an important area of information relevant to the scientific basis of anesthetic practice, which could not be elucidated in the absence of computational techniques.

REFERENCES:

Ackerman, J.J.H., Grove, T.H., Wong, G.G., Gadian, D.G., Radda, G.K. 1980. "Mapping of metabolites in whole animals by ^{31}P NMR using surface coils." Nature 283:167-170.

Chance, B., Eleff, S., Leigh, J.S., Jr. 1980. "Noninvasive, nondestructive approaches to cell bioenergetics.: Proc Natl Acad Sci USA 77:7430-7434.

Chance, B., Eleff, S., Leigh, J.S., Jr., Sokolow, D., Sapega, A. 1981. "Mitochondrial regulation of phosphocreatine/inorganic phosphate ratios in exercising human muscle: A gated ^{31}P NMR study." Proc Natl Acad Sci USA 78:6714-6718.

Delpy, D.T., Gordon, R.E., Hope P.L., Parker, D., Reynolds, E.O.R., Shaw, D. and Whitehead, M.D. 1982. "Noninvasive investigation of cerebral ischemia by phosphorus nuclear magnetic resonance" Pediatrics 70:310-313.

Dong, W.K., Bledsoe, S.W., Eng, D.Y., Heavner, J.E., Shaw, C.-M., Hornbein, T.F., Anderson, J.L. 1983. "Profound arterial hypotension in dogs: Brain electrical activity and organ integrity." Anesthesiology 58:61-71.

Ellis, R.J., Wisneiwski, A., Potts, R., Calhoun, C., Loucks, P., Wells, M.R. 1980. "Reduction of flow rate and arterial pressure at moderate hypothermia does not result in cerebral dysfunction." J Thoracic Cardiovasc. Surg. 79:173-180.

Fukishima, E., Roeder, S.B.W. 1981. "Experimental pulse NMR, a nuts and bolts approach." Addison-Wesley, Reading, Massachusetts.

Gadian, D.G. 1982. "Nuclear Magnetic Resonance and Its Application to Living Systems", Clarendon Press, Oxford.

Glonek, T., Kopp, S.J., Kot, E., Pettegrew, J.W., Harrison, W.H. and Cohen M.M. 1982. "P-31 Nuclear magnetic resonance analysis of brain: the perchloric acid extract spectrum" J Neurochem. 39:1210-1219.

Harper, A.M. 1966. "Autoregulation of cerebral blood flow: Influence of the arterial blood pressure on the blood flow through the cerebral cortex.: J Neurol Neurosurg Psychiat 29:398-403.

Hossman, K.-A. 1982. "Treatment of experimental cerebral ischemia." J Cerebral Blood Flow and Metab 2:275-297.

Kolkka, R., Hilberman, M. 1980. "Neurologic dysfunction following cardiac operation with low-flow, low-pressure cardiopulmonary bypass." J Thorac Cardiovasc Surg 79:432-437.

Michenfelder, J.D., Theye, R.A. 1977. "Canine systemic and cerebral effects of hypotension induced by hemorrhage, trimethaphan, halothane, or nitroprusside." Anesthesiology 46:188-195.

Morawetz, R.B., Crowell, R.H., DeGirolami, U., Marcoux, F.W., Jones, T.H., Halsey, J.H. 1979. "Regional cerebral blood flow thresholds during cerebral ischemia." Fed Proc 38:2493-2494.

Myers, R.E., Yamaguchi, M. 1976. "Effects of serum glucose concentration on brain response to circulatory arrest." J Neuropathol Exp Neurol 35:301.

Myers, R.E. 1979. "A unitary theory of causation of anoxic and hypoxic brain pathology." In, Advances in Neurology, Vol. 26. Cerebral Hypoxia and Its Consequences, (Fahn, S., Davis, J.N., Rowland, L.P., eds.), pp. 195-213, Raven Press, New York.

Rehncrona, S., Rosen, I., Siesjo, B.K. 1981. "Brain lactic acidosis and ischemic cell damage: 1. Biochemistry and neurophysiology." J Cereb Blood Flow Metabol. 1:297-311.

Selkoe, D.J., Myers, R.E. 1979. "Neurologic and cardiovascular effects of hypotension in the monkey.: Stroke 10:147-157.

Shoubridge, E.A., Briggs, R.W., Radda, G.K. 1982. "31-P NMR Saturation transfer measurements of the steady state rates of creatine kinase and ATP synthetase in the rat brain." FEBS Letters 140:288-292.

Siesjo, B.K. 1978. Brain Energy Metabolism. John Wiley, Chicester.

Stockard, J.J., Bickford, R.G., Myers, R.R., Aung, M., Dilley, R.B., Schauble, J.F. 1974. "Hypotension-induced changes in cerebral function during cardiac surgery." Stroke 5:730-746.

MEASURING PULMONARY BLOOD FLOW WITH AN 8085

J.W. BELLVILLE, L. ARENA, O. BROVKO AND D.M. WIBERG

1. INTRODUCTION

Pulmonary bloodflow is an important indicator of a patient's physiologic state during the clinical course of anesthesia, while recuperating from myocardial infarction and many serious diseases. We wished to measure it non-invasively.

We rejected the method using metabolic gases such as CO_2 essentially for the reasons stated by Butler in his review (1). We also rejected methods that are too slow to analyze, that is, they cannot be done on-line such as that of Homer and Denisyk (2).

Zwart's Soluble Gas Method (3) is a relatively new non-invasive method that appears to be cheap and convenient. It is a soluble gases technique and can be directly implemented using a standard anesthesia machine or a ventilator. For most other soluble gas techniques to be truly non-invasive, one requires estimates of the mixed venous concentrations to apply Fick's principle (4). Zwart's method and ours does not.

A small amplitude sinusoidal inhaled concentration of halothane is introduced with a relatively high frequency (3 min. period). Because of the large time constant of the body tissues this causes the sinusoidal amplitude in the mixed venous concentrations to be damped to very small levels. Consequently, one can model the whole body circuit as just a compartment representing the lungs. That is:

$$P_A(\omega) = (1 + \frac{\lambda \dot{Q}^{-1}}{\dot{V}}) (j\omega \tau_L + 1)^{-1} P_I(\omega)$$

where:

$P_A(\omega)$ = the alveolar concentration (%) transform
ω = angular frequency (min^{-1})
λ = blood to gas partition coefficient
$\dot{Q}$ = cardiac output (ℓ/min)
$\dot{V}$ = ventilation (ℓ/min)
j = $\sqrt{-1}$

$$\tau_L = \left(\frac{\lambda Q + \dot{V}}{C_I} \right) - I$$

C_I = the equivalent ideal part lung capacity (liters)

$P_I(\omega)$ = the inhaled anesthetic concentration (%) transform

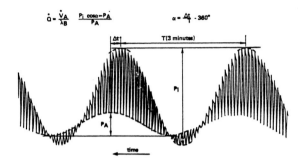

Figure 1. Implementation of Zwart's method of determining pulmonary blood flow over 3 minutes. Note the amplitude of P_A and P_I and the phase shift Δt.

And, consequently, the cardiac output estimate (See figure 1)

$$\dot{Q} = \frac{\dot{V}}{\lambda} \left(\frac{|P_I|}{|P_A|} \cos \phi - 1 \right)$$

where:

$|x|$ = the amplitude of sinusoidal time function x
ϕ = the phase lag between the inhaled and alveolar gas.

This method is equivalent to a spectral technique, so that nonvarying hemodynamics and steady state conditions are required. Error sources such as distorted (sinusoidal) inhaled concentration, measurement noise (cardiogenic oscillations included), stochastic nature of lung perfusion, nonsteady state and varying hemodynamics, lung inhomogeneity, variability of blood/gas partition coefficient, and small fractional mixed venous returns still exist in this method as with most classical soluble gas techniques.

We have extended Zwart's method by dithering the inhaled halothane (forane or ethrane). This then reduces to a simple problem in system identification and a new estimate is obtained after each breath.

The monitor has been built, and is currently undergoing extensive laboratory and clinical testing. Initial modeling and algorithmic development have been reported in detail elsewhere (5,6), as has an extensive error analysis (6,7). Here the development of an actual hardware device from a mathematical model is reported. A more complete treatment is given in (8).

The pulmonary perfusion monitor operates on the soluble gas principle so that the amount of any inert blood-soluble gas taken up by a subject is proportional to the amount of fresh blood flowing through the lungs, provided that the blood contains no soluble gas initially. The amount of the gas taken up at each breath is measured by subtracting the amount of the gas exhaled from the amount inhaled.

The solubility of the gas in blood must not be too low, (λ_b < 30), or the amount of gas taken up per breath is difficult to measure. Also, the solubility of the gas must not be too high, (such as the solubility of acetone) because then most of the gas is taken up by tracheal and bronchial tissue rather than the blood. For clinical use, the gas must be non-flammable, easily handled, easily measured, etc. At present ethrane is used because it also serves as the anesthetic so that no other connection with the patient is needed. However, in applications other than surgery, the pulmonary blood flow monitor can also function at trace (non-anesthetic) levels of ethrane or other suitable gases, i.e. concentrations below .1%.

Multiple breaths of the soluble gas contaminate the fresh blood entering the lungs because the soluble gas is recirculated. For this reason, the direct Fick method needs an invasive measurement of venous blood. Zwart's (9) modification and our dither method (5) obviates this measurement by applying the soluble gas inhaled concentration as a sinusoidal waveshape or square wave in time.

The parameter estimation technique is that of Wiberg (10) which is essentially a modification of the extended Kalman filter. Details of this algorithm applied to the pulmonary perfusion monitor can be found in Brovko (6).

2. THE MODEL

Inhaled and end-tidal soluble gas pressure $P_I(t)$ and $P_A(t)$ are measured. End-tidal gas is the last portion of exhalation, in which the gas partial pressures are most nearly in equilibrium with arterial gas partial pressures. The breath time t is necessarily discrete, but traditionally a continuous time compartmental model has been used to model gas uptake and recirculation. This traditional model is:

$$C_I \frac{dP_A}{dt} = \left[(1-x)\dot{V}+(1-y)\lambda_b\dot{Q}_o\right] P_A + (1-y)\lambda_b \sum_{j=i}^{N} \dot{Q}_j P_j + (1-x)\dot{V}P_I \quad (1)$$

$$C_j \frac{dP_j}{dt} = \lambda_b\dot{Q}_j \left[(1-y)P_A + y\sum_{k=1}^{N}P_k\dot{Q}_k/\dot{Q}_o - P_j\right] \quad j=1,2,\ldots,N \quad (2)$$

where:

C_I = Equivalent gas volume of the gas exchanging part of the lung;

C_j = Equivalent gas volume of the jth body compartment;

λ_b = Blood-gas partition coefficient;

x = Fraction of physiologic dead space in the lung;

y = Fraction of cardiac output shunted across the lung;

$P_A(t)$ = End-tidal (alveolar) gas partial pressures;

$P_I(t)$ = Inhaled gas partial pressures

$P_j(t)$ = Partial pressure in the jth body compartment;

$\dot{Q}_j(t)$ = Perfusion of the jth body compartment; thus, $\sum_{j=1}^{N}\dot{Q}_j(t) = \dot{Q}_o$, volume per unit time;

$\dot{V}$ = Ventilation, volume per unit time;

N = Number of body compartments.

It was found that the factors x and y have a **great** influence on accuracy of measurement $\dot{Q}_o$ (10). This is the largest error source and invalidates the quantitative accuracy for subjects with lung disease states or other abnormalities in which a good estimate of x or y is not available. However, **relative** pulmonary blood flow changes can still be measured in these subjects, which in many clinical situations is perhaps of greater importance than the quantitative accuracy. Also, constants x and y can be measured if it is necessary or if it is suspected they are abnormal.

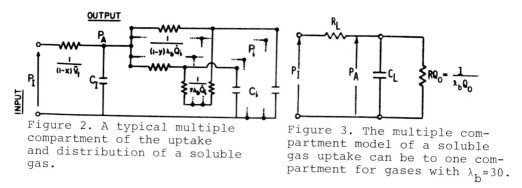

Figure 2. A typical multiple compartment of the uptake and distribution of a soluble gas.

Figure 3. The multiple compartment model of a soluble gas uptake can be to one compartment for gases with $\lambda_b \approx 30$.

For inputs in the frequency range of interest, it was found that the uptake model can be very accurately described by four body compartments (N=4). However, one body compartment (N=1) gives errors of less than 3%, and is used in most of our simulation studies and experiments. Equation (1) is a one compartment model of the lung. Actually the lung is a distributed gas exchanger. The associated time constant is actually a lumped approximation to this (See Figs. 2 and 3).

The algorithm takes measurements of P_I (t), P_A (t), and $\dot{V}(t)$, and computes an estimate of $(1-y)\lambda_b \dot{Q}_o$ based on the model (1) and (2). Initial estimates for C_I and C_j are fitted to the data. The blood-gas partition coefficient λ_b is considered known and constant. The model and the algorithm are stored in the computer.

3. HARDWARE DESIGN

The design philosophy of the pulmonary perfusion monitor is to combine maximum versatility for laboratory use with the greatest simplicity for clinical applications. Calibration and commands are self-explanatory and diagnostic messages are displayed if the software or hardware fails. For clinical applications the monitor has been built into a standard anesthesia machine. The anesthesia machine also houses the transducers for the measurement of ventilation and inhale-exhale concentration of anesthetic gas.

The main tasks to be performed by the pulmonary perfusion monitor are (i) modulation of the inspired gas concentration, (ii) measurement of the inspired-expired anesthetic gas concentration, and (iii) implementation of the parameter

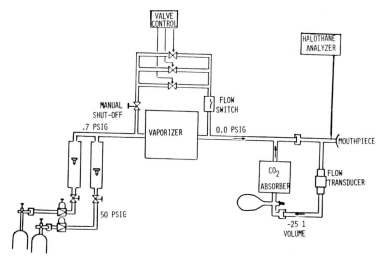

Figure 4. Diagram of anesthesia machine and bypass valving.

estimation routine. Different parts of the monitor perform these various tasks. These parts are discussed here in the order given above.

The computing unit containing the display and the command keyboard is located on the upper part of the anesthesia machine at eye level. The gas flowmeter and the gas analyzers are in the lower part, below the anesthesia gas lines.

The inspired gas concentration is modulated using a gas bypass across the ethrane vaporizer. Three solenoid valves, driven by the 8085 CPU, control the variable bypass flow. The flow through each valve can be individually adjusted to realize a variety of waveforms. A manual control also regulates the flow through the three solenoid valves and acts as a multiplicative factor. The manual control also has the function of valve override. When the shut-off valve is closed, the monitor can be used as an ordinary anesthesia machine.

The solenoid valves used in this application are designed for low current and low heat generation. As a safety measure, the action of the valves can only reduce the gas concentration. Additionally, a flow switch which senses the flow in the bypass loop generates an error signal in case of valve failure and is included in the gas control circuit.

The measurement of the anesthetic gas concentration presents contrasting requirements. The gas analyzer must be able to measure small variations of concentration around a relatively large constant value. It must have both high sensitivity and large dynamic range. Also,it must not be as expensive nor as large as a mass spectrometer. A compact hydrogen flame ionization detector, specially built for this kind of application, has recently become commercially available from WTI in Holland. Main features of this instrument are (i) sensitivity (0.00001 ml/ml), (ii) high level of stability, (iii) rapid response time (0.2 sec), (iv) small amount of sample needed (3.0 ml/min), (v) simple calibration, (vi) built-in vacuum pump, (vii) accuracy of 5% of full scale, and (viii) transport delay of 0.6 sec, variable during an operation, but corrected by the software.

The tidal volume is calculated by rectangular integration of the flow signal during the expiratory phase. A constant temperature linearized anemometer (T.S.I. model 1054 B) is used to measure the mass flow of expired gas.

The data processing unit was chosen on the basis of the computation load. For this application a word size of 32 bits was chosen to minimize numerical instability in the estimation algorithm. However, the time constraint for an on-line operation is satisfied with an 8-bit processor. Simulations showed that a single 8085 system could handle both the data collection and the pulmonary blood flow estimation routines. The system reached its final single-processor configuration shown in Figure 6.

The Space Byte CPU, used in the final configuration of the data processor, is almost a complete computer on a single board. It contains most of the interfaces for hard copy, CRT terminal and disk operation. This board also contains a 3K resident monitor which provides most of the basic software used by the estimation routines. The data processor is built according to the industry standard "S-100" bus. A large supply of add-on modules are available for this configuration. The only custom made units in the pulmonary blood flow monitor are

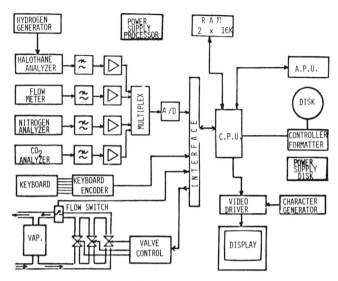

Figure 5. Block diagram of the complete system including anesthesia machine, gas sensors, interface, computer and display.

the four-channel signal conditioner, the keyboard encoder and the solenoid valve driver.

To increase the flexibility of the monitor, the operating system is not stored in EPROMs but on floppy disks. Each time the monitor is used, the operating system is loaded into a large RAM memory by a self-starting bootstrap sequence. It is thus possible to change the operating system by simply loading a new magnetic disc.

Four analog inputs connect the gas and flow transducers to the data processor. Each channel has an independent gain and bias control to match the range of the analog input to the characteristic of the A/D converter. This solution simplifies the calibration procedure and reduces the quantization noise.

The analog signals are sampled and digitized at a rate of 50 samples per second. The input bandwidth is then restricted to 25 Hz. This is not a limitation for the gas concentration signal whose bandwidth is approximately 10 Hz. It is a limitation for the flow signal whose bandwidth is about 5 KHz and must be then low-pass filtered. It is convenient to choose the sampling rate as high as possible because this allows the use of simpler integration routines, i.e. rectangular instead of trapezoidal. A high sampling rate also reduces the aliasing and has less stringent pre-filtering requirements. The upper limit of the sampling rate is determined by the computation power of the processor. The sampling interval is controlled by a 7555 chip which is connected to a high priority (7.5) interrupt. A standard S-100 module, Cromemco D+7A I/O, is used for A/D conversion. To meet the real time requirement and to increase the numerical accuracy, a floating point Arithmetic Processing Unit (APU) is used to perform most of the computations for both the estimation and the preprocessing routines. The APU performs 41 different floating point operations and does automatic floating point normalizations.

Graphic capability is realized by means of a programmable character generator which is under software control. The use of this module reduces the software overhead. The character generator board has its own memory and works (in combination with the video driver board) as an independent unit without the use of external system memory or any DMA activities. The central processor is free to execute different tasks while the video display is being refreshed. The monitor display is a 12-inch high resolution unit. The natural choice of mass storage to go with the Space Byte CPU was the ICOM FD-3700 disk drive with the FC-360 controller formatter. The ICOM drives use an 8-inch IBM compatible 256K diskette. It is thus possible to store the data of the day-long study on one disk.

The valve controller circuit has two functions. First it converts the TTL logic signals to a power level sufficient to drive the solenoid valves. Second, it generates the pulsed signals required by the valves from the computer command.

A single one-byte command controls the three valves. The bit pattern of the command word selects the valve to be operated. The duration of the current pulse is determined by a monostable circuit activated by the processor output strobe.

The keyboard decoder shares a digital port with the solenoid valve decoder. An interrupt line is used to signal the CPU when a character is typed in. This solution is preferred to a "polled" configuration because it saves time.

4. SOFTWARE DESIGN

As was the case for the hardware, the constraints on the software were that no particular computer skills were to be required from the operator and that the monitor operating system had to be flexible enough to allow its use both in the laboratory and in clinical applications.

Effective use of logic processors requires that the software be intimately related to the hardware. Higher level languages are more powerful but their translation into object code is not as efficient as a program written directly in machine language. For this application it was important to choose a programming language which minimized both the size of the program and the execution time. Assembly language was therefore a natural choice.

The monitor operating system occupies about 24,000 bytes of memory, shared in equal parts by the estimation routines and the housekeeping routines. The software package can be divided into the following parts: (1) user prompt routines, (2) preprocessing, (3) estimation, (4) valve control, (5) graphics, and (6) utility routines.

To start the system, a RESET command initializes the TRAP service routine by writing a JUMP to the on-board loader sequence. The bootstrap command activates the TRAP interrupt which causes the operating system to be transferred from disk into core. Once the loading of the operating system is complete, the execution of the program starts automatically.

An interactive sequence takes the operator through the initialization, hardware check, calibration and command setting. At the end of the prompt sequence a "READY" message informs the operator that the system is correctly initialized and then the file number can be entered and the START key pressed. When the START key is pressed a new disk file is opened and the current set of parameters is stored, the sampling clock is enabled and the collection of data begins.

412

Warning messages are given in the case of (1) duplicate file name, (2) hardware failure in the disk drive, (3) incorrect disk positioning, (4) disk full.

In calibration mode the output of the flowmeter and the gas analyzer is continuously sampled and displayed. The values of the bias and multiplicative factors used to convert, in software, the signals from A/D units to flow and gas concentration units are also displayed.

The preprocessing routines perform the following operations: (1) sampling of analog signals from gas and flow analyzers, (2) A/D conversion, (3) calculation of inspired and expired gas concentrations, tidal volume and breath time, (4) detection of inspiratory and expiratory phases, and (5) compensation for the delay between the flow and gas analyzers. Detection of inspiratory and expiratory phases are especially critical, and flow artifacts due to coughing, swallowing, etc. are eliminated by threshold comparisons.

The estimated values of pulmonary perfusion are displayed on the CRT as shown in Figure 8. This format was chosen in an effort to convey the information in the most effective way for clinical use. On the Y axis are values of blood flow in liters/minute, on the X axis the breath number. The screen contains a maximum of 60 breaths. When a full screen is completed the graphic wraps around.

During the execution of the estimation routines the collection of data is interrupted but no information is lost. The perfusion estimation is performed in 200 msec. during the initial part of the inhale phase, when no samples are collected either for the calculation of the tidal volume or the calculation of the gas concentration. The tidal volume is calculated during the exhale phase and the end-inspired and end-expired gas concentrations are calculated when the collection of data has already been restored.

5. RESULTS

Experiments were performed for two main reasons, a) to compare the estimated values of pulmonary perfusion to values of cardiac output measured with an invasive technique so that the hardware and software could be evaluated and b) to evaluate the acceptance of this monitor in the clinical environment, especially in the operating room.

More than 140 measurements were performed on the healthy volunteers, patients undergoing surgery, and dogs. Reference methods were thermal dilution and, in the dog, electromagnetic blood flow.

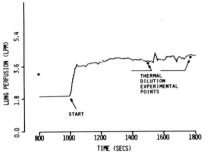

Figure 6. Thermal dilution cardiac outputs and continuous pulmonary blood flow estimates in 67 year old female (see text).

In Figure 6 are shown the results from the pulmonary perfusion monitor in a 67 year old female undergoing surgery. The anesthetic gas was ethrane and you can see the several thermal dilution estimates as compared to the continuous on-line pulmonary perfusion estimates. The pulmonary perfusion monitor was initialized shortly after a thermal dilution cardiac output showed 2.4 liters. The algorithm rapidly converged and agreed well with the two Swan-Ganz catheter thermal determinations. Both thermal dilution estimates correlated well with the continuous pulmonary blood flow monitor.

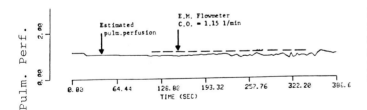

Figure 7. Output from an electro-magnetic flow meter and from the pulmonary perfusion monitor.

Studies were done on dogs with electromagnetic flow meters around the ascending aorta. There was generally good correlation between electromagnetic flow meter reading and the estimated pulmonary perfusion (Figure 7).

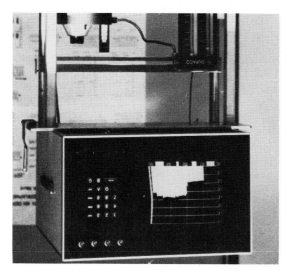

Figure 8. The pulmonary blood flow monitor with the computer and display at eye level. The anesthesia machine flow meters can be seen in the lower left while in the lower right corner is the gas vaporizer. Beneath the cabinet is located the computer controlled valve-rig.

6. SUMMARY AND CONCLUSION

The first prototype of the pulmonary perfusion monitor has led to the identification and solution of numerous problems connected with the implementation of this soluble gas technique.

Our experimental experience has shown that the accuracies of pulmonary perfusion estimate is dependent in large measure on accuracies of the parameters measured. The newer estimation technique which measures the exact amount of gas taken up gives consistently better results.

The error analysis has shown that the correct representation of the lung capacity in the model of the gas uptake is of great importance. We plan therefore in a new version of the monitor to incorporate means of estimating periodically the lung capacity from another soluble gas. This then would be an additional state and be estimated on-line by the computer algorithm.

The vulnerability of the model to deviations in lung capacity or dead space represents the most serious problem of this monitoring technique. The arbitrary, although educated choice of the parameter sets can induce errors on the estimated pulmonary perfusion. We are now extending this model to the use of four gases for estimating parameters within the model such as dead space, functional, residual capacity and capacity of the lung; this will improve the pulmonary perfusion estimate.

7. REFERENCES

1. Butler, J. Measurement of cardiac output using soluble gases. In: Handbook of Physiology, Sec. 3: Respiration, Vol. II, American Phys. Society, pp. 1489-1503.

2. Homer, LD, Denisyk, B. 1975. Estimation of cardiac output by analysis of respiratory gas exchange . J. Appl. Physiol. 39:159-165.

3. Zwart, A, Van Dieren, A. Monitoring and control aspects during halothane anesthesia. Progress Report 4, 1974 Inst. Med. Phys. Da Costakode 45, Utrecht, Netherlands, pp. 70-82.

4. Fick, A. 1870. Uber die Messugn des Bkitquantums in der Merzventrickeln Sitzber, Physik. Med. Ges. Wurzberg. 36.

5. Brovko, O, Wiberg, DM, Arena, L, Bellville, JW. 1981. The extended Kalman filter as a pulmonary blood flow estimator. Automatica 17:1213-1220.

6. Brovko, O. 1979. The extended Kalman filter as a pulmonary blood flow estimator. Ph.D. Thesis, Dept. of System Science, University of California, Los Angeles.

7. Brovko, O, Zwart, A, Wiberg, DM, Bellville, JW, Arena, L. 1979. Sensitivity of Ljung's algorithm for estimating pulmonary blood flow. Proc. 18th IEEE Conf. on Decision and Control.

8. Arena, L. 1981. A monitor for noninvasive estimation of pulmonary blood flow. Ph.D. Thesis, Dept. of System Science, University of California, Los Angeles.

9. Zwart, A, Bogaard, JM, Jansen, JRC, Versprille, A. 1978. A noninvasive determination of lung perfusion compared with direct Fick method. Pfluger Arch. 375:213-217.

10. Wiberg, DM, Brovko, O. 1979. Some factors affecting the rate of convergence during on-line parameter estimation. Proc. 9th IFIP. Conf. on Opt. Techniques.

8. ACKNOWLEDGEMENTS

This work was supported in part by Grant GM 23732 awarded by the National Institute of Health, General Medical Sciences.

A MICROCOMPUTER-BASED CHARTING SYSTEM FOR DOCUMENTATION OF
HEAMODYNAMIC, RESPIRATORY PARAMETERS AND DRUG ADMINISTRATION
DURING CARDIAC ANAESTHESIA.

S.G. van der Borden, O. Prakash, S.H. Meij

INTRODUCTION

The practice of documentation of respiratory and heamodynamic
parameters during an anaesthetic procedure has proven to be of
great value. Documentation of anaesthetic records can be achieved
by either manual or automatic methods. Manual record keeping is
done by entering into the chart, the relevant parameters every
15 minutes. Manual record keeping was found to be laborious and
time consuming specially during an acute episode. During this
period, important vital information was often missed and forgotten.
In such situations conventional record keeping by hand has proved
to be unsatisfactory and unreliable. If one is looking for precise
documentation then automatic recording system is preferable.

GENERAL IDEA

Due to intensive manual handling of heart lung machine during
extracorperal circulation, it was not easy to keep an upto-date
record of heamodynamics and other events by hand. In 1980 it was
decided to use microprocessor-based recording system for
convenience and reliability. A prototype version of microprocessor-
based recording system was introduced in the operating room. It
proved popular and three more systems were introduced for routine
use. At the same time, an idea was generated to develop similar
system for anaesthesia department.

DESIGN CONSIDERATION

To accelarate the acceptance of the Automatic Charting System (ACS)
(fig 1) by the user, the chart produced by the "ACS", lookes
almost the same as the original handwritten anaesthesia chart.

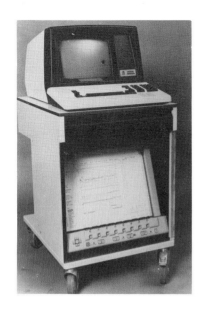

FIG 1. Anaesthesia Charting
System (ACS)

In this way the information documented on the chart can easily be recognized by the user. The information entered into the recordkeeping system consists of both alpha and numeric data, like numbers and text, a alphanumeric keyboard has to be used. A typewriter like keyboard was chosen for this purpose with additional function keys to minimize commands entered into the system.

For verification of all the information entered into the system, a video display is used which gives a continuous overview of all the documented information

Reliability and accuraccy of the chart depends mainly on the plotter used for the recordkeeping system. Despite the high cost of a plotter which offers both reliability and accuraccy, we have selected a commercial available color plotter which can plot on an A3 format.

SYSTEM DESCRIPTION

The "ACS" automatically documents, collects and presents trends, of heamodynamic and respiratory parameters on a minute to minute basis and documents manually entered data via a keyboard e.g. administration of drugs etc.

The "ACS" forms an extension of the routinely used monitors for heamodynamic and respiratory parameters. These monitors preprocesses the bio-signals from the patient e.g. ECG, bloodpressure, airway pressure, airway flow.

Both monitoring systems are microprocessor-based equipped with a RS 232C serial output port for transmission of measured and derived parameters.

The "ACS" is connected to both monitoring systems via the RS 232C

serial ports and receives, the preprocessed heamodynamic and
respiratory parameters for further documentation. (Fig. 2)

D A T A   F L O W   D I A G R A M

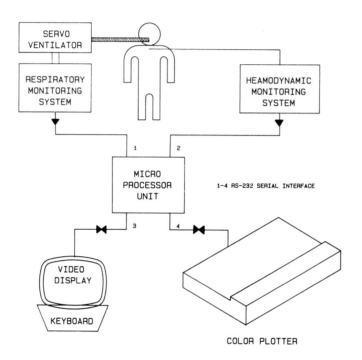

FIG. 2.   Data flow diagram shows the Anaesthesia Charting System
          connected to the other monitoring devices in the
          operating room.

Two other RS 232C serial ports are available on the "ACS" to
communicate with the video terminal and the color plotter. The
terminal is used for viewing the display of all the current
available parameters and messages. The keyboard is used for
manual inputs for drugs and bloodgas values into the system.

HARDWARE FOR THE "ACS"

The "ACS" consist of a commercially available terminal (Beehive
DM1S) for display and manual input of data and a color plotter
(Hewlett Packard 7221C) and a microprocessor control unit
(based on Intel 8080 microprocessor). The microprocessor control
unit contains a central processor unit, 4 serial interfaces,
32 kilobyte of RAM for storage of data.

SOFTWARE FOR THE "ACS"

The program is written in assembly language for the Intel 8080
microprocessor and stored in Eprom. The program is driven by
a menu displayed on the screen. The system responds with a small
menu or message on the display indicating the kind of entry
the system expects.

The program can be divided in 4 parts, each perform the following
tasks:

1. handling of data received from the monitoring systems and
   data entered via the keyboard
2. data output to the video display of the terminal
3. data computation and storage for the plotting program
4. data output to the plotter for plotting of the anaesthesia
   chart.

The format of the program can perform multi-tasks and the 4
main programs seem to run parallel to each other. This results
in immediate response desired by the user.

VIDEO DISPLAY

On the video display an overview is given of:

1. information automatically entered into the system, like
   heamodynamic and respiratory parameters.
2. information entered via the keyboard;e.g. name, date, blood-
   gas values, drugs, etc.
3. information of system status;e.g. plotter On or Off.

The screen is refreshed with new information every second.

FUNCTION KEYS

Fifteen function keys are provided to reduce the amount of keyboard input to a minimum and to perform certain task like switching the plotter on or off. Another example is the input of a drug given. This can be accomplished by entering the function key which says 'drug input' and then press a number which can be read from the display indicating the amount of the drug given. Additional drugs which are not shown in the menu, can be entered via the keyboard.

CHART PLOTTING

Like the original handwritten chart, the plotted chart is divided in different fields (fig 3.) such as a patient general information area e.g. patient's name, date, age etc., other fields are for trend curves, general remarks, drug administered, or fluids given or happening of an important event, bloodgas values, urine output and blood/fluid balans.

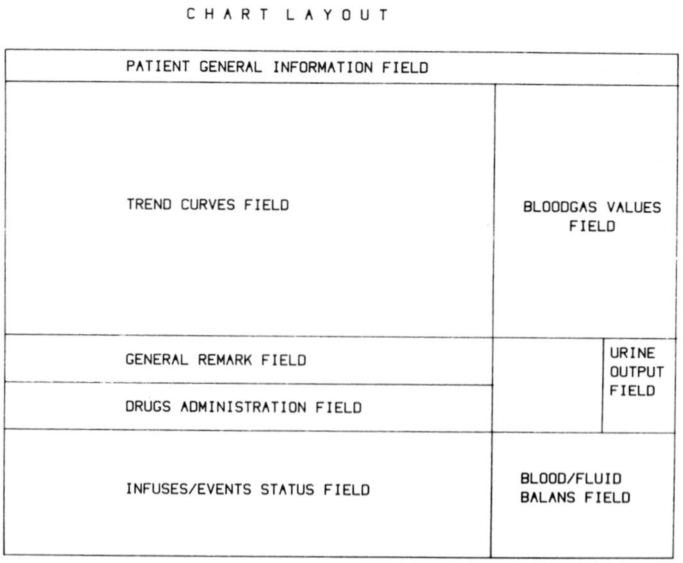

CHART LAYOUT

PATIENT GENERAL INFORMATION FIELD		
TREND CURVES FIELD	BLOODGAS VALUES FIELD	
GENERAL REMARK FIELD		URINE OUTPUT FIELD
DRUGS ADMINISTRATION FIELD		
INFUSES/EVENTS STATUS FIELD	BLOOD/FLUID BALANS FIELD	

FIG 3. shows the division of the chart

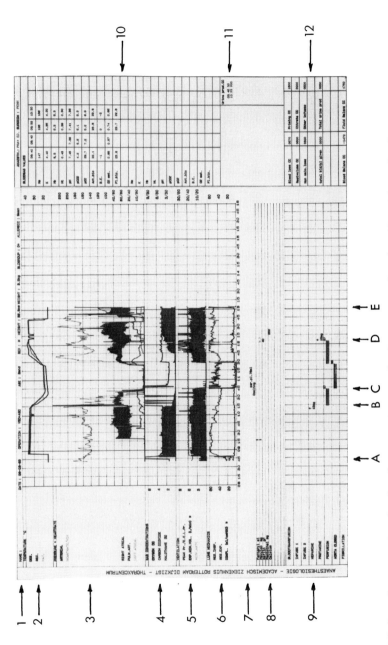

FIG 4. shows a typical chart output of the Anaesthesia Charting System.

1. general information 2. temperatures (oes./nas./rect.) 3 heartrate + Arterial, Right atrial and Left atrial pressures 4. gasconcentrations (O2, CO2, Halothane) 5. ventilation (airway pressure, respiratory rate, expired minute volume) 6. lungmechanics (resistance, compliance) 7. general remarks 8. drug administration 9. i.v. fluids + events 10. blood gas values 11. urine output 12. values of fluid/blood balance calculation.
A. start induction B. start perfusion C. start open heart surgery D. stop perfusion
E. end operation.

An example of a plotted chart is given in figure 4. This example demonstrates a report of an open heart surgery in a small child. Black and white chart shown here is actually plotted in different colours.

This system allows monitoring and recording at the same time. The heamodynamic and respiratory data on the plotter chart are updated every 2 minutes, with a plot resolution of one minute. Up to 8 hrs of trend can be plotted on one chart. Provisions are made to extend plotting on a new chart for another 8 hours. Manual input information is plotted immediately after assignement of valid information entered by the microprocessor system.

STORAGE/COPY

The "ACS" features a 32K of RAM to store all automatic measured parameters and manual input up to 16 hours of information. At the end of the record keeping a copy can be made for duplication of the original chart.

CONCLUSION

The system is in operation for nearly two months. Users and designers are in constant touch for further refinement of the system. The cost of the system is prohibitive for general use. It is expected that the cost will come down in the near future for general acceptance among the users.

COMPUTER CONTROL OF INTRAVENOUS ANESTHESIA

T. H. STANLEY, M.D.

In the last decade numerous intravenous compounds have become popular as alternatives to sodium thiopental as induction agents[1-5] and to all of the inhalation agents as maintenance anesthetic agents.[6-17] In this chapter I will discuss the difficulties of using intravenous agents and the likely impact of the computer and computer technology of the future on intravenous anesthesia.

Differences Between Administration of Intravenous and Inhalation Anesthetics:

In contrast to the inhalation anesthetics, it is difficult to measure, determine and maintain a constant depth of anesthesia utilizing intravenous agents.[18-20] In order to help determine what are adequate levels or blood concentrations of intravenous agents, numerous investigators have been measuring tissue, blood and urine concentrations of these agents; thus a new group of investigators called pharmacokineticists has evolved.[18-20] The pharmacokineticist of intravenous anesthetic agents is not really different from the expert on uptake and distribution who evolved during the development of inhalation anesthetics. However, the pharmacokineticist's subspecialty is still evolving and the tools of his trade still developing. Thus, the clinical relevance and reliability of many of the pharmacokinetic techniques are still unconfirmed. One major difference between intravenous and inhalation anesthesia which has enormous clinical significance and which will mandate computer involvement in future techniques of intravenous anesthesia is the fact that metabolism is an important component of intravenous anesthesia and is not in inhalation anesthesia. Although certain inhalation anesthetics (halothane, methoxyflurane) are metabolized, the clinical importance of this drug (anesthetic) treatment from the point of view of anesthetic induction, maintenance and recovery is minimal. Of course, the picture is entirely different with intravenous agents. With the later, besides solubility in water, blood and tissues, plasma and tissue lipid and protein binding and regional and total blood flow, drug disposition, biotransformation, receptor-drug-complex interactions and various routes of excretion have major influences on blood and brain concentrations and thus depth and kind of anesthetic depression.

Another major difference which effects the administration of intravenous agents to a greater extent than inhalation agents is volatility. That intravenous agents are not volatile markedly changes the methods and thus the speed with which they can be measured in blood. Numerous studies have demonstrated that end-tidal expired concentrations of inhalation anesthetics are virtually the same as plasma concentrations. Using gas chromatography and mass spectroscopy it is thus possible to virtually continuously measure end tidal concentrations of inhalation anesthetics in our modern operating rooms.[21] Such is not the case with intravenous agents and therefore numerous pharmacokinetic profiles in a variety of tissues, including brain, liver, lung, etc., are reported in the literature.[18-20] From these profiles the clinician is supposed to determine the ideal rate of infusion of an intravenous compound at all times after beginning an anesthetic procedure. Whether this is practically possible and whether it is important in the overall clinical effectiveness of intravenous anesthesia has really yet to be determined.

The Computer Impact on Intravenous Anesthesia:

It is probably at this point in the history of anesthesia, and more specifically in the history of intravenous anesthesia (which is now), that the computer will make its most important impact in terms of anesthetic delivery. Indeed, there are already intravenous anesthetic delivery systems based on the pharmacokinetics of at least two compounds, etomidate and fentanyl, which are now in development (Peters M, personal communication). Probably other machines which are in fact, mini computers designed to administer the appropriate dose of an intravenous compound based on average pharmacokinetics and average ideal infusion rates also exist at the present time. However, one of the serious and perhaps major questions to be asked at this juncture is what effect will these devices have on the clinical application of intravenous anesthesia. Although not documented, it is certainly the feeling of most anesthesiologists in the United States that continuous intravenous infusion techniques are difficult at best and certainly very different than the techniques they

are accustomed to. Perhaps this is related to the fact that anesthesiologists in the United States have not been trained to deal with machines
designed to continuously infuse an intravenous compound. Most of us
growing up in the various schools of anesthesia in the USA have been
attuned to turning dials that change oxygen, nitrous oxide, halothane,
isoflorane, and enflurane concentrations, but certainly not dials that
would regulate a continuous infusion of sodium thiopental, fentanyl or
other intravenous anesthetic agents. Although continuous infusion of
anesthetic adjuvants (sodium nitroprusside, nitroglycerin) and cardiac
inotrophic agents has certainly become more popular of late, it appears,
at least to this author at this time, that the continuous intravenous
infusion of an intravenous anesthetic agent, especially when dictated by
a machine, is different.

Is there really a difference in "black box" directed anesthesia and
anesthesia of the past? I think it is probably too soon to really say.
Are these mini computers that are just beginning their development phase
going to have a large impact on intravenous anesthesia and, secondarily,
anesthesia as a whole? This question is also unanswerable at the present
time. The reason why these questions are, in my opinion, unanswerable
is simple, and that is that the science of pharmacokinetics is still a
new and untested science and, as such, its real impact on anesthesiology
as a whole and on intravenous anesthesia in particular is unknown. Indeed,
it is difficult to know at the present time just how much variation in
blood concentration there will be after administration of a bolus or
continuous infusion of, for example, the opioid fentanyl. In addition,
the importance of regional blood flow changes induced by a variety of
disease states including obesity, diseases of the liver, kidney, etc.,
and the effects of these changes on "average" pharmacokinetic profiles
and thus computer directed changes in infusion are unknown. Finally,
the effects of numerous simple demographic factors such as previous drug
history, history of alcohol and caffeine intake and smoking on intravenous
anesthetic blood and brain concentration requirements are unknown at the
present time. Even if a uniform group of patients, in terms of drug
history, other disease states, blood volume, etc., could be obtained,
exactly how much variation in terms of intravenous anesthetic blood
concentration occurs after a given bolus or infusion of fentanyl and
most other agents is unknown. Will the computer be able to come to our

assistance in these peculiarities of intravenous anesthesia? I am sure it will! In what way and form? These are the important questions to be answered in the next five to ten years.

Another crucial difference between intravenous anesthesia, at least intravenous opioid anesthesia, and inhalation anesthesia, is that the fundamental mechanisms producing anesthesia are probably different. Adequate opioid anesthesia is dependent upon saturation of a certain percentage of specific opioid receptors[22] which, although dose dependent, is difficult to clinically determine even with the use of sophisticated electroencephalographic technology. The same is probably true with many, if not all, intravenous anesthetics. Furthermore, surgical stimulation with inadequate levels of at least certain intravenous anesthetics can result in very unstable circulatory dynamics and other dangerous clinical conditions which may often not be easily or rapidly corrected. These situations are much easier dealt with using standard inhalation anesthetics via the employment of significantly higher concentrations of the anesthetics (over pressure) until conditions are corrected. Perhaps by integrating many clinical signs and symptoms into the overall known or average pharmacokinetic profile of a given drug, a sophisticated computer system designed for a specific intravenous anesthetic technique will be able to automatically increase or decrease infusion rates faster than the clinician can do so. It is possible in so doing that these devices of the future may be able to predict and determine the onset of inadequate depths (and more than adequate depths) of anesthesia before or as they are occurring and therefore guarantee adequate levels of anesthesia at all times.

There are a number of investigations which now document that continuous infusions of fentanyl, alfentanil and ketamine, for example, dramatically reduce the total dosage of these agents required in any given operation and apparently maintain ideal plasma concentrations to insure adequate depth of anesthesia.[23-25] In these studies the incidence of hypertension, tachycardia and other disturbing changes in cardiovascular dynamics is significantly less during continuous infusions of the agents, as compared to multi-bolus type techniques. As a result, postoperative recovery is significantly faster.[25]

Intravenous Anesthetics of the Future and the Computer:

The anesthetics of the future are not going to be like the anesthetics of the past. It appears clear that the opioids and perhaps the new central serotonin receptor blockers, for example, are markedly different from inhalation anesthetics. What do I mean by "markedly different"? As mentioned above, with agents such as halothane, enflurane and iso-florane, if inadequate anesthesia is present a clinician simply has to use a much higher concentration (over pressure) for a short time to depress cardiovascular stimulation and rapidly return hemodynamics to desired levels. This is not as easy with agents like the opioids, the benzodiazepines and other new intravenous compounds. These and perhaps other new intravenous agents do not act as myocardial or cardiovascular depressants.[3,13] In addition, these compounds probably do not act as non-specific central nervous and other organ system depressants, but rather act at specific central nervous system receptors to produce seda-tion, amnesia, analgesia and anesthesia. These are, of course, one of their advantages. As a result of acting at specific receptors, compounds like the opioids and other new intravenous agents can not easily deal with sympathetic activation once it has occurred. Rather, clinicians must use compounds that vasodilate or effect heart rate (the peripheral manifestations of sympathetic activation) rather than directly depressing the sympathetic nervous system. The new intravenous agents therefore dictate that the right dose be used at the right time. If not, then other agents will be rapidly required to correct clinical conditions. One can easily imagine the use of a potpourri of drugs, one attempting to correct the unwanted actions or "over shoot" of the other. Indeed, this author believes this practice is already common place today and may likely get worse in the near future.

Thus it is very imperative to have the right dosage. Fascinating new data accumulated by Westenskow D and Pace N (unpublished data) suggest that the use of anesthetic adjuvants (other agents), which this author has always felt was less than desirable, may not be all that terrible. The reason for this is that with microcomputer regulated infusions of sodium nitroprusside, for example, and continuous systolic, diastolic, and perhaps in the future cardiac output and heart rate data input, use of these adjuvants may be limited and correction of unbalanced hemodynamics extremely rapid. Thus, it would appear that by use of new intravenous agent directed computer technology and measurements and integrations of a variety of well defined as well as still undefined physiologic symptoms and signs, it may be possible to minimize anesthetic polypharmacy and optimize clinical conditions rapidly and virtually automatically.

An alternative to the above approach would be the ability to rapidly measure and integrate blood levels of intravenous agents into a computer programmed patient knowledge bank. The knowledge bank, operation to be performed, surgeon and other clinical information would allow automatic computer directed infusion rates of all anesthetics and anesthetic adjuvants. With this an anesthesiologist would be assured of having a sufficient blood level, and sufficient central and peripheral nervous system binding of all appropriate agents. This may be quite an idealized concept at this time but one which is probably not that far away from clinical reality.

In conclusion, it appears clear to this investigator that the computer will be needed to close the loop, so to speak, in intravenous anesthesia much sooner than it will be needed in more common inhalation anesthetic techniques. All of this does not preclude, in my opinion, the use of manual anesthesiologist override at any moment, but certainly the ideal would be to rarely have need of such manual override in the administration of intravenous anesthetic compounds. It would appear that the easiest place to begin working with this kind of intravenous anesthetic administration would be in the area of muscle relaxants. It seems to me that establishment of continuous computer interaction with the variety of methods used to clinically quantitate neuromuscular function at the present time would be easy. Automated computer control of train-of-four, electromyography and various twitch and tetanus devices available to quantitate neuromuscular function would seem, on the surface, to be easy to accomplish. A continuous system of administering and evaluating responses to administration of various neuromuscular agents may be the simplest and easiest intravenous agent modality with which to develop experience that can be used in future intravenous anesthesia administration. I wonder if such devices exist at the moment? It would appear that if they don't, they should be in at least an evolutionary stage of development.

REFERENCES

1. Nauta J, Stanley TH, de Lange S, et al: Anaesthetic induction with alfentanil: Comparison with thiopental, midazolam and etomidate. Can Anaesth Soc J 30:53-60, 1983
2. Nauta J, de Lange S, Koopman D, et al: Anesthetic induction with alfentanil: A new short-acting narcotic analgesic. Anes Analg 61: 267-272, 1982
3. McClish A: Diazepam as an intravenous induction agent for general anesthesia. Can Anaesth Soc J 13:562-575, 1960
4. Dundee JW: The ideal intravenous anesthetic(s). In: Aldrete JA, Stanley TH, eds. Trends in intravenous anesthesia. Chicago Year Book, 1980, pp 127-142
5. Stanley TH. Pharmacology of intravenous non-narcotic anesthetics. In: Miller RD, ed. Anesthesia. New York, Churchill Livingstone, 1981, pp 451-486
6. Lowenstein E, Hallowell P, Levine FH, et al: Cardiovascular response to large doses of intravenous morphine in man. N Engl J Med 281: 1389-1393, 1969
7. Hasbrough JD: Morphine anesthesia for open-heart surgery. Ann Thorac Surg 10:364-369, 1970
8. Lowenstein E: Morphine "anesthesia" -- A perspective. Anesthesiology 35:563-565, 1971
9. Arens JF, Benbow BP, Ochsner JL: Morphine anesthesia for aorto-coronary bypass procedures. Anesth Analg 51:901-907, 1972
10. Stanley TH, Webster LR: Anesthetic requirements and cardiovascular effects of fentanyl-oxygen and fentanyl-diazepam-oxygen anesthesia in man. Anesth Analg 57:411-416, 1978
11. Stanley TH, Berman L, Green O, et al: Fentanyl-oxygen anesthesia for coronary artery surgery: Plasma catecholamine and cortisol responses. Anesthesiology 51:S139, 1979
12. Stanley TH, Philbin DM, Coggins CH: Fentanyl-oxygen anesthesia for coronary artery surgery: Cardiovascular and antidiuretic hormone responses. Can Anaesth Soc J 26:168-171
13. de Lange S, Boscoe MJ, Stanley TH, et al: Comparison of sufentanil-O_2 and fentanyl-O_2 for coronary artery surgery. Anesthesiology 56: 112-118, 1982
14. Stanley TH, de Lange S, Boscoe J, et al: The influence of chronic preoperative propranolol therapy on cardiovascular dynamics and narcotic requirements during operation in patients with coronary artery disease. Can Anaesth Soc J 29:319-324, 1982
15. de Lange S, Stanley TH, Boscoe MJ: Alfentanil-oxygen anesthesia for coronary artery surgery. Br J Anaesth 53:1291-1296, 1981
16. de Lange S, Boscoe MJ, Stanley TH, et al: Antidiuretic and growth hormone responses during coronary artery surgery with sufentanil-oxygen and alfentanil-oxygen anesthesia in man. Anesth Analg 61: 434-438, 1982
17. Stanley TH: Pharmacology of intravenous narcotic anesthetics. In: Anesthesia. Miller R, ed. New York, Churchill-Livingstone, 1981, pp 425-450
18. Bovill JG, Sebel PSL: Pharmacokinetics of high dose fentanyl. A study in patients undergoing cardiac surgery. Br J Anaesth 52:795-802, 1980
19. Bovill JG, Sebel PS, Blackburn CL, et al: The pharmacokinetics of alfentanil (R 39209): A new opioid analgesic. Anestheisology 57:439-443, 1982

430

20. Stanski DR, Hug CC: Alfentanil -- A kinetically predictable narcotic analgesic. Anesthesiology 57:435-438, 1982
21. Eger EI: Anesthetic Uptake and Action. Baltimore, Williams & Wilkins
22. Stanley TH, Leysen J, Niemegeers CJE, et al: Narcotic dosage and central nervous system opiate receptor binding. Anesth Analg (In press)
23. de Lange S, de Bruijn, Stanley TH, et al: Alfentanil-oxygen anesthesia: Comparison of continuous infusion and frequent bolus techniques for coronary artery surgery. Anesthesiology 55:A42, 1981
24. McLeskey CH: Alfentanil-loading dose/continuous infusion for surgical anesthesia. Anesthesiology 57:A68, 1982
25. White PF: Continuous infusion vs intermittent bolus administration of fentanyl or ketamine for outpatient anesthesia. Anesthesiology 57: A329, 1982